THE ADULT ATTACHMENT PROJECTIVE PICTURE SYSTEM

The Adult Attachment Projective Picture System

Attachment Theory and Assessment in Adults

Carol George
Malcolm L. West

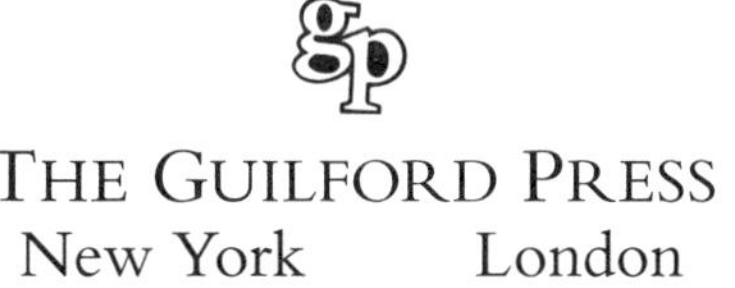

THE GUILFORD PRESS
New York London

A Division of Guilford Publications, Inc.
72 Spring Street, New York, NY 10012
www.guilford.com

Printed in the United States of America

This book is printed on acid-free paper.

Last digit is print number: 9 8 7 6 5 4 3 2 1

The authors have checked with sources believed to be reliable in their efforts to provide information that is complete and generally in accord with the standards of practice that are accepted at the time of publication. However, in view of the possibility of human error or changes in behavioral, mental health, or medical sciences, neither the authors, nor the editor and publisher, nor any other party who has been involved in the preparation or publication of this work warrants that the information contained herein is in every respect accurate or complete, and they are not responsible for any errors or omissions or the results obtained from the use of such information. Readers are encouraged to confirm the information contained in this book with other sources.

Library of Congress Cataloging-in-Publication Data

George, Carol.
The adult attachment projective picture system : attachment theory and assessment in adults / Carol George and Malcolm L. West.
p. cm.
Includes bibliographical references and index.
ISBN 978-1-4625-0425-1 (alk. paper)
1. Attachment behavior. 2. Attachment disorder. 3. Adulthood—Psychological aspects. 4. Behavioral assessment. I. West, Malcolm L. II. Title.
BF575.A86G46 2012
155.9′2—dc23

2011047662

About the Authors

Carol George, PhD, is Professor of Psychology at Mills College in Oakland, California. She has been at the forefront of developing attachment assessments for children and adults, including the Attachment Doll Play Projective Assessment, the Caregiving Interview, and the Adult Attachment Interview. Dr. George has authored numerous research articles and book chapters on adult and child attachment and caregiving, and is coeditor, with Judith Solomon, of the book *Disorganized Attachment and Caregiving.* She teaches courses in development and attachment, co-directs a master's-degree program in infant mental health, and trains and consults on the application of attachment assessment in research and clinical settings.

Malcolm L. West, PhD, is retired Professor of Psychiatry at the University of Calgary in Alberta, Canada. Dr. West worked as a clinician and researcher throughout his career. His research has used attachment theory in clinical research, including cardiac rehabilitation patients, depression in women, and suicidal behavior in adolescents. In addition to the Adult Attachment Projective Picture System, Dr. West has developed self-report assessments of attachment in adults and adolescents. He is coauthor, with Adrienne Sheldon-Keller, of the book *Patterns of Relating: An Adult Attachment Perspective.*

Acknowledgments

A number of colleagues and friends contributed to the early development of the Adult Attachment Projective Picture System (AAP), for which we are extremely grateful. We thank Adrienne Sheldon-Keller, Odette Pettem, and Sarah Rose for their commitment to the AAP. We thank Diane Benoit for her invaluable suggestion to add the *Corner* stimulus to the AAP set and for administering the AAP in the first setting outside of our own laboratory. We could not have completed the validity study without our talented research assistants, who also helped us, not only with recruitment and data collection, but with what probably seemed to them endless hours of transcription of the AAP and the Adult Attachment Interview. Alexandra Sanderson singlehandedly coordinated the Calgary subsample. The Mills College research team—Sara Baskin, Paloma Hesemeyer, Katie Holzer, Rebecca Jackl, and Megan McConnell—coordinated the California subsample.

We are indebted to the many individuals who have attended the AAP training seminars. Responding to their insightful questions helped us to refine the AAP coding system and the attachment concepts on which the AAP is built.

We thank Robert S. Marvin for his review of our work. We appreciate the encouragement and patience of our publisher, The Guilford Press. The grant support from the Social Sciences and Humanities Research Council of Canada and from Mills College is gratefully acknowledged.

Finally, in the most heartfelt way, we thank our spouses, David George and Riva West. They have been our secure base throughout this project.

Preface

This book is concerned with what we feel is a basic need in the assessment of adult attachment status: a "user-friendly" and construct-valid measure. Over the last decade, we have worked to develop such a measure, the Adult Attachment Projective Picture System (AAP). In addition to attachment classification status, the AAP coding system evaluates core attachment constructs and processes that are not assessed by other adult attachment measures. The AAP provides an efficient means to "observe" attachment representation under conditions that activate the attachment system and is amenable for use in a wide range of research and clinical settings, including neurobiological research and the evaluation of clinical treatment effectiveness.

One of our goals in writing this book was to provide a foundation in attachment theory that is needed to understand the development and use of the AAP in assessing attachment. Obviously, a book of this nature can be neither a text on attachment theory nor a classification and coding manual. Our intention is to illustrate a way of thinking about qualitative differences in attachment organization and to show that this way of thinking leads to characterizations of adult attachment patterns that accord well with the contemporary developmental Bowlby–Ainsworth model of attachment. Using the AAP as a framework, we evaluate and expand on attachment constructs throughout the book and present a new way of thinking about the centrality of mental representation in understanding attachment in adults.

Part I addresses the autobiographical narrative and its place in attachment theory and assessment. These chapters cast the process underlying narrative intelligibility as the action of ineradicable affective memories. This analysis of affective memories brings us to Bowlby's concept of the inner working model as a mechanism of continuity across the lifespan. Here our efforts illuminate what it means at the representational level to be secure, dismissing, preoccupied, or unresolved, using the well-established attachment group nomenclature of the Adult Attachment Interview (AAI).

Part II presents the "nuts and bolts" of the AAP for readers who want to "see" how the AAP works. Chapter 3 discusses the development and validation of the AAP. This process required us to re-evaluate the meaning of "coherency" in attachment assessment. Theory, research, and clinical applications almost unilaterally focus on AAI discourse coherency—and its psychoanalytic cousin, reflective capacity—as the single most important dimension of attachment representation (Fonagy, Steele, & Steele, 1996; Hesse, 2008; Main, Kaplan, & Cassidy, 1985). This attachment axiom has received so much attention that it has obscured thinking about how the core concepts in attachment relate to adults. Coherency and reflective capacity address the relative integration of attachment representation in an interview, but they *do not inform us directly* about any of these core concepts. We conceive of the integration of the core attachment concepts as *attachment coherency*. We demonstrate through the development and validation process how the AAP provides a unique understanding of the underlying patterns of attachment coherency that define adult attachment patterns.

Chapters 4 and 5 provide an overview of the AAP coding system. Chapter 4 describes AAP story content coding: *agency of self, connectedness in relationships, synchrony*, and the assessment of self–other boundaries. These dimensions are necessary to clarify the ways and the extent to which attachment security and insecurity are defined by a system of concepts; it requires that patterns of attachment be couched in terms of several variables simultaneously. Chapter 5 is devoted to attachment defensive processes, which serve as the overarching frame of reference for classifying patterns of attachment. With the exception of an occasional nod to the role of defense in attachment, this is an area that essentially has been neglected by attachment theory and research. This chapter, therefore, expands on the concept of defense in attachment theory, including operationally defining defense for application in the AAP. Chapters 4 and 5 are intended only as a coding overview. Coding the AAP requires training. Readers who are interested in learning more about the AAP system are encouraged to contact us through the AAP website, *www.attachmentprojective.com.*

Part III is dedicated to the discussion of individual differences in patterns of adult attachment "in action." At the representational level, attachment group placement communicates important basic information about memory and appraisal of attachment experience, emotions, affect regulation, and expectations of the self and others. We summarize childhood history, provide in-depth interpretation of verbatim AAP transcripts, and highlight the similarities and differences between the AAP and AAI approaches for each case. Chapters 6 through 9 present a comprehensive analysis of the prototypical features and individual differences of the four major adult attachment classifications groups. Chapters 6, 7, and 8 are dedicated to presentations of the AAP for the organized attachment groups—secure, dismissing, and preoccupied—by illustrative full-case presentations.

Chapters 9 and 10 address new horizons in attachment based on extending attachment theory and research using the AAP. Chapter 9 builds on the concept of unresolved attachment, delineating for the first time in the field a comprehensive conceptualization and operational definition of attachment trauma. Similar to the chapters dedicated to the organized classification groups, this discussion in Chapter 9 is accompanied by illustrative case examples.

The context for discussing attachment in action in Chapter 10 is using the AAP in neurobiology research. Dr. Anna Buchheim, a collaborating author on this chapter, has raised the bar for neurobiological attachment research using the AAP with precision and creativity. These studies not only address the validity problems in measuring attachment faced by other neurobiological researchers, but also present for the first time individual differences in brain pattern imaging associated with unresolved attachment.

Our second goal was to produce a book that would be useful to a wide audience. The chapters serve as summaries and expand on new ideas in attachment theory that will interest both the novice and expert reader. The chapters in Part II will be especially useful to researchers or clinicians interested in knowing more about how attachment theory is applied in assessment. Readers who are already deeply trained in attachment theory and assessment procedures can use the coding nuances and case descriptions to further their knowledge regarding different patterns in and among classification groups. Clinicians will appreciate the standardized coding and classification system that fosters standardized evaluations, not only about classification group, but regarding the unique attachment strengths and challenges that clients bring to therapy.

The seed idea to write a book presenting the AAP as a viable adult attachment methodology was developed quite a few years prior to the book's publication. We wanted to ensure before this book went to press that the AAP had good psychometric properties. Establishing strong convergent validity with the international "gold standard" of adult attachment measures, the AAI, was especially important. We also wanted to make sure that independent researchers were successful in establishing convergent validity and predictive validity. The AAP coding and classification system was refined in connection with its use in a series of training workshop meetings and symposia on adult attachment assessment that we have conducted over the past decade.

We now present the AAP in its entirety. It supports the idea that attachment theory, as a system of concepts, is a big system. As Ainsworth (1964) articulated, attachment involves patterns that require integrating several variables simultaneously; attachment is not adequately described using a single or discrete set of orthogonal dimensions. We also hope that introducing the AAP in this way will make attachment theory more amenable for clinical application, which lags far behind attachment research. We invite the readers of this book to join us in using the AAP as a new lens in our continued discovery of the contributions of attachment to adult development and mental health.

CAROL GEORGE
MALCOLM L. WEST

Contents

PART I

Background

1

Narrative versus Non-Narrative Assessment of Adult Attachment

Early in her career Mary Ainsworth was intimately involved in personality assessment and the Rorschach technique. In speaking about the differences between tests of personality and the Rorschach, Ainsworth (Klopfer, Ainsworth, Klopfer, & Holt, 1954) put forth formulations that are insightful today with regard to the narrative versus non-narrative methods of assessing adult attachment. She pointed out that typical personality tests attempt to place all tested individuals on a continuum with respect to one or more variables. By contrast, the Rorschach attempts to describe (rather than measure) the individual qualitatively in terms of patterns of interrelated variables. Whereas personality tests achieve their results by adding up the "true–false" scores or summating scores of the component scales, such a summation procedure is inapplicable to the Rorschach method. Instead, the Rorschach evokes a great variety of responses and provides a way of classifying and interpreting these responses. Ainsworth clearly applied her early thinking on this subject to her work in attachment. She emphasized that attachment is a qualitative and organizational construct, not a dimensional construct (Ainsworth, Blehar, Waters, & Wall, 1978).

All of the foregoing considerations confront us when we consider the two patently different approaches to the assessment of adult attachment. One approach originates in developmental attachment research and is based on the evaluation of mental representations of attachment evidenced by the attachment narrative. This approach is the foundation of the Adult Attachment Projective Picture System (AAP). The other approach originates in social personality research and is based on social cognitive self-report questionnaires (see Crowell & Treboux, 1995, and Crowell, Fraley, & Shaver, 2008, for an overview of this work). Both approaches assert that they are derived from the Bowlby–Ainsworth model of attachment; both articulate adult relationships using similar terminology. Despite broad similarities, there are vast differences in the conception of the attachment construct and in the application of "adult attachment" theory. Because of these differences, attempts to integrate these approaches without acknowledging their independent origins and goals have resulted in conceptual and empirical confusion (George & West, 1999; Waters, Crowell, Elliott, Corcoran, & Treboux, 2002).

The rapidly increasing interest in attachment in relation to adult mental ill health makes it especially important, before we introduce the AAP, that we are clear about the conceptual differences between the developmental and social personality approaches. Perhaps because of the rising interest in and growing acceptance of the attachment construct by theorists and clinicians alike, the definitional trend of this construct is toward a disconcerting sprawl. Definitional boundaries have become blurred and all intimate relationships (e.g., social bonding) are beginning to be treated as synonymous with attachment relationships (see Chapter 10). In preparation for the discussion of how the developmental and social personality approaches explain adult attachment, we first review the conceptual and methodological foundations of each approach in an attempt to establish their conceptual boundaries. It is recognized that the whole problem of the conceptual boundaries of attachment is controversial and thus one runs a considerable risk of being criticized for some degree of arbitrariness. This risk is offset by the gain in sharpening and clarifying the issues around which our current thinking and application of the AAP seem to cluster. In addition, what follows here provides some background on major attachment referents. Cassidy and Shaver's (2008) theoretical and research summary of the relevant attachment literature is a valuable source of discussions of attachment concepts.

ADULT ATTACHMENT: THE DEVELOPMENTAL PERSPECTIVE

The developmental perspective of adult attachment is intricately tied to the fundamental tenets of Bowlby's attachment theory (1969/1982) and to individual differences in attachment as explicated by Ainsworth (Ainsworth et al., 1978) and Main (Main & Solomon, 1990). Bowlby conceived of the essential aspects of relationships in terms of innate behavioral systems. For Bowlby, the key to understanding attachment was to delineate a model that explained how the activation of the attachment behavioral system and accompanying attachment behavior served the evolutionary function of protection, survival, and reproductive fitness. The child's attachment (more precisely, the bond between child and caregiver that is developed as the product of the attachment behavioral system) was considered primary because it was the first relationship-based behavioral system that contributed to the child's survival and child and parent fitness (i.e., transmission of parent's genes to future generations). But Bowlby emphasized as well that, with development, relationships are defined not only by the attachment system, but also by the developmental integration of attachment with other relationship-based behavioral systems such as the affiliative and sexual systems (see also Hinde & Stevenson-Hinde, 1991; Weiss, 1982; West & Sheldon-Keller, 1994).

Over the course of almost three decades, attachment theory and research have defined how the child's qualitatively different experiences of receiving protection and care from the attachment figure are organized into discrete behavioral and mental representational patterns: secure, avoidant, ambivalent, and disorganized (Ainsworth et al., 1978; Main & Solomon, 1990). Beginning with Ainsworth's seminal work, attachment researchers have demonstrated that these qualitatively different patterns are related especially to corresponding differences in maternal sensitivity and responsiveness (de Wolff & van IJzendoorn, 1997) and maternal protection (George & Solomon, 1996, 2008; Solomon & George, 1996, 2011a, 2011b).

One of Bowlby's most significant contributions to our understanding of attachment and our work with the AAP was his transformation of the concept of mental representation, the mental schemes that organize behavior and thought (see Chapters 2 and 5). In his first volume, *Attachment*, Bowlby (1969/1982) drew upon ethology to reformulate the psychoanalytic concept of mental representation as the innate cognitive underpinnings of biologically based behavioral systems (see also Hinde, 1982). In his third volume, *Loss*, Bowlby (1980) used cognitive theory to again reformulate mental representation into a model of defensive exclusion. Drawing upon research in information processing, he explicated the mechanisms and conditions surrounding defensive processing and the organization of feeling, thought, and behavior in relation to attachment experience. In order to protect personal integrity and biological homeostasis, defensive exclusion filters and often changes affect-laden information about attachment that would otherwise produce anxiety, suffering, and pain. Important to our discussion here, this view of mental representation is the basis for how developmental attachment theorists measure attachment and how the meanings of different organizations of attachment relationships are ascribed. Indeed, following Bowlby (1969/1982), these theorists argued that the attachment system itself is never directly observable. Rather, internal working models of attachment are revealed by activating the attachment system and then viewing behavioral and representational responses through the lens of a particular assessment methodology.

These fundamental assumptions of attachment theory, in concert with Bowlby's belief that attachment was important across the lifespan, paved the way for a developmental model of adult attachment. Based on analyses of adults' descriptions of their childhood experiences with attachment figures in the Adult Attachment Interview (AAI; George, Kaplan, & Main, 1984/1985/1996), Main and Goldwyn (1985/1988/1994; Main, Goldwyn, & Hesse, 2003; Main et al., 1985) identified four categories of adult attachment analogous to the categories of child attachment: secure-autonomous, dismissing, preoccupied, and unresolved with respect to loss or abuse. Although behavioral expressions of the four infant attachment groups change over the course of childhood (and presumably adulthood as well; see, e.g., Cassidy, Marvin, et al., 1987–1992; Main & Cassidy, 1988; Marvin, 1977; Schneider-Rosen, 1990), these groups are characterized by the same core representational features across the lifespan (George & West, 1999; Solomon, George, & De Jong, 1995; West & George, 1999, 2002).

Briefly, to be securely attached means that the individual is confident that he or she can rely on attachment figures, and when older, also on internal representations of attachment to *provide safety and protection*. The result is a relatively undefended *behavioral and psychological integration* of attachment experience, memories, and affect. This allows the individual to function in attachment relationships flexibly; that is, he or she is able and willing to integrate the needs, feelings, and perspectives of both the partner and the self in a goal-corrected partnership that succeeds in contributing to one's safety and well-being (following Bowlby, 1969/1982). To be insecurely attached means that the individual is not confident that he or she can depend on attachment figures or internal representations of attachment to provide the kind or degree of protection necessary for immediate physical or psychological safety. The result is the development of costly behavioral strategies and patterns of defensive exclusion, the goal of which is to override personal anxieties and fear so that the individual can maintain integrity of self and remain "connected" in relationships. Because there is some degree of protection risk associated with insecure attachment, the individual cannot achieve full psychological integration of attachment experience, memories, and affect. Under the most severe circumstances (e.g., child maltreatment, relationship violence), insecure attachment leaves the individual distressed and potentially dysregulated as the result of conscious and/or unconscious appraisals of failed protection and abandonment (see also Solomon & George, 2011a).

Mental representation and defensive exclusion are especially important to our discussion of the two theoretical streams of adult attachment. Evidence based on evaluations of individual differences in "current states of mind" (Main & Goldwyn, 1985/1988/1994; Main et al., 2003) and analyses of attachment status in terms of defensive processing (George & Solomon, 1996; Solomon et al., 1995) suggest that because secure attachment is relatively integrated (i.e., coherent) and undefended, mental representations of secure individuals are characterized by positive internal evaluations of self as worthy of protection and care. By contrast, the mental representations of insecure individuals (detached, preoccupied, or unresolved) are marked by attachment anxiety. Because of their anxieties, these individuals must rely on partial or full defensive exclusion in attempts to block from consciousness painful evaluations of the self as unworthy of protection and, to some degree, as vulnerable and unsafe (George & Solomon, 2008; George, West, & Pettem, 1999; Solomon et al., 1995) that develop from chronic experiences of parental compromise or failure to provide comfort, protection, and care. In other words, according to attachment theory, *all individuals judged insecurely attached are by definition characterized to some degree by negative (i.e., unworthy) internal evaluations of the self.*

ADULT ATTACHMENT: THE SOCIAL PERSONALITY PERSPECTIVE

Bowlby maintained a general vision that intimacy was in some way related to attachment (Bowlby, 1988). As compared to the methodical care with which he mapped out the link between attachment and psychopathology, he and other early attachment theorists (e.g., Ainsworth, 1989) failed to specify how such core concepts as the attachment behavioral system and concepts of protection and safety were related specifically to adult intimate or romantic relationships. From the beginning, the bridge between attachment theory and adult romantic and intimate relationships had nevertheless been established. On the surface, the social personality and developmental perspectives of attachment appear to be grounded in the same underlying phenomena. This impression is maximized by the fact that both views define adult attachment in relation to categorical patterns of attachment. In contrast to Bowlby's goal of explaining resiliency and risk, social personality researchers have extrapolated concepts from attachment theory explicitly at first to explain loneliness and then generalized to explain adult romantic love (Hazan & Shaver, 1987). Identified by the personality typology term, "adult attachment style," attachment was transformed into a model of intimacy in romantic relationships.

Modeled on Ainsworth's three-category classification system of infant behavior in the Strange Situation, Hazan and Shaver (1987, 1990) defined a priori three prototypic categories of adult attachment. Adults who identified themselves as feeling confident and comfortable being close to others were defined as secure. Adults who identified themselves as unable to trust others, anxious about being pushed toward intimacy, and feeling uncomfortable around others were defined as avoidant. Adults who identified themselves as reluctant to get close to others but desiring closeness, and worried about their partner's commitment to them in the relationship were defined as ambivalent.

The conceptual question that must be addressed here is whether the concept of adult attachment style is equivalent to attachment as defined by Bowlby and Ainsworth. Although scant empirical energy has been spent on this issue, social personality theorists made their case for equivalence on the basis of two basic lines of thinking: sample distributions and mental representation. The first line of thinking emphasized the fact that sample distributions in adults of secure, avoidant, and ambivalent self-identifications paralleled attachment classification distributions for infants (Shaver & Clark, 1996). This argument for construct validity is not one that is typically endorsed by methodologists (Nunnally, 1978). Even if the proportion argument was sound, the studies in which the similarities between the infant and adult data emerged are, importantly, very different. Specifically, Bowlby (1969/1982) emphasized that the attachment system can be observed only under conditions where attachment is activated. There is no reason to believe that attachment style measures, assessed using paper-and-pencil tests (and often administered to groups of adults collectively), activate the attachment system.

A final concern with the proportions argument is that adults may identify with a particular adult attachment style on the basis of other factors, including identity, personality, intimacy, or representations of interpersonal relationships that are not completely overlapping with attachment (de Haas, Bakermans-Kranenburg, & van IJzendoorn, 1994; Levitt, 2005). Taking this point a bit further, we find it interesting that validation for the social personality model of adult attachment was derived almost completely from traditional-age college students in short-term relationships. Based on the behavioral systems perspective we outlined earlier, there is no reason to believe that attachment style in fact reflects attachment; instead, participants' responses may be confounded by sexual or affiliative relationships that are, according to developmental theory, heightened during this phase of the lifespan (see also Hinde & Stevenson-Hinde, 1991).

The attachment style model emphasizes that young people shift their attachments from parents to peers in adolescence (Zeifman & Hazan, 2008). Contrary to this thinking, Berndt (1996, 2004) discussed how individuals in this phase of development increasingly seek informational, instrumental, companionship, and esteem-building support from their peers, but there is no evidence in the literature to date that documents an age-appropriate shift in attachment figures during this period of development. Normative development in adolescence and emerging adulthood (18–25, conceived in contemporary developmental models as a late stage of adolescence), is defined by exploring the sexual system and practicing with pair bonds. Emotional loneliness in adolescence and emerging adulthood has been found to be higher than in any developmental period during the lifespan (Iacovou, 2002; Rokach, 2000), suggesting that the attachment transfer from parents to peers is incomplete in a vast number of adolescents who are postponing committed relationships. Smith and George (1993), for example, found that while the exploratory system of traditional-age college students was organized around peers, parents nonetheless remained their primary source of protection and security. Only highly insecure adolescents (unresolved on the AAI) reported shifts in attachment-figure preferences from parents to peers. This suggests that a shift in adolescents who are not in committed relationships may be driven by feelings of failed parental protection (Solomon & George, 1996; West, Rose, Spreng, & Adam, 2000), situations that have been documented in even young children as forming "attachment-like" relationships (e.g., Freud & Dann, 1949).

For all of the above reasons, therefore, self-reports of attachment style likely assess young adults' sexual or affiliative relationships, not long-term couple-attachment relationships (see Ainsworth, 1989).

The second, and more important, line of thinking used to claim construct validity centers on the concept of mental representation. In the social personality view of attachment style, mental representation is defined in terms of cognitive attribution. Following the tradition of assessment in social cognition, this approach emphasizes mental representation in terms of self-report responses to predefined inventories (Collins & Read, 1990; Crowell et al., 2008; Feeney & Noller, 1990; Hazan & Shaver, 1987). Attachment style is designated on the basis of a person's conscious self-evaluation; classification is based on what the individual designates or *claims* to be true about self and others in intimate relationships.

In the developmental view, representational approaches to classification of adult and child attachment status are based on evaluations of patterns of mental processes. The emphasis is on the organization of thought in terms of the individual's "state of mind" and, more recently, defensive exclusion (George & Solomon, 2008; George et al., 1999; Solomon et al., 1995). Thus ultimately in the developmental view, *little real consideration is given to what the individual claims to have happened or his or her assertions regarding current or past situations or relationships*. Indeed, this emphasis on unconscious defensive processes has led to strong construct and discriminant validity. Researchers have shown that attachment as measured by the AAI, for example, is related to other construct-validated assessments, including measures of child and adult attachment (e.g., Bakersman-Kranenbrug & van IJzendoorn, 2009) and adult caregiving (George & Solomon, 2008).

Given the differences between these two approaches, it is not surprising that researchers have not found a significant correspondence between developmental patterns of attachment (i.e., attachment status) and attachment style (see Crowell & Treboux, 1995; Crowell et al., 2008). For example, in a study of the relations between AAI outcomes and data from questionnaires on attachment style in a sample of 83 mothers, de Haas et al. (1994) concluded: "The self-report questionnaires for attachment style and memories of parental behavior were therefore found to be not suitable for obtaining information about attachment working models as assessed by the AAI" (p. 471). As Crowell and Treboux (1995) argued, the consistent failure to demonstrate equivalence in these forms of classification raises questions as to whether these approaches describe the same construct.

Indeed, the matter has now been more or less settled in favor of this position; social personality researchers generally agree that the two methodologies are not comparable (Crowell et al., 2008). Studies using self-report questionnaires designed to assess adult and romantic attachment have also shown little or no relation between these two phenomena. Woodhouse, Dykas, and Cassidy (2009), who used a self-report questionnaire to assess secure base, found no relation between this core attachment construct and romantic attachment. Bifulco, Moran, Jacobs, and Bunn (2009) found that family system characteristics relevant to adolescent attachment risk were unrelated to the mother's attachment style. The results of studies such as these support the conclusion that the sexual and attachment systems have different goals (security vs. coitus) and thus it is probably no accident that the sexual relationship is not isomorphic with attachment in normal adults.

Bartholomew, following a somewhat different approach than previous researchers in this area, developed an adult attachment typology to describe intimate reciprocal interaction (Bartholomew & Horowitz, 1991; Scharfe & Bartholomew, 1995). Bartholomew's approach combined two fundamental aspects of contemporary attachment research (infant attachment categories and Bowlby's [1969/1982, 1980] formulation of self and other mental representations of attachment) with Millon's (1969) model of personality. As a result, Bartholomew defines attachment "in terms of the intersection of two underlying dimensions of internal working models—positivity of models of the self and positivity of models of hypothetical others—resulting in four attachment patterns" (Scharfe & Bartholomew, 1995, p. 394). Dimensions of positivity were then expanded to include the dimensions of avoidance and dependency (Bartholomew & Horowitz, 1991). Thus Bartholomew's conceptualization of adult attachment style was derived from a predefined model that included four classification prototypes; each prototype describes a different combination of positive and negative evaluations of self and other. The descriptions for each prototype were formulated by extrapolating from research reports using the AAI and Hazan and Shaver's measure as they fit each predefined personality category. The prototype in which individuals described self and other as positive, and in which individuals were neither avoidant of nor dependent on others, was labeled secure. The three other prototypes in which individuals described negative evaluations of self, other, or both, and in which individuals reported problems with avoidance and/or dependency were labeled insecure.

Although Bartholomew's prototypes have been shown to be related empirically to some adult personality variables (Crowell & Treboux, 1995; Crowell et al., 2008; Shaver & Clark, 1996), the larger issue of construct validity that we raised earlier remains: To what degree does Bartholomew's adult attachment typology reflect Bowlby's construct of attachment? There are no published studies comparing the developmental and Bartholomew models; however, given their conceptual divergence, correspondence between these attachment style categories and adult attachment status would be unlikely. We believe this to be true particularly because the construction of these prototypes ignored mental or defensive processes. Westen (1992) stated:

> Social-cognitive models now often assume that a schema can be 'tagged' with affect of one valence or another; however, matters are far more complex. A person's schema . . . may include dozens of specific and generalized representations, which may not only have conflicting affective qualities among them but also within them. These encoded affective valuations will influence information processing and behavior in complex and interactive ways. . . . [one cannot assume] that the representation that becomes conscious is the one that receives the most activation, because a strongly activated representation may be too painful to acknowledge and may thus leave its mark though a defensively transformed derivative. (p. 384)

We find Westen's statement to be especially relevant to Bartholomew's interpretation of avoidant adult attachment. According to Bartholomew's scheme, a defining criterion of individuals judged avoidant is positive evaluation of self and a negative evaluation of other. From a defensive processing point of view, it is more likely that the conscious, positive evaluation of self reflects a self-serving bias and not a positive underlying internal working model of self. Indeed, we reiterate that, according to Bowlby's model, attachment insecurity is accompanied by negative internal evaluations of self. Self-serving bias, the tendency for an individual to portray him- or herself in a positive light to others, is a well-researched topic in social psychology; however, this concept has been ignored in Bartholomew's model.

FEARFUL AVOIDANCE AND CLINICAL RISK

Bartholomew's model of adult attachment style is the only social personality model that has been used systematically to address issues of clinical risk. According to Bartholomew, the underpinnings of risk are fearful avoidance, the prototype defined as a combination of negative evaluation of self with negative evaluation of other. "The fearful prototype is characterized by avoidance of close relationships because of a fear of rejection, sense of personal insecurity in relationships, and a distrust of others" (Bartholomew & Horowitz, 1991, p. 228). Studies have found fearful avoidance to be associated with problems in social interactive style and negative personality attributes such as problems with self-disclosure, intimacy, self-confidence, passivity, and the tendency toward exploitation (Bartholomew & Horowitz, 1991; Scharfe & Bartholomew, 1995). Fearful avoidant men tend to be more destructive in response to conflict interaction with their partners (e.g., ignore the problem, threatening to leave the relationship) than men with secure, dismissing-avoidant, or preoccupied attachment styles (Scharfe & Bartholomew, 1995). Fearful avoidance has also been found in greater proportions than other insecure attachment styles in battering men and in women survivors of sexual abuse (for overview, see West & George, 2002). Thus, according to Bartholomew's model, pathological risk is an extreme form of fearful avoidant attachment.

Although fearful avoidance fits nicely in a four-cell typology of adult attachment and views of adult avoidance coincide nicely with 1980s attachment models of risk, an increasing number of attachment theorists no longer view avoidance as a *primary* contributor to risk (Lyons-Ruth & Jacobvitz, 2008; Solomon & George, 1996, 2000, 2011a, 2011b). Main (1990) cogently argued that avoidance is a secondary behavioral strategy that serves the attachment goal of maintaining proximity while allowing the infant to ignore or minimize distressing activation of the attachment system that arises due to the parent's rejection of attachment needs. As a consequence, except under severe conditions of distress or threat, the infant can maintain proximity to the attachment figure because bids for physical contact and proximity are replaced by strategies that both decrease proximity (moving away, avoiding eye contact, displaced attention to objects) and the expressed need for the attachment figure (crying or calling). Solomon and George (1996; George & Solomon, 2008) have further argued that, in terms of protection, avoidant strategies are "good enough" under normal circumstances (i.e., in the absence of loss, abuse, or threat to self). That is, the rejecting or distance-promoting strategies that mothers and children in avoidant relationships utilize still allows the mother to protect the child from physical danger and threat.

Following Bartholomew's model, fearful avoidance may indeed explain the self-reported behavior (i.e., product of conscious thought) of some individuals who are at clinical risk for individual or relationship-based problems. It is unlikely, however, that a form of avoidance of relationships explains the attachment-related mechanism and defensive processes underlying risk and psychopathology because, ultimately, avoidance maintains attachment relationships. As we explicate with AAP case examples in Chapter 9, contemporary attachment theory and research suggest that risk for relationship pathology is rooted in a more profound form of relationship insecurity, attachment disorganization, and dysregulation (Solomon & George, 2011a).

Although we inevitably chafed against the limitations inherent in self-report questionnaires, we have developed and validated scales to measure the features of attachment for both adolescents and adults. A brief summary of the results of this project for adolescent attachment is presented because it illustrates an orientation toward scale development that is organized around the conceptual specification of the constituent elements of attachment rather than simply around seeking statistically significant precipitates that are then rationalized to "support" attachment concepts. Too often, in other words, scale development starts from a "naïve," non-construct-oriented approach as if no relevant attachment theory were extant. This approach is dictated more by post hoc statistical manipulations such as factor analysis than by conceptual considerations. Our approach is not simply empirical but follows Loevinger's (1957) construct-oriented and Jackson's (1971) sequential analysis approaches to scale development in which scales are derived a priori from theoretical considerations.

Because we were aware from related research that young adults organize their expectations of relationships in a manner that reflects a functional distinction between attachment and affiliation (friends, romantic partners), we first paid careful attention in the instructions to the identification of the individual's attachment figure. As noted by Crowell et al. (2008), this is a unique feature of our instruments. In the adolescent study, the majority of the participants (91.5%) identified their mother as their attachment figure.

We next identified two criteria distinguishing attachment relationships—availability and goal-corrected partnership. In general, attachment provides a unique relationship with the attachment figure who is perceived as available and responsive and who is turned to for emotional support. We included, as a separate scale, an assessment of the extent to which the adolescent considers and has empathy for the needs and feelings of the attachment figure and called this scale *goal-corrected partnership*. Bowlby (1973) identified anger directed toward the attachment figure as a reaction to the frustration of attachment needs and desires. We included *angry distress* as a scale to tap negative affective responses to the perceived unavailability of the attachment figure.

Following identification of these characteristics of adolescent–parent attachment, we developed scales for each of them and validated the scales in a large normative sample (n = 691) and a sample of 133 adolescents in psychiatric treatment. All scales demonstrated satisfactory internal reliability and agreement between scores for adolescents (n = 91) from the normative sample who completed the scales twice. Significantly, the three scales showed high convergent validity with the AAI. Specifically, adolescents classified as secure scored significantly different than other participants on *availability*, participants classified as preoccupied had significantly different scores on the scale *angry distress*, and participants classified as dismissing scored significantly different on the scale *goal-corrected partnership* (see West, Rose, Spreng, Sheldon-Keller, & Adam, 1998).

We included a description of this study because it provides evidence that a construct-oriented method of defining and measuring developmental attachment in adolescence can yield a self-report questionnaire with good psychometric properties and strong convergent validity with the AAI. But, as noted above, self-report questionnaires have inherent restrictions including the inability to include open-ended probes, the problem of socially desirable responses, and the inability to further explore contradictory responses. Measurement problems of this sort have pushed us to undertake the development and empirical validation of the AAP in adolescent populations.

CONCLUSION

We are at a point now in the assessment of adult attachment where choices of what to retain and what to leave out are not only possible but actually necessary. Despite the failure to demonstrate a reliable correspondence between attachment style and attachment status, measures of adult romantic attachment have strong internal validity, and the patterns identified by these measures predict a wide range of phenomena. Yet we have argued here that this approach, in focusing solely on self–other cognitive schemas and their underlying avoidance and anxiety dimensions, was never intended to capture the essential features of attachment relationships as described by Bowlby.

Finally, and very important to our work with the AAP, it also seems true that the social personality venture was dictated by a striving toward easy-to-use and-score measures of adult attachment that required no special training for administration and classification. This effort does reflect what seems to us to be one of our basic needs in the assessment of adult attachment—our need for an expedited way to activate the attachment system in the evaluation of an individual's attachment status. As we describe in Chapter 3, one of the main goals in developing the AAP was to provide researchers and clinicians with a construct-valid measure of developmental adult attachment status. Like the AAI, the AAP emphasizes evaluation of unconscious defensive processes. Like the self-report measures, however, the AAP is "user friendly" in terms of resources and training; administration, transcription, and the classification process itself are all expedited.

2

Defining Attachment Stories as Representational Precipitates

The AAP classification and coding system is based on evaluation of an individual's narrative, the window to attachment representation. Narration has a long history in attachment assessment, drawing from its gained prominence as a fundamental mode of explanation in psychoanalysis. The narrative mode was first emphasized by Spence (1982), whose book, *Narrative Truth, Historical Truth,* was dedicated to the effort to establish narratives as the form through which an individual's life may be apprehended. Schafer (1992) and Ammaniti and Stern (1994) describe narrative as a fundamental mode of interpretation in psychoanalysis. Schafer (1992), for example, in his *Retelling a Life*, holds that analysands' life histories are open narratives whose story lines, like a literary text, are collaboratively created during the analytic process.

Paralleling the contemporary accent on story lines in psychoanalysis has been the intensive study of coherence in the assessment of adult attachment status using the AAI (George et al., 1984/1985/1996; Main & Goldwyn, 1985/1988/1994; Main et al., 2003). Temporal quality (i.e., that is the sense of time and place where something important happened) is central to the construction of a coherent narrative as applied to the telling of actual life experience during the AAI. To speak of narrative coherence is simply to accent the historical nature of the internal working model, or as we discuss later, a re-finding of affective memories.

It has been possible to draw inferences regarding individual's current working models of attachment from the narrative patterns of how past attachment experiences with parents and other primary attachment figures are described. Within the capacity for narrative, wide individual differences with respect to the ability to perceive meaningful connections in the whole attachment history are recognized. Underlying these differences in autobiographical perception is the assumption that individuals' attachment-related experiences are available to them in the relative coherence of their present organization. The closer individuals are to perceiving the unity among these attachment experiences and the influence of these experiences on the current "self," the more coherent their personal attachment stories. We see, then, that autobiographical competence in this sense plays a crucial role in the attachment concept of narrative.

Despite the interest in narration as a mode of explanation in the recent literature of psychoanalysis and attachment, Bowlby (as cited in Holmes, 1993) opposed this trend. He viewed it as an attempt to contrive a psychology without an empirical basis by limiting attention to the hermeneutic understanding of how experience is endowed with meaning. Bowlby stated his position rather forcefully as follows: "I believe that our discipline can be put on to a scientific basis. A lot of people think you can't or don't know how to. There are people who think psychoanalysis is really a hermeneutic discipline. I think that's all rubbish quite frankly" (quoted in Holmes, 1993, p. 145). We may suppose that Bowlby was inclined to dismiss narration on the grounds that it was empirically "sloppy" and, in terms of the fundamental principles of attachment theory, it served no basic psychological or biological need. In other words, attachment experience as mediated by narrative appears to be the hermeneutic alternative to his thesis that attachment is a biologically wired-in behavioral control system.

We can perhaps reconcile these two points of view by noting that the coherence of the attachment narrative comes up ultimately against the constraints of affective memories. Furthermore, in contemporary attachment theory, reconciliation is also addressed by recent models that posit similarities between attachment narrative coherence and neurological coherence (Siegel, 1999). Bowlby (1973) regarded affects as primary (in the sense that affects are biological phenomena essential to survival) and observed "man's emotional expressions are as much a product of his evolution as are his anatomy and physiology" (Bowlby, 1991, p. 402). In Modell (1990), we find the same emphasis on affects as fundamental to human existence. Modell stated, "It is affects that provide meaning and significance to our past . . . affects are at the crossroads of biology and history" (p. 82). Neuroimaging studies (Damasio, 2003; Ruby & Decety, 2004) also indicate that affects are an integral aspect in the creation of meaning and representation and are of evolutionary value as internal signals essential for survival. For example, separation fear, as Bowlby (1973) observed, is one such affect signal. In summary, *we now understand* that affects that are imprinted on memory set the bounds for privately created narratives and, in turn, narrative coherence is ultimately derived from the embodied internal working model and its affective memories.

Bowlby's (1969/1982; 1973) account of internal working models, into which representations of emotionally significant aspects of attachment experience are integrated, is especially relevant in this regard. We propose here that individuals make sense of attachment situations, including the AAP situation, by using their affective responses to guide their search for meanings. Before discussing the working model of attachment as a particular instance of an affective category within memory, we first review the traditional understanding of this concept.

THE TRADITIONAL UNDERSTANDING OF THE WORKING MODEL OF ATTACHMENT

Attachment writing about the working model of the self and others has adhered basically to Bowlby's theory and the language of information processing that it dictates. This theory is as elegant as any in psychoanalysis. It uses only a few simple principles to explain a wide range of different phenomena—individual differences in attachment patterns, defensive processes, continuity, and change. Because extensive accounts of Bowlby's theory of the development of the internal working model of self exist in the attachment literature (e.g., Bretherton, 1985, 2005; Bretherton & Munholland, 2008), we confine our discussion here to a brief examination of his major ideas.

In Bowlby's (1969/1982, 1973, 1980) view, the working model of the self and attachment relationships constitute a dynamic configuration, the elements of which are so closely intertwined that the concept of self barely retains its integrity. For Bowlby, everything of consequence to the self—its coherence and continuity—is closely tied to the attachment environment surrounding the individual. Although it is therefore difficult in Bowlby's writing to draw lines of demarcation between the individual's self and the person's attachment environment, four major conceptions of the working model of the self that have contemporary currency nonetheless emerge.

First, Bowlby emphasized the role of actual attachment experiences in determining the child's inner mental world. With experience, representations of "ways-of-being-with" the caregiver, to use Stern's (1985) term, form the building blocks of more or less durable working models of self and of attachment figure(s). Bowlby stressed that a working model of the self is derived from common variations in how a caregiver responds to a child's attachment behaviors. These variations form patterns of responsiveness that strongly influence the child's concept of self. Bowlby (1973) put it this way: "the model of the attachment figure and the model of the self are likely to develop so as to be complementary and mutually confirming" (p. 204).

Main et al. (1985) and Stern (1985) expressed a similar point of view. Thus for Stern, the early core of the sense of self consists of "representations of interactions that have become generalized." Main et al. stated, "Knowledge of self and of other will be embedded in event-based relationships from the outset" (p. 75). This model of "the self in relation to attachment" suggests that the structure of the internal working model of self consists of affective memories of actual attachment relationships.

Second, unlike Cicchetti and Schneider-Rosen (1986) who used self-cognition and self-affect to refer to different phenomena, Bowlby emphasized that affects embedded in the working model of the self are rarely without ideational content. Indeed, when affects do not have mental content, they are experienced as a danger to the integrity of the self.

Third, Bowlby (1973, 1980) believed that the working model of the self is from the beginning an organismic whole that may subsequently split into multiple models as a defensive reaction to child–caregiver experiences that cannot be assimilated or integrated, experiences that were often traumatic or that threatened the attachment–caregiver bond. Main (1991; Hesse & Main, 2006) stressed that these experiences have a high potential to disrupt the child's ability to maintain a coherent model of attachment figures and of the self. Bowlby described how the child developed multiple models of self and attachment figures in order to safeguard the integrity of the self. This idea of multiple models suggests that information about one model of the self is defensively excluded from another model of the self (Bowlby, 1980). In this regard, Bowlby acknowledged his indebtedness to Winnicott's (1965) twofold organization of the self: the true self and the false self. Like Winnicott, Bowlby's notion of multiple models assumes that some models of the self are unconscious.

Fourth, as is well known, Bowlby preferred the term "working model" to "representational model" because he felt that the word *working* connoted something more dynamic than a mere static cognitive representation; a working model can always be updated. The term "working" was used to connote the potential for examining and integrating new attachment experiences into the model of self or reworking old attachment experiences based on the present. In adulthood, a number of what Bowlby (1969/1982) called major or radical changes in the attachment environment may lead to a process of conscious updating and revision of the model of self.

Fifth, like Freud's (1895/1954) effort in a *Project for a Scientific Psychology* to describe mental structures in terms of brain physiology, Bowlby (1969/1982) believed that the internal working model was not a metaphor but, in principle, an organization of processes in the brain. However, the impoverished computational model of the brain available to Bowlby precluded the possibility of achieving this goal. Only infrequently at this time were efforts made by researchers such as Hebb (1980) to connect these two areas. Today, likely inspired by recent advances in neuroscience, there has been a rising interest in bringing the processes of the internal working model into closer relation with neuroanatomical processes, thereby exposing the extent to which the two areas overlap. Numerous neuroimaging studies show the beginnings of the assembly of different brain structures and brain dynamics that may eventually permit us to think of the internal working model in a way that is compatible with Bowlby's (1969/1982) notion that the brain constructs them (see Chapter 10). At the very least, the evidence does suggest a fresh approach to the nature of memory and the internal working model within the framework of new neurobiological knowledge. As outlined below, Edelman's (1992) theory of memory as recategorization indicates that the internal working model must be conceived as generative and not as a static replica of attachment experience.

To summarize, the implication of Bowlby's theory is that the child actively uses what he or she anticipates about the consequences of attachment events to construct a model of the self as worthy of seeking and receiving care and protection from attachment figures. When, as with a rejecting or inconsistently responsive caregiver, the relationship is disturbed, the child will likely experience him- or herself as incompetent (at least in the sphere of attachment) and unlovable. By contrast, when events have led the child to anticipate the caregiver's availability, understanding, and responsiveness, the child will consequently experience him- or herself as competent and valuable. In short, Bowlby emphasizes that the empathic responsiveness of the caregiver to the child's attachment behaviors integrates or fragments the working model of the self.

In this view of the working model, early experiences are embedded in memory in a model of attachment relationships that has a continuous and discrete existence within our minds. In characterizing the working model as the primary feature of the adult attachment system, Bowlby worked within the information processing models of brain functioning that were predominant in the last century and which lead to great success in the development of computer technology. But information processing models that posit a stored model that is isomorphic with past experience have not provided useful tools for deciphering the puzzle of working models, affects, and memories. Of particular significance in this regard has been Edelman's (1992) concept of "memory as categorization" as set forth in his book *Bright Air, Brilliant Fire*. Reviving Freud's (1895/1954) term *Nachtraglichkeit*, or the idea that memory is the retranscription of subsequent experience, Edelman argued that the brain does not store memories. Rather, it establishes potentials for rediscovering previous categories in current situations. In Edelman's words, "Recategorical memory is dynamic, transformational, associative, and distributed—its procedures are *representative* of categorizations, but are not necessarily representations" (p. 270).

A NEW APPROACH TO UNDERSTANDING THE WORKING MODEL OF ATTACHMENT

In Edelman's (1992) theory, stored models do not evoke affects and behaviors; rather, the reverse happens. Motoric stimuli, including behaviors and affects, form the basis for *perception and learning*. Through motoric activity we participate in and test new environments; this stimulates a perceptual search for applicable mental categories. These mental categories, once recovered, provide the basis for what Modell (1990) called a "*retranscription* of memory in a new context" (p. 64). To the extent that there are mental models, they are constantly recreated as a synthesis of old categories and new experiences. These synthesized models are a characteristic of the present and not stored in memory; rather, their *effects* are incorporated as potentials for influencing renewed models in future experiences.

Following Edelman's (1992) theory, the working model of attachment becomes a particular affective category within memory. Modell (1990) stated, "Affect categories reflect the memory of a unique constellation of experience (whether veridical or not); they can be thought of as units of experience of the past brought into present time" (p. 66). The affective category of attachment is refound when current behaviors or feelings stimulate a perception of continuity with and similarity to past attachment-related experiences.

This view of memory as having the potential to re-find categories is in keeping with neuroimaging studies that support the embodiment of meaning. In research on specific sites in the prefrontal cortex and appraisals of one's own and others' actions, three major sites that support this type of intersubjective awareness emerge: the orbitofrontal prefrontal cortex that enters into the facilitation of new adaptive responses and the suppresion of habitual responses; the anterior cingulate prefrontal cortex, often considered to be related to the signaling of conflict in information processing; and the dorsolateral prefrontal cortex, the substrate of memory that permits the consideration of alternative courses of action (see Chapter 10). As a result of this recent evidence, it is now possible to think about the actual mental processes underlying the internal working model in ways that are commensurate with neurophysiological processes.

This conceptualization of working models as affective categories offers several advantages over the "engineering model" of Bowlby (1969/1982) and the "algorithm model" of traditional attachment theory mental representation of attachment (e.g., Main et al., 1985). At the risk of overgeneralization, we attempt a concise comparative summary. In the traditional view of working models, early attachment experiences create an internalized model, containing expectations about behaviors and affects associated with attachment relationships. This internalized model has historical continuity and is used by the individual to guide behaviors and affects in new attachment-relevant situations. The model establishes, for the individual, rules or procedures for responding to attachment stimuli. The affective content flows from these rules. The working model precedes, and indeed determines, the perception of a current attachment-relevant experience.

In the updated view of working models proposed here, behaviors and affects that were once associated with attachment form the basis for the perception of potential recategorization of experiences to include both old and new attachment-relevant information. There is no discrete model maintained in the memory, but rather a *potential* to reclassify or recategorize past experiences in the light of current experiences. Perception of attachment-related behaviors and affects *precedes* rediscovery or re-creation of the affective category derived from attachment experiences. Affects are not merely part of the content of the working model; they are the mechanism for reactivating in the present the category established in the past. Working models are dynamic, associative, affective categories that have the potential to be rediscovered and reformed in new situations.

Consistent with this model of memory, we may view Main's (Hesse & Main, 2000) discussion of lapses in narrative coherence attending traumatic events as "disorders" of categorization, memory, and integration. With a new emphasis on a "brain" metaphor of the mind, these narrative lapses are understood as arising from the individual's inability to differentiate internal cognitive processes from old perceptions. The essential point is that whether reactivated affective memories support or diminish narrative coherence depends on the degree to which they are recategorized. Anything that interferes with recategorization such as dissociation will prevent the disconfirmation of an affective category.

SUMMARY

To step outside of neurophysiological theory and back into the reality of the AAP response process, the conceptualization of working models as affective categories offers a useful way to understand the AAP response process. In Chapter 3, we propose that the AAP opens up and renders amenable to interpretation those personal elements of attachment distress that, ordinarily, individuals transform or keep locked away (i.e., excluded from conscious awareness). In responding to the instructions to make up a story about what is going on in the picture, individuals make sense of the various depicted attachment situations by using their perceptual and affective responses to impart meaning to the picture stimuli. The external attachment "pull" of the AAP picture stimuli prompts a search of the internal for applicable mental concepts. In their effort to give meaning to and find meaning in each picture stimulus, a shifting balance of adaptive and defensive processes is evidenced in adults' story responses. Depending on the relative ascendance of adaptation and defense, the final story product may range from a thoughtful and reflective response to an automatic, unreflective, and even disorganized one. We describe this range of representational functioning during the AAP story-telling task in the chapters that follow, and we ultimately use these descriptions in the assignment of an attachment group classification.

PART II

Development, Validation, and Coding of the AAP

3

The Development and Validation of the AAP

This present chapter describes the development and validation of the Adult Attachment Projective Picture System. This discussion precedes a discussion of the details of the coding and classification system (see Chapters 4 and 5) to provide the reader with basic overarching information about the AAP.

The core of representational assessments is the view that narrative descriptions of experience are individuals' subjective constructions of their lives guided by internalized mental representations. In the course of development, and particularly in instances of compromised care, the personal and affectively charged elements in these "stories" are distorted in attempts to keep certain aspects of attachment-related distress carefully deflected. Experience and affect are transformed in order to be acceptable to consciousness and sometimes "locked away" and defensively excluded from conscious attention and memory. We discuss an attachment theory approach to defensive exclusion in Chapter 5. The point for the present discussion is that the goal of representation-based assessment is to uncover distortions and unlock walled-off elements in order to see through individuals' carefully constructed defensive maneuvers and thereby render the themes contained within their stories amenable to interpretation.

Historically, although attachment theory is grounded in naturalistic observation (Ainsworth, 1964; Bowlby, 1951), some of the earliest assessments of attachment were representational. Bowlby was intrigued by the notion of using projective methodology to examine children's responses to separation and loss (Bowlby, 1973; Klagsbrun & Bowlby, 1976). Since attachment theory's "move to the level of representation" (Main et al., 1985) in the 1980s, researchers have developed interpretative schemes that draw upon the individual's ability to use symbolic representation and to organize knowledge conceptually (Bretherton, 2005; Waters & Waters, 2006). These mentalizing elements can be elicited from representation-based assessments beginning in the preschool years. Many representational assessments for children follow semiprojective methodologies for which researchers have developed rating scales for attachment-relevant constructs (e.g., sensitivity) or classification schemes (secure, avoidant, ambivalent, disorganized). The assessment stimuli include pictures or story stems that the children enact and narrate using family dolls. Detailed discussion of these forms of assessment for children is beyond the scope of this volume. The reader is referred to Solomon and George (2008) for a comprehensive review of representational and behavioral child attachment measures.

Representational assessment of adult attachment originated with the AAI (George et al., 1984/1985/1996), which is considered to be the "gold standard" measure for researchers and clinicians following the developmental attachment tradition. The AAI is a quasi-clinical interview during which individuals describe their childhood experiences with attachment figures using a series of standardized questions and probes that are designed to elicit memories of attachment figures in contexts that generate attachment distress, including separation, physical and psychological hurt, rejection, loss, and abuse. Individuals' accounts of experience vary in the extent to which their stories reveal unity or coherence among the network of attachment memories. Each interview is examined for one of three primary attachment patterns as analogous to the infant attachment groups—secure/autonomous, dismissing, and preoccupied—and for evidence of an unresolved state of mind regarding loss through death or abuse. The structured open-ended questioning of attachment-oriented themes has been demonstrated to be a valuable design feature of the AAI. This form of questioning encourages individuals to create their life story in a "conversation" with the interviewer that provides a picture of childhood attachment experiences and the meanings that surround these experiences. Readers interested in learning more about the AAI are referred to Hesse's (2008) discussion of AAI development, validation, and use.

Unlike the AAI, the AAP was not designed to elicit autobiographical narrative; rather, it systematically activates attachment by presenting a standardized set of projective attachment stimuli. Individuals are asked to create narrative "stories" about drawings that depict attachment scenes. Like the AAI, the responses to the AAP stimuli are conceived as the product of individuals' internal working models of attachment.

Our picture system approach follows the semiprojective assessment already in use the field to assess attachment in children, in particular the Attachment Doll Play Assessment (Solomon et al., 1995). The common denominator of projective methodology (i.e., free-response task) is the access to conscious and unconscious thoughts and emotions through verbal responses to a standardized set of ambiguous visual stimuli (Hilsenroth, 2004). The administration technique is unstructured. Unencumbered by administrative directives, individuals are encouraged to respond freely, guided only by a few basic standardized, open-ended questions. As such, projective methodology is not contaminated by the self-serving biases that plague self-report measures, have a lower risk of the exaggerations and minimizations of experience found in clinical interviews, and are economical and easy to use (Hilsenroth, 2004). The narratives provide a rich picture of interpersonal and behavioral dimensions, revealing patterns of unconscious and automatic defensive processing that lead to reliable interpretation when interpretive rules follow standardized guidelines (Leichtman, 2004). Although criticized by some assessment experts as subject to interpretive bias, and poor validity and reliability, large-scale studies of reliability (interrater, test–retest reliability) and predictive validity demonstrate that the projective technique is a valid form of assessment (Hilsenroth, 2004; Meyer, 2004; Wood, Nezworski, & Stejskal, 1996), especially when interpretation has a strong theoretical foundation (McClelland, Atkinson, Clark, & Lowell, 1953).

PICTURE STIMULI SELECTION PROCESS

The scenes that comprise the stimuli for the AAP were selected to capture three core features of attachment theory as defined by the Bowlby–Ainsworth model. The first feature is observing attachment under conditions that activate the attachment system. Bowlby's seminal attachment trilogy (1969/1982, 1973, 1980) stressed the importance of observing attachment in contexts that threaten or compromise physical or psychological safety. Strictly speaking, of course, the internal working model of attachment is not directly observable, and assessment must activate the system in order to "see" the variations in its representational manifestations. A study of the "contents" and vicissitudes of attachment representation is inferred directly during assessment. The importance of activating attachment during assessment is somewhat controversial. Bowlby clearly described its importance; Ainsworth integrated these ideas directly into her naturalistic observation format and designed the Strange Situation to be a mini-drama of attachment activating events (Ainsworth, 1967; Ainsworth et al., 1978). Recently, the question of how to assess attachment in children based on scripts and in adults based on measuring conscious social cognitions has raised the issue of how to interpret attachment "data" when the system is not activated. The recent script literature acknowledges the overlaps among attachment group distinctions, for example, when individuals know the scripts of security but may not themselves be secure (Waters & Waters, 2006). More problematic is evaluating attachment groups or dimensions based on social cognitive responses to generic questionnaire items that bear only semantic resemblance to actual activating events (Maier, Bernier, Pekrun, Zimmerman, & Grossmann, 2004). Therefore, in developing the AAP stimulus set, we followed Bowlby's model and selected scenes that portray major attachment life events—separation, solitude, fear, and death.

The second feature is the availability of an attachment figure. This feature is one of the defining constructs in attachment theory (Ainsworth et al., 1978; Bowlby, 1969/1982). Ainsworth showed that attachment security was related to the attachment figure's direct availability and responsiveness. Compromises in availability are associated with the development of avoidant and ambivalent-resistant forms of organized insecure attachment. Unable to achieve proximity successfully through direct signaling, these insecure children must rely on alternative mechanisms to achieve proximity and the caregiver's attention when distant or distracted (George & Solomon, 2008; Main, 1990; Solomon & George, 1996). The hallmark of disorganized attachment is the child's subjective experience of attachment figure abandonment and unavailability (George & Solomon, 2008; Solomon et al., 1995). Solomon and George (2000) developed the concept of "abdication of the caregiving system" to describe the caregiving failures that leave the child feeling helpless and vulnerable and having to take responsibility for his own attachment needs.

West and Sheldon-Keller (1994), expanding on Weiss (1982), pointed out that there are qualitative differences over the lifespan in the form of the kind of attachment figure availability required to assuage distress.

In infancy and early childhood, attachment figures need to be physically present and accessible. By adolescence and throughout adulthood, individuals predominantly use "psychological" or representational proximity to replace in many situations the physical access to attachment figures required by children (see also Allen, 2008; Main et al., 1985).

Following this theoretical foundation, the AAP picture stimuli depict attachment figure availability in two forms. One form explicitly portrays the proximate availability of an attachment figure by drawing characters in dyadic pairs. We call these stimuli the dyadic pictures. The other form portrays individuals alone. We call these stimuli the alone pictures. In the absence of a visible cue, availability must be created by describing an internalized or physically present attachment figure, a task consonant with the abstract thought that characterizes adult mental representations of attachment (see Main et al., 1985). We define the attachment figures created in alone responses in terms of the *internalized secure base* and *haven of safety*, respectively (see Chapter 4).

The third feature captures attachment theory's lifespan view. Bowlby and Ainsworth laid the foundation for thinking about attachment contributions to development and mental ill-health beyond infancy (Ainsworth, 1989; Bowlby, 1969/1982). We integrated this lifespan view in the AAP stimulus set by including characters that depict childhood to old age.

The drawings that comprise the AAP picture system were originally selected based on pictures in children's story books and coffee-table books thought to depict attachment situations. A large set of drawings was developed and presented to undergraduate college students to rate for attachment pull (see West & Sheldon-Keller, 1994, for a detailed description of the stimulus selection process). The initial AAP stimulus set was composed of three scenes. These scenes depicted solitude (*Child at Window*), nighttime separation (*Bed*), and separation in the context of illness or death (*Ambulance*). Other scenes were later added to the set to enhance the AAP's ability to activate attachment by presenting a broader spectrum of attachment events.

THE TASK

The AAP stimulus set is comprised of eight line drawings. The first stimulus serves as a warm-up for the AAP task; it is not an attachment scene. The seven other stimuli depict theoretically derived attachment scenes. The drawings contain only sufficient detail to identify an event; facial expressions and other potentially biasing details are absent. The characters were drawn to capture a diverse range in cultural background, gender, and age. The AAP stimuli are presented in Figures 3.1–3.8. The scenes include *Neutral*—two children play with a ball; *Child at Window (abbreviated as Window)*—a child looks out a window; *Departure*—an adult man and woman stand facing each other with suitcases positioned nearby; *Bench*—a youth sits alone on a bench; *Bed*—a child and woman sit opposite each other on the child's bed; *Ambulance*—a woman and a child watch ambulance workers load a stretcher into an ambulance; *Cemetery*—a man stands by a gravesite headstone; and *Child in Corner (abbreviated as Corner)*—a child stands askance in a corner.

The AAP is administered in a private setting. It can be used alone or as part of an assessment battery. If used with other assessments, the rule of thumb for research and clinical work is to administer developmental attachment measures before any other assessments that day. We often use the AAI in our work; therefore, we needed to know whether there was an administration effect for these two measures. We found no order effects in a subsample in which we counterbalanced the administration of the AAP and the AAI in the same session. Our own preference when these measures are administered in tandem is to give the long and ardu-

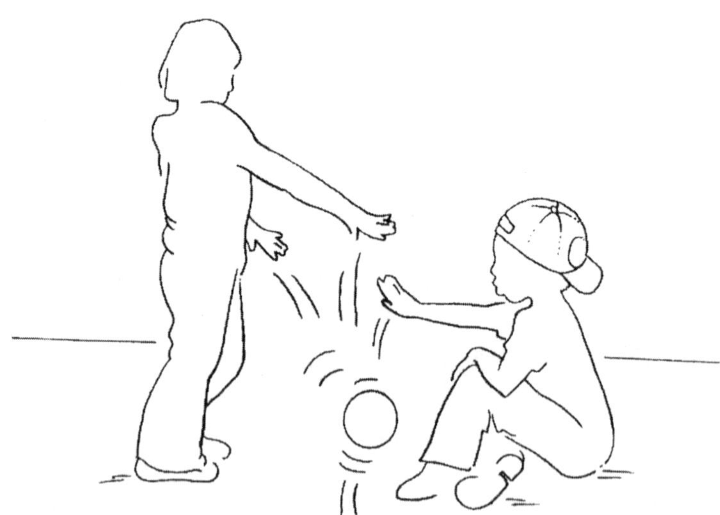

FIGURE 3.1. *Neutral.* Copyright 1997 by Carol George, Malcolm L. West, and Odette Pettem. Reprinted by permission.

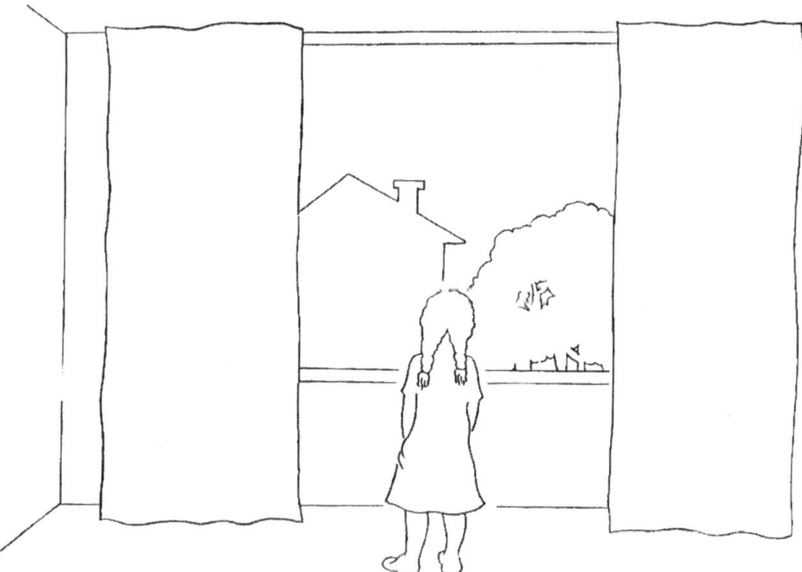

FIGURE 3.2. *Child at Window.* Copyright 1997 by Carol George, Malcolm L. West, and Odette Pettem. Reprinted by permission.

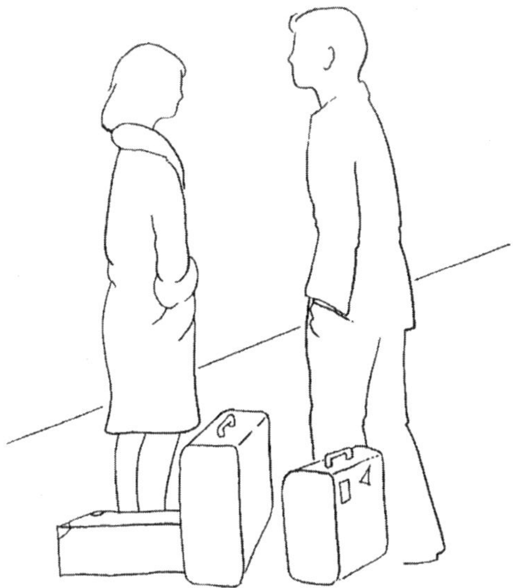

FIGURE 3.3. *Departure.* Copyright 1997 by Carol George, Malcolm L. West, and Odette Pettem. Reprinted by permission.

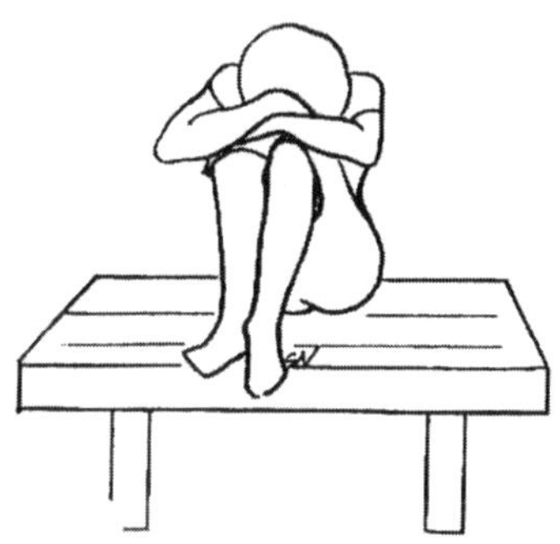

FIGURE 3.4. *Bench.* Copyright 1997 by Carol George, Malcolm L. West, and Odette Pettem. Reprinted by permission.

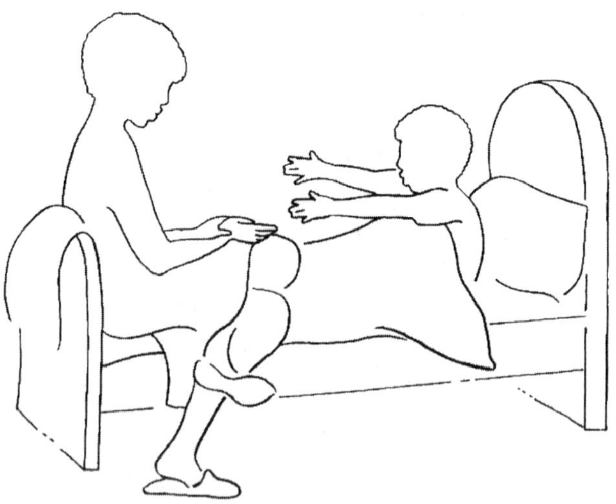

FIGURE 3.5. *Bed.* Copyright 1997 by Carol George, Malcolm L. West, and Odette Pettem. Reprinted by permission.

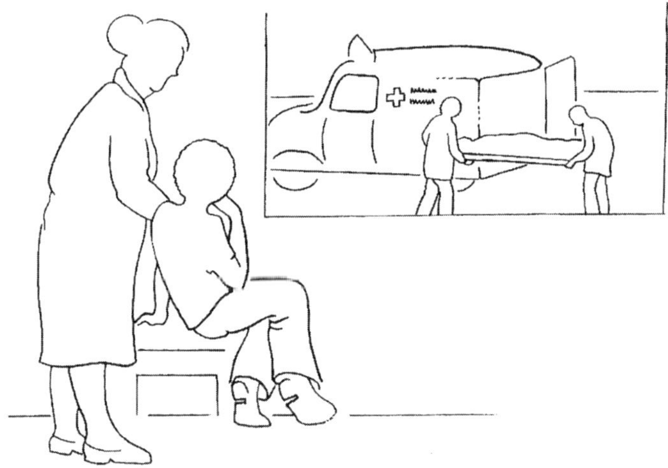

FIGURE 3.6. *Ambulance*. Copyright 1997 by Carol George, Malcolm L. West, and Odette Pettem. Reprinted by permission.

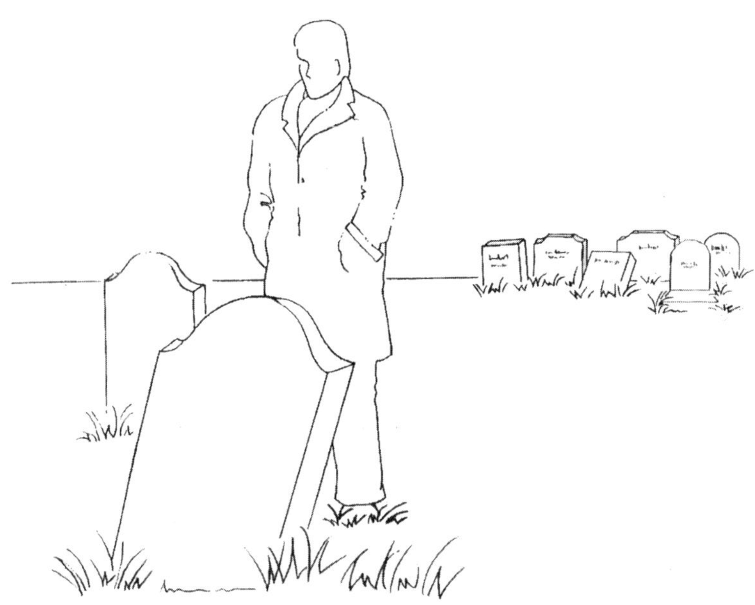

FIGURE 3.7. *Cemetery*. Copyright 1997 by Carol George, Malcolm L. West, and Odette Pettem. Reprinted by permission.

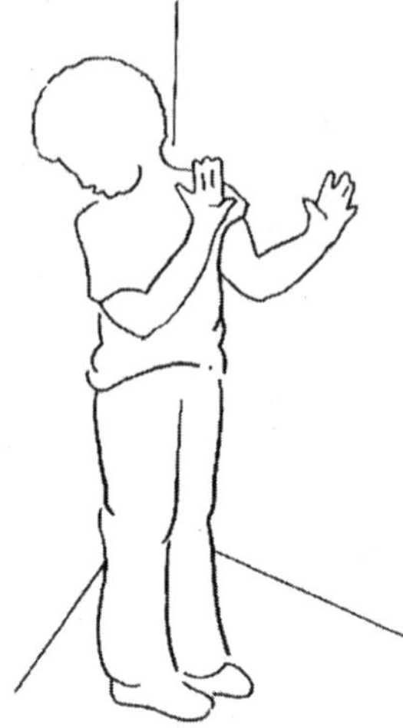

FIGURE 3.8. *Child in Corner.* Copyright 1997 by Carol George, Malcolm L. West, and Odette Pettem. Reprinted by permission.

ous AAI first. We find that the shorter and simpler AAP is a good way to "wrap up" the attachment portion of an assessment battery.

The AAP administration method combines apperceptive projective free-response and semistructured interview techniques. This approach has strong demonstrated success in adult and child attachment assessment (e.g., Bretherton, Ridgeway, & Cassidy, 1990; George & Solomon, 2008; Solomon et al., 1995). The interviewee is seated across from the administrator. The interviewee is handed each stimulus to hold while responding. The task begins with the *Neutral* warm-up scene.[1] The administrator begins by stating the instructions: "Describe what is happening in the picture, what led up to the events, what the characters are thinking or feeling, and what will happen next." One need not look far for the implications of the task instructions. At once, the individual is confronted with a paradox. The stimuli are clearly pictorial and at one level define the task as a purely perceptual one. The instructions simultaneously encourage a subjective response in that they require individuals to use their imagination as well as conscious and unconscious memories and mental concepts of attachment. Performance anxieties are eased by

[1] Variations of administration using more than one warm-up stimulus are described in Chapter 10.

assuring the interviewee that there are no incorrect answers. Throughout the task, the administrator waits comfortably for the interviewee to complete the response, using the above questions to prompt storytelling as needed. Once a response is completed, the administrator hands the interviewee the next picture stimulus and proceeds similarly through the remainder of the picture set.

The AAP is administered only using the full set of picture stimuli in the order designated above. Unlike some free-response assessments, the administrator may not select stimuli or alter the presentation order. We designed the presentation order so that less distressing stimuli are presented early on during the AAP, progressing to increasingly threatening attachment scenes. This design order parallels the design of other developmental attachment assessments (Strange Situation, doll play story stems, AAI).

Our conceptualization of the the AAP stress activation progression is supported in a neuroimaging study that examined attachment activation in the fMRI scanner. Buchheim, Erk et al. (2006; see also Chapter 10) reported increased activation of the right inferior frontal cortex over the course of the AAP task, an area of the brain that is associated with the process of suppressing unwanted emotion and reappraising unwanted emotions in unemotional terms. This study also found increasing activation in medial temporal regions of the brain (amygdala, hippocampus) for individuals with unresolved attachment. In summary, these results point to increased involvement of emotion control processes as the attachment stimuli portray increasingly threatening events.[2]

The AAP is tape-recorded and coded later from a verbatim transcript. The standard administration time is approximately 25 minutes. AAP transcripts are typically two to three pages long, sometimes longer in the case of clinical clients. Coding and classification is done by a trained reliable judge and typically takes between one-half and 2 hours.

Administrators do not need to have a background in attachment theory, assessment technique, or the AAP coding and classification system. The AAP has been administered by a range of different individuals, including women, men, undergraduate research assistants, experienced researchers, and clinicians, and has been administered in

[2] An interesting observation related to presentation order is when individuals' responses to the initial AAP stimuli include dysregulated attachment themes. This is an atypical response that we interpret as individuals' hypersensitivity to events as highly threatening. This type of responsiveness appears more frequently in research with clinical samples and in psychotherapy clients than in typical samples.

languages other than English (e.g., French, German, Japanese, Italian). Administration training typically requires three to four supervised practice cases. Ethical use of the AAP is important for the validity of the instrument and protection of research participants, clients, and patients. It is assumed, and we have indeed found, that most individuals who are asked to respond to the AAP have a positive attitude and are cooperative. Interviewees typically do not get upset during the AAP experience. No debriefing or follow-up is typically required. It is important to remember, however, that the pictures are powerful stimuli. In some situations, the administrator may detect some reluctance or distress in the individual's response to the task. Interviewers are trained to follow the probes carefully and not debrief or engage in caretaking during the task. Debriefing may be necessary if the interviewee is highly emotionally distressed during the task. On rare occasions, the interviewee asks to stop. We have developed clear guidelines to help administrators identify defensive resistances as compared to cues that would require terminating the administration session. If an interviewee is highly distressed, the AAP should be curtailed and re-administered on another day. This strategy is rarely needed with the AAP, which makes it amenable for use in stressed populations in which other attachment measures, especially the AAI, may be too stressful or prohibited (Buchheim & George, 2011; Szanjberg & George, 2011). These guidelines have been approved by national and international internal review boards that oversee research with human participants.

Training in the coding and classification of the AAP is also part of its ethical use. Evaluation to determine the individual's attachment response and representation cannot be done intuitively, even if one is trained in other attachment assessments. More information about training and use is available on the AAP website: *www.attachmentprojective.com.*

VALIDATION OF THE AAP

We have dedicated the past decade to validating the AAP. Beginning with Ainsworth's seminal work with the Strange Situation (Ainsworth et al., 1978), developmental attachment theory primarily uses a taxomic measurement approach; children and adults are placed into secure or insecure classification groups. This is not the only approach to measuring attachment, and some argue the merits of adding dimensional or other approaches to augment our understanding of the attachment construct (Fraley & Spieker, 2003; Solomon & George, 2008; Solomon et al., 1995; Waters & Beauchaine, 2003). However, with the exception of the Attachment Q-sort methodology (van IJzendoorn, Vereijken, Bakermans-Kranenburg, & Riksen-Walraven, 2004; Waters, 1995; Waters & Deane, 1985), nontaxonomic approaches are poorly validated or define new constructs that are only tangentially related to the Bowlby–Ainsworth model of attachment (Crowell et al., 2008; Riggs et al., 2007). Therefore, we chose to follow the taxonomic tradition for validating the AAP and developed a classification scheme that discriminates among the four major adult attachment groups: secure, dismissing, preoccupied, and unresolved. Our approach led to the development of a set of unique assessment dimensions that permit examination of mechanisms that contribute to individual differences, which Waters and Beauchaine (2003) pointed out has been virtually ignored in the field of attachment. Recent research focusing on analyses of the AAP dimensions both supported the taxonomic classification approach and yielded new information about the underlying mechanisms of attachment. The "nuts and bolts" dimensions of our classification scheme are discussed in subsequent chapters, including the application of the AAP dimensions to case interpretation. Here we present our development and validation research that establishes the AAP as a valid taxonomic adult attachment classification measure.

We approached development and validation in three stages. The initial version of the AAP classification scheme was based on evaluations of 13 transcripts of men and women recruited from the community through newspaper advertisement. This work used a form of the AAP that included only six attachment stimuli; we had not yet developed the *Corner* scene. We examined the verbatim AAP transcripts of the attachment stimuli stories from a number of different aspects, including looking for attachment themes, specific content features, and descriptive images. This process led to developing a set of AAP content coding dimensions that we thought would differentiate among attachment group classifications. We also examined narrative discourse patterns, following the well-established AAI tradition. Our primary goal when we began this endeavor, and one that we maintained throughout our work, was to validate the AAP by establishing concurrent predictive validity for four attachment groups as designated by the AAI. Nine of the individuals in this initial group had completed the AAI prior to administration of the AAP. AAIs were classified blind by the first author. We checked our AAP classifications against the AAI classifications and then used our knowledge of the AAI classification to refine the AAP classification system on a case-by-case basis. At this point, we added the *Corner* picture, a stimulus that extended the AAP attachment themes to include potential abuse[3] as well as coding rules for evaluating defensive processes.

The next step was to examine the validity of our classification scheme using two new samples and the eight-picture stimulus set. We continued to test for concurrent validity with the AAI and also sought to establish interjudge reliability. The first sample included a subsample of 25 mothers drawn randomly from a large ongoing study of infant risk conducted by Dr. Diane Benoit, which included a control sample of mothers of infants who were not at developmental risk. Dr. Benoit, a trained, reliable AAI judge without any knowledge of our AAP coding scheme, classified the AAIs and had members of her research team administer the AAP. The AAP development team (Drs. George, West, and Pettem) classified the AAP transcripts blind to AAI classification and infant risk status. The second sample included 24 women who had participated in a large-scale study of depression (West & George, 2002). AAIs were coded blind by the first author. Interjudge reliability was examined by comparing the independent classifications of the two other members of the development team, one of whom (Pettem) was blind to clinical group status.

The validity analyses based on these two samples demonstrated acceptable validity for the AAP. Interjudge reliability in this phase of developing the AAP (n = 49) was 87% agreement for four-group classifications (i.e., secure, dismissing, preoccupied, unresolved; kappa = .82, $p < .000$) and 97% agreement for secure versus insecure classifications (kappa = .73, $p < .000$). There was 92% AAP/AAI convergent agreement for four-group classifications (kappa = .89, $p < .000$) and 97% convergent agreement for secure versus insecure groups (kappa = .80, $p < .000$).

THE AAP VALIDATION STUDY

The third step in our validity research was to design a large scale psychometric investigation that added AAP test–retest reliability, discriminant validity, and AAI reliability to our research design.[4] This study consisted

[3] We are indebted to Dr. Diane Benoit for this suggestion.

[4] This study was supported by grants awarded to Dr. West from the Social Science and Humanities Research Council of Canada and funding awarded to Dr. George from the Barrett Foundation and Mills College.

of a sample of 144 participants represented by two subsamples of individuals, one from Calgary, Alberta, Canada ($n = 73$) and the other from northern California ($n = 71$). Adults between the ages of 18 and 65 were recruited from September 2002 to August 2003 from community and college settings using newspaper and Internet advertisement. Individuals with insufficient fluency in English were excluded from participation. Further exclusion criteria included a diagnosis of psychosis, or organic brain or central nervous system disorder. Three participants were judged Cannot Classify (CC) on the AAI and dropped from the validity sample. These exclusion criteria were necessary for this psychometric study because the attachment classifications derived from the AAI and the AAP are based largely on language discourse rating criteria that would be unduly biased by cognitive or psychiatric impairment or a poor ability to use the English language.[5] Dropping CCs from the analysis was necessary because it is atypical in community samples and there is no well-established understanding of this classification group (Hesse, 2008; we explore this issue further in Chapter 9).

One of the strengths of our validity sample was that it included both female and male participants, which adds significantly to the scarcity of adult attachment validation data for males. Of the 144 participants, 100 were female and 44 were male. The mean age for females was 36.2 years ($SD = 15.2$) and for males was 26.4 years ($SD = 8.9$). The males participating in this study were on average significantly younger than the females ($t = 4.88$; $p < .000$). There was a significantly greater number of Canadian female participants than U.S. women ($n = 58$) in the sample and there was a significantly greater number of U.S. men ($n = 29$) than Canadian men ($n = 15$) in the sample. The mean level of education was 14.7 years. The Alberta sample was uniformly Caucasian. The racial composition of the California sample was as follows: 49% Caucasian, 10% African American, 4% Hispanic, 12% Asian/Filipino, and 25% failed to specify.

Individuals participated in one-on-one sessions in a private office. Participants signed consent forms prior to beginning a session. During the session, research assistants first administered the attachment mea-

[5] The use of the AAP with individuals with cognitive and psychiatric impairment is being explored by researchers and clinicians. The first author is currently involved in research using the AAP with individuals with cognitive impairment. No results from this study are available at this time. Studies using the AAP with psychiatric patients have shown the AAP to be a valid measure for both out- and inpatients (Buchheim, Erk, et al., 2006; Buchheim & George, 2011)

sures, counterbalancing AAP/AAI administration in order to minimize potential administration order effects. A verbal intelligence measure was administered following the attachment measures. Other questionnaires were either filled out by participants at the end of the laboratory session or were mailed to the participants for completion in advance of the laboratory session. Approximately 12 weeks later (range 8–15 weeks), 69 individuals (48%) returned to complete the AAP a second time. Only the AAP was administered during the return testing session.

Measures

Adult Attachment Projective Picture System

The AAP picture system used in this study was the now standard eight-picture stimulus set. As in previous studies, AAPs were audiotaped and transcribed for later verbatim analysis. Three trained and reliable judges, blind to all information about the participants, independently coded the AAP transcripts. All transcripts were classified by at least two judges. $\text{Judge}_{\text{AAP}}1$ classified the entire set of AAPs; $\text{Judges}_{\text{AAP}}$ 2 and 3 classified subsets of AAPs that overlapped with $\text{Judge}_{\text{AAP}}1$. $\text{Judge}_{\text{AAP}}$ 2 classified 74 cases; $\text{Judge}_{\text{AAP}}$ 3 classified 135 cases.

Adult Attachment Interview

The most recent (third edition) version of the AAI (George, Kaplan, & Main, 1996) was used in this study. This version includes more questions and probes about trauma than in the earlier versions of the AAI. AAIs were classified blind by two reliable judges. The total number of AAIs was 130; 14 were dropped because of technical problems. $\text{Judge}_{\text{AAI}}1$ classified all of the AAIs in the sample; $\text{Judge}_{\text{AAI}}2$ classified 30 transcripts ($n = 30$; 21%) in order to establish interjudge reliability. AAI interjudge reliability was 85% agreement for four-group classifications (kappa = .72, $p < .000$; phi = 1.26, $p < .000$) and 87% agreement for secure versus insecure classifications (kappa = .63, $p < .000$; phi = .64, $p < .000$).

Balanced Inventory of Desirable Responding

The Balanced Inventory of Desirable Responding (BIDR; Paulhus, 1998) is a 40-item social desirability assessment inventory that uses a 7-point Likert scale to assess two subscales: self-deception and impression management. The self-deception scale is designed to assess defensiveness toward personal threats and positively biased responding that the respondent believes to be true (e.g., "I am a completely rational person"). The impression management scale is designed to measure responding that seeks to create a favorable impression on others (e.g., "I never take things that don't belong to me"). Each scale has 10 true-keyed and 10 false-keyed items. This measure has established acceptable validity (e.g., Holden, Starzyk, McLeod, & Edwards, 2000; Lanyon & Carle, 2007).

Verbal Intelligence

The vocabulary and similarities subtests from the Wechsler Adult Intelligence Scale—Revised (WAIS-R; Wechsler, 1981) were used to measure verbal intelligence. The verbal intelligence scales were selected from the WAIS because AAP responses and the coding system are language based.

Symptom Check List–90—Revised

The Symptom Check List–90—Revised (SCL-90-R; Derogatis & Cleary, 1977) is a validated and widely used measure of current levels of distress. The 90 questions yield separate scales related to nine symptom dimensions: somatization, obsessive–compulsive, interpersonal sensitivity, depression, anxiety, hostility, phobic anxiety, paranoid ideation, and psychoticism. Participants are asked to rate the extent to which they felt distressed by the problem within the last 7 days on a 5-point scale ranging from extremely (0) to not at all (4). In addition to the symptom dimensions, the SCL-90-R also yields three composite scales: the Global Severity Index (GSI), an overall index of distress averaged across the nine dimensions; the Positive Symptom Total (PST), the number of symptoms endorsed; and the Positive Symptom Distress Index (PSDI), an index of severity of endorsed symptoms.

Results

Analyses of AAP and AAI classifications showed no administration order effects and we did no further analyses based on administration order. The AAP classification distribution of the 144 participants[6] was as follows: 25 (17%) were autonomous (F); 37 (26%) were classified as dismissing (Ds); 30 (21%) were preoccupied (E); and 52 (36%) were unresolved (U). This distribution was satisfactory for our study, which

[6] Not all measures were available for all participants.

sought to establish test characteristics and not population characteristics. The mean ages for each classification group were F, 28.27 years; Ds, 30.92 years; E, 38.57 years, and U, 34.12 years. Preoccupied participants were significantly older than autonomous participants ($F_{3,144}$ = 2.80, $p < .05$). Age, gender, national residency, and years of education were not related to attachment classification.

Interjudge reliability for the AAP was calculated for both four-group (F, Ds, E, U) and two-group (secure vs. insecure) classifications. The classification matrices for the four-group and two-group classifications of $\text{Judge}_{\text{AAP}}1$ as compared with $\text{Judges}_{\text{AAP}}2$ and 3 are shown in Tables 3.1–3.4. Analyses using the kappa statistic demonstrated significant AAP interjudge reliability. There was 90% agreement between AAP Judges 1 and 2 on four-group classifications and 85% agreement between AAP Judges 1 and 3. There was a 99% and 92% respective concordance rate for two-group classifications for the two pairs of AAP judges.

TABLE 3.1. AAP Interjudge Classification Reliability between $\text{Judge}_{\text{AAP}}1$ and $\text{Judge}_{\text{AAP}}2$: Four Adult Attachment Classification Groups

	$\text{Judge}_{\text{AAP}}2$				
$\text{Judge}_{\text{AAP}}1$	F	Ds	E	U	Total
F	**1**	1	0	0	2
Ds	0	**13**	0	2	*15*
E	0	1	**19**	1	*21*
U	0	1	1	**34**	*36*
Total	*1*	*16*	*20*	*37*	*74*

Note. Kappa = .85, $p < .000$; phi = 1.41, $p < .000$.

TABLE 3.2. AAP Interjudge Classification Reliability between $\text{Judge}_{\text{AAP}}1$ and $\text{Judge}_{\text{AAP}}3$: Four Adult Attachment Classification Groups

	$\text{Judge}_{\text{AAP}}3$				
$\text{Judge}_{\text{AAP}}1$	F	Ds	E	U	Total
F	**34**	4	0	1	*39*
Ds	3	**43**	1	1	*48*
E	1	1	**14**	4	*20*
U	0	4	0	**24**	*28*
Total	*38*	*52*	*15*	*30*	*135*

Note. Kappa = .79, $p <.000$; phi = 1.38, $p < .000$.

TABLE 3.3. AAP Interjudge Classification Reliability between Judge$_{AAP}$1 and Judge$_{AAP}$2: Secure versus Insecure Adult Attachment Classification Groups

	Judge$_{AAP}$2		
Judge$_{AAP}$1	Secure	Insecure	Total
Secure	**1**	1	2
Insecure	0	**72**	72
Total	*1*	*73*	*74*

Note. Kappa = .66, $p <.000$; phi = .702, $p < .000$.

TABLE 3.4. AAP Interjudge Classification Reliability between Judge$_{AAP}$1 and Judge$_{AAP}$3: Secure versus Insecure Adult Attachment Classification Groups

	Judge$_{AAP}$3		
Judge$_{AAP}$1	Secure	Insecure	Total
Secure	**34**	5	*39*
Insecure	5	**91**	*96*
Total	*39*	*96*	*135*

Note. Kappa = .82, $p < .000$; phi = .82, $p < .000$.

Convergent predictive validity was calculated for the four-group and two-group classifications by comparing AAP and AAI classifications ($n = 130$). Classification disagreements among the three AAP judges and between the two AAI judges were independently resolved through consensus. Convergent agreement was examined using the kappa statistic. Analyses demonstrated significant convergent agreement between AAP and AAI (see Tables 3.5 and 3.6). Convergent agreement on AAP/AAI four-group classifications was 90%. Convergent agreement on AAP/AAI two-group classifications was 97%.

Test–retest reliability was determined for the 69 participants (48%; 39 females, 30 males) who returned for Time 2 testing. The kappa statistic was used to evaluate Time 1 and Time 2 AAP concordance for four- and two-group classifications. Test–retest reliability for four-group classifications was 84% and 91% for two-group classifications (see Tables 3.7 and 3.8). Stability from Time 1 to Time 2 was 82%, 96% for individuals judged dismissing, 62% for individuals judged preoccupied, and 80% for individuals judged unresolved. Of the 11 participants whose classifications changed over the retest period, seven were shifts between

TABLE 3.5. AAP/AAI Convergent Validity: Four Adult Attachment Classification Groups

	AAI				
AAP	F	Ds	E	U	Total
F	**19**	0	0	1	*20*
Ds	0	**30**	3	1	*34*
E	2	1	**26**	1	*30*
U	1	3	2	**40**	*46*
Total	*22*	*34*	*31*	*43*	*130*

Note. Kappa = .84, p <.000; phi = 1.49, p < .000.

TABLE 3.6. AAP/AAI Convergent Validity: Secure versus Insecure Adult Attachment Classification

	AAI		
AAP	Secure	Insecure	Total
Secure	**19**	1	*20*
Insecure	3	**107**	*110*
Total	*22*	*108*	*130*

Note. Kappa = .89, p < .000; phi = .89, p < .000.

TABLE 3.7. AAP Test–Retest Reliability: Four Adult Attachment Classification Groups

	AAP retest				
AAP	F	Ds	E	U	Total
F	**14**	1	0	2	*17*
Ds	0	**23**	1	0	*24*
E	0	2	**5**	1	*8*
U	3	0	1	**16**	*20*
Total	*17*	*26*	*7*	*19*	*69*

Note. Kappa = .78, p <.000; phi = 1.32, p < .000.

unresolved and organized classifications (four changed from unresolved to organized/resolved and three changed from organized/resolved to unresolved).

The discriminant validity analyses (MANOVAs) showed that AAP classifications were not influenced by verbal intelligence and social desirability. The results are presented in Table 3.9.

TABLE 3.8. AAP Test–Retest Reliability: Secure versus Insecure Adult Attachment Classification Groups

	AAP retest		
AAP	Secure	Insecure	Total
Secure	**14**	3	*17*
Insecure	3	**49**	*52*
Total	*17*	*52*	*69*

Note. Kappa = .77, $p < .000$, phi = .77, $p < .000$.

TABLE 3.9. Discriminant Validity: Verbal Intelligence and Social Desirability

	AAP classification group										
	F (n = 25)		Ds (n = 37)		E (n = 30)		U (n = 52)				
	Mean	*SD*	Mean	*SD*	Mean	*SD*	Mean	*SD*	*F*	*df*	*p*
WAIS Verbal	12.4	1.95	13.45	2.06	13.25	2.34	13.25	2.31	.86	3	.46
WAIS Similarities	11.50	1.97	13.00	2.63	13.43	2.52	13.00	2.68	2.05	3	.11
BIDR IM	7.45	3.58	6.95	3.89	8.73	4.10	8.73	4.14	1.89	3	.13
BIDR SDE	2.45	2.38	3.41	3.31	3.67	4.16	2.06	2.21	2.40	3	.07
BIDR Total	9.19	4.02	10.35	5.42	12.40	6.26	10.78	4.99	1.21	3	.31

We were also interested in examining differences among attachment groups on symptomology reported on the SCL-90-R GSI, PSDI, and PST. This measure is normed separately for women and men. The results were analyzed separately for gender using one-way analysis of variance. Analysis of PSDI scores for women was controlled for age because of a significant correlation between these two variables. We ran two sets of analyses. One compared the SCL-90-R scores of secure versus insecure adults; the other compared the scores of unresolved versus resolved/organized adults. Drawing from the attachment literature on risk (Cassidy & Shaver, 2008), we predicted that the scores for secure individuals would be lower than the scores for insecure individuals, and the scores for unresolved individuals to be higher than resolved/organized individuals. The results of these analyses are shown in Table 3.10. The results showed no differences on SCL-90-R symptoms between women or men on either of these dimensions. These results suggest several things. One is that there were a lot of distressed women and men in this "community" sample. It is likely that many studies assume that these types of sample recruited from the general population are symptom free but, as Bakermans-Kranenburg and van IJzendoorn (2009) also emphasized, this assumption is not necessarily correct. We must stop and ask, "Who are the individuals who volunteer for a psychological study on 'relationships'?" We have found that it is not uncommon for individuals who volunteer for psychology studies to feel they have something to contribute or have "issues" they want to discuss. This may have led to an overabundance of insecure and troubled individuals in our sample, which was advertised as a "relationship" study. We present in Chapter

TABLE 3.10. SCL-90-R GSI, PDSI, and PST Scores for Women and Men

	GSI Mean (*SD*)	PDSI Mean (*SD*)	PST Mean (*SD*)
		Women	
Secure (*n* = 15)	54.48 (12.03)	55.55 (10.92)	54.95 (11.74)
Insecure (*n* = 82)	55.55 (10.92)	50.99 (7.92)	56.07 (10.32)
Organized (*n* = 63)	53.75 (9.64)	51.11 (7.82)	50.35 (7.37)
Unresolved (*n* = 34)	53.09 (8.52)	53.71 (10.22)	53.24 (8.74)
		Men	
Secure (*n* = 6)	59.67 (17.26)	50.83 (9.93)	62.17 (14.99)
Insecure (*n* = 36)	59.72 (13.19)	55.56 (9.36)	61.69 (9.74)
Organized (*n* = 25)	58.84 (14.78)	55.12 (9.94)	61.12 (10.74)
Unresolved (*n* = 17)	61.00 (11.96)	54.53 (9.02)	61.65 (10.24)

9 a new model of unresolved attachment that broadens the conceptualization of risk in attachment theory, following Bowlby's (1980) model of mourning. Utilizing this new approach in thinking about psychiatric risk samples may provide a better understanding of risk patterns in community and clinical samples than the standard comparisons we tested here.

OTHER AAP VALIDITY STUDIES

Concurrent Validity with the AAI in the German Language

Interjudge reliability and predictive concurrent AAP/AAI validity has been independently established for the AAP for use in the German language. This work also established the validity for using the AAP with psychiatric patients and to examine neurological patterns of attachment in a functional magnetic resonance imagery (fMRI) environment (Buchheim, Erk, et al., 2006; Chapter 10). The data comprise interviews from 74 females participating in several studies that included psychiatric patients and nonpatient controls (see Buchheim & George, 2011). Twenty-eight AAPs were administered in the fMRI environment (11 borderline inpatients, 17 controls), and 46 were administered using the procedure described above (5 controls, 21 borderline outpatients, 20 anxiety inpatients) and the AAI was administered 6 weeks later. Two reliable judges classified the AAPs, one using the German language transcripts and the other using English translations. The translator and the English-language judge were blind to all information about the participants. AAIs were classified by two reliable AAI judges who had established interjudge AAI reliability in other German samples. One AAI judge was blind to all information about the participants.

AAP interjudge reliability was reported only for four-group classifications. There was 98% agreement between the judges (kappa = .97, $p < .000$). AAP/AAI convergence for four classification groups was 84% (kappa = .71, $p < .000$), 91% for secure versus insecure (kappa = .70, $p < .000$), and 88% for unresolved versus resolved (kappa = .75, $p < .000$). These results establish the validity of the AAP in German-speaking samples for clinical and healthy participants. This reported AAP agreement is especially notable because the two AAP judges were coding and classifying independently in German and English.

Predictive Validity Studies

Independent studies using the AAP supports the validity of this measure. The AAP has been used in basic and clinical research, including studies of mothers' attachment in rel rising interest in and growing acceptance ofation to their children's adjustment and risk (Béliveau & Moss, 2005), adolescent development and maltreatment (Aikins, Howes, & Hamilton, 2009; Webster & Hackett, 2007, 2011; Webster, Hackett, & Joubert, 2009; Webster & Knoteck, 2007), foster care (Webster & Joubert, 2011), adult immigration (Van Ecke, 2006; Van Ecke, Chope, & Emmelkamp, 2005), depression (West & George, 2002), posttraumatic stress symptomology (Benoit, Bouthillier, Moss, Rousseau, & Brunet, 2010), and emotional development in psychiatric patients (Subic-Wrana, Beetz, Langenbach, Paulussen, & Beutel, 2007). Recent innovative research has used the AAP to examine the neurological and biochemical substrates of attachment in community and psychiatric samples (Buchheim, Erk, et al., 2008a; Buchheim, Erk et al., 2008b; Buchheim, Erk, et al., 2006; Buchheim & George, 2011; Buchheim et al., 2009; Warren et al., 2010; see Chapter 10). The AAP has been used to inform clinical practice (Finn, 2011; Lis, Mazzeschi, Di Riso, & Salcuni, 2011; Smith & George, in press) and child custody evaluation (George, Isaacs, & Marvin, 2011; Isaacs, George, & Marvin, 2009)

SUMMARY

We have been especially mindful of the issue of construct validity from the inception of the AAP. Our goal was to establish predictive concordant validity with the AAI, the only other well-validated developmental assessment of adult attachment in the Bowlby–Ainsworth tradition. Throughout the validation process, the AAP has demonstrated impressive agreement with the AAI, the gold-standard assessment in developmental adult attachment research. We can specify several reasons for this strong convergence. We briefly describe these reasons here, providing a bridge to describing the coding, classification, and application of the AAP that follows in subsequent chapters.

First and foremost, we emphasize that we did not start developing the coding and classification scheme "from scratch." We both had a strong foundation in attachment theory, and both authors had independently already developed and validated a number of other attachment assessment measures with other collaborators (e.g., AAI, George et al., 1984/1985/1996; Main & Goldwyn, 1985/1988/1994; Main et al.

2003; Attachment Doll Play Procedure, Solomon et al., 1995; Caregiving Interview, George & Solomon, 1996, 2008; Reciprocal Attachment Questionnaire, West, Sheldon, & Reiffer, 1987; Adolescent Attachment and Unresolved Attachment Questionnaires, West et al., 2000; West et al., 1998). We drew heavily from theory and integrated several ideas from our other measurement approaches. We found that adding the evaluation of defensive processes that George and Solomon originally conceived and validated for the analysis of their Attachment Doll Play Procedure (Solomon et al., 1995) and their maternal caregiving system assessment (George & Solomon, 1996, 2008) to be essential to our success in differentiating among the insecure adult classification groups (see Chapters 4 and 5 for discussions of defensive exclusion and AAP content coding).

Another reason for the strong AAP concurrent validity is that we were guided during our individual development phase by evidence from AAI research that had established validity for assessing attachment status based on narrative patterns. This led us to develop the AAP as a narrative-based assessment, rather than adopting some other format such as a questionnaire or a thematic approach as in the Rorschach. Interestingly, however, in contrast to the "sin qua non" role of narrative coherence for analyzing the AAI, narrative coherence does not contribute meaningful information toward classification. There are clearly differences in these two different kinds of narrative assessments. The AAI is an autobiographical task that depends first and foremost on the ability and willingness of the interviewee to engage in a cooperative conversation with the interviewer. Grice's philosophical narrative maxims, the fundamental guidelines Main used to develop the evaluation of coherence for the AAI, are conversation rules. The AAP is not an autobiographical task, and the structure does not take a conversational form. The administration instructions release the interviewee from the constraints of interpersonal discourse. Main's AAI interpretations of Grice's maxims added little to interpreting the AAP. But what was useful about AAI coherence in relation to the AAP was pointing out how narrative structure and content that heretofore was predominantly used only in clinical interpretation could be systematically described and examined empirically.

Rather than discourse coherence, the AAP assesses how the narrative response reveals *attachment coherence*, which we define as the representational integration of attachment and caregiving, that is, coherence in the relationship. *Attachment-coherent* doll-play stories characteristically portray children's needs clearly, attachment figures as sensitively attuned and protective, and an integrated, capable self, rather than restriction, confusion or a disorganized self (Solomon et al., 1995).

Descriptions of attuned and integrated responses combined with the mother's desire to achieve flexibility and balance between her caregiving system and her child's attachment needs are the hallmark of caregiving security (George & Solomon, 2008; Solomon & George, 1996).

These integrative elements in the narrative responses of adults and children provide the conceptual foundation for the evaluation of *attachment coherence* in the AAP, defined as the flexible integration of the attachment and caregiving systems and the portrayal of an autonomous and integrated self. The degree to which individuals achieve *attachment coherence* in the AAP depends on the shifting balance between adaptive processes and defensive exclusion in their efforts to give meaning to and find meaning in each picture stimulus.

This brings us back to defensive processes. Defense limits *attachment coherence.* George and Solomon's research has demonstrated that insecure attachment and caregiving (organized-insecure and disorganization) involves heightened defensive exclusion of the "normal" operation of the attachment system (George & Solomon, 1996, 2008; Solomon et al., 1995). Because the purpose of defensive exclusion is to suppress direct expression of attachment thoughts and feelings, assessment attends to defensive substitutions or what is unleashed when defensive exclusion breaks down. All of the features of attachment coherence (and incoherence) are described in the chapters that follow, delineated as we describe more fully the details of the AAP coding scheme and the AAP "meaning" associated with each of the different attachment groups.

Another factor that we believe contributed to the success of the AAP/AAI concordance rate is our restriction to developing a scheme that identifies only the major attachment categories (F, Ds, E, and U). The AAI classification scheme identifies subgroups within each major classification group (e.g., five forms of the secure classification group), analogous to Ainsworth's original group descriptions for the Strange Situation (Ainsworth et al., 1978). The field of attachment, however, rarely specifies category subgroups in research or clinical application, and in Chapter 10 we discuss how new classification groups and subgroups have emerged from empirical need rather than theoretical relevance. For most research purposes, the classification groups are collapsed for statistical analysis (i.e., secure vs. insecure; organized vs. disorganized). The taxonomic approach is based on identifying major groupings, a task that has been successfully established for the AAP through our validity work. Classification subgroups presumably provide some evidence of different underlying patterns within a particular classification group. But these underlying patterns have never been clearly explicated in attachment theory, other than to say that different subgroup patterns exist.[7] The attachment meaning of some of these subgroups is poorly understood, such as the irrational fear of death associated with the dismissing classification group (Ds_4 subgroup on the AAI).

Finally, following Ainsworth's lead stressing the importance of "patterns of attachment" (Ainsworth et al., 1978), and the subsequent success of this approach in developing other attachment assessments, the AAP coding dimensions elucidate several different kinds of representational processes that we combine as patterns in order to derive a classification. Classification assignment follows explicitly schematized rules that define how to think about these patterns within a hierarchically integrated series of decision points.

The work that we described in this chapter establishes the AAP picture system as a valid measure for assessing adult attachment. Validation work is never finished. We hope that others will pick up this task in their research groups and clinical practice.

[7] We have had some success in identifying subgroups in our later work, but this has never been our goal. Rather, we have found that our defensive exclusion approach to classification is helpful in examining the underlying mechanisms, especially defensive processes that differentiate individuals among classification groups and individuals placed in the same attachment group.

4

The Attachment Self

The AAP Attachment Content Coding Dimensions

In the following we consider the first major coding category of the AAP—attachment content analysis. This chapter identifies three content dimensions and specifies their referents in AAP responses. The first dimension is *agency of self*, which describes integrated and functional forms of agency. The second dimension comprises two AAP content features that are central to attachment and reciprocal intimate relationships: *connectedness* and *synchrony*. The third dimension is *personal experience*, which differentiates between distinct and blurred multiple representations of self.

AGENCY OF SELF

Attachment-based agency of self has two perspectives. One is turned outward, either to seeking attachment figures to provide a haven of safety or to the story character taking action in the world. The other is turned inward, a form of agency that comprises mental activity that makes the self the object of inner work and elaboration. The formation of these perspectives reflects individuals' efforts to deal with the challenge of describing the events and emotions in response to the attachment stimuli. It should be further emphasized here that the stimuli confront individuals with attachment events they might otherwise defensively set aside. For example, the *Bench*, *Cemetery*, and *Corner* scenes confront individuals with aloneness, loss, and potential threat, and the AAP task requires addressing these issues. In addition, as we explained in Chapter 3, the four alone picture stimuli were designed specifically to activate distress in the absence of visibly "accessible" attachment figures. The fact that characters are portrayed as alone amplifies the intensity of attachment activation in these stimuli, an AAP design feature that has been confirmed by developmental attachment neurological research (see Chapter 10). Facing distress and threat alone, agency of self in the story response connotes that characters have available to them the active means to solve problems or implement productive change. In its outward form, agency of self is demonstrated by the story character's ability to make things happen in the world. Agency in this form may be understood to encompass what White (1959) referred to as the efficacy of the self, in contrast to a sense of helplessness or futility. In its inward form, agency of self is demonstrated by the inner capacity of a self that is autonomous and capable of renewal, extension, flexibility, and integrative balance. It is the self that uses solitude without succumbing to loneliness to create new meanings out of the ramifications of past attachment experiences. The selection of different forms of agency of self in their AAP responses tells us a good deal about what kinds of agency are available to individuals in their everyday attachment situations.

The AAP defines three forms of agency of self that are coded only for responses to the alone picture stimuli: internalized secure base, haven of safety, and the capacity to act. We define these forms of agency in the next sections, accompanied by examples from AAP stories.

Internalized Secure Base

Internalized secure base is an attachment construct that we developed based on our work with the AAP. It assesses the main character's willingness and ability to engage in self-reflection occasioned by solitude, in contrast to being lonely, bored, or restless (George & West, 2001, 2008, 2009; George, West, & Pettem, 1997–2007). We briefly pause to clarify how internalized secure base fits within the framework of attachment theory.

Ainsworth used the concept of the secure base to describe how the attachment relationship fosters exploration (Ainsworth et al., 1978).

Exploration is guided by its own behavioral system, one that is antithetical to attachment because it leads the child away from the attachment figure (Bowlby, 1969/1982). Exploration is motivated by curiosity and discovery of the unknown; it also can engender worry, anxiety, and fear. The courage to explore requires an attachment figure that literally serves as the child's "secure base." In infancy, exploration is encouraged by the physical proximity and accessibility of the attachment figure. In the developmental phase of attachment that Bowlby (1969/1982) called the "goal-corrected partnership," beginning in the preschool years, the child begins to form enduring internalized models of attachment that will serve as the representational foundation of the attachment figure's accessibility throughout the life span (Ainsworth, 1989; Allen, 2008; Bretherton, 1985; Bretherton & Munholland, 2008; Main et al., 1985; Marvin & Britner, 2008). Developmental achievements, including the capacity for abstract reasoning, result in more highly differentiated internal representations of attachment. The secure base effect is no longer maintained exclusively by physical proximity to attachment figures; it is increasingly maintained by drawing on internalized attachment figures (Weiss, 1982; West & Sheldon-Keller, 1994). This internalization of attachment figures informs and shapes the mental representation of self (Bowlby, 1969/1982; Sroufe & Fleeson, 1986).

We developed the concept of internalized secure base to describe a feature of the internal working model of the self that promotes self-exploration. Exploration of the self, like exploration of the environment, proceeds from security that is derived largely from the individual's internal relationship to the attachment figure. As such, the internalized secure base permits an individual to explore and think about the inner world of the self—including thinking about undesirable or threatening facets of the self and past attachment experiences—without marked interference from defensive processes. Bowlby (1980) stated that adults developed a self system "that, being capable of self-perception, becomes capable also of conceiving of the self as an agent; and further, that the integrity of that system is provided through its constant access to a more or less continuous store of personal memories" (p. 60). In this statement, Bowlby seems to emphasize that the coherence of the self is enhanced when the self extends its agency through the self-development of new meanings.

In Chapter 2 we described how the creation of new meanings is rooted in the recategorization of old memories. Recategorization is an indispensable process to the coherence of the self, since new meanings cannot be created without it. From these considerations, it would seem that in adulthood the integrity of the mental representation of self depends less on validation from an attachment partner than in childhood because it is largely self-generated through the creation of private meanings. At the same time, it has long been recognized that the child's ability "to progress to conceptualizing the mind as potentially a private domain" (Hobson, 1994, p. 579) rests on the paradoxical fact that this ability is in part determined by the quality of the early child–caregiver relationship (Main, 1991). This point is reminiscent of Winnicott's (1965) paradox that the true self, which underpins autonomy from the environment (i.e., the capacity to be alone), initially requires the supportive presence of the parent. As adults, the internalized secure base is, as it were, the growing point of our attachment experiences. Inner elaboration may convert these experiences into something quite different, and we need to allow for the development of private meanings for which recategorical memory prospects.

Superficially, the internalized secure base concept may appear similar to other representational constructs that have been related to adult attachment security and caregiver sensitivity, for example, "earned security" (Main, 1995), "reflective capacity" (Fonagy, Steele, & Steele, 1991; Slade, Grienenberger, Bernbach, Levy, & Locker, 2005), and "mind-mindedness" (Bernier & Dozier, 2003; Meins, Fernyhough, Fradley, & Tuckey, 2001). The internalized secure base concept is unique, however, because it is a process that emphasizes the individual's ability to use solitude as a spur to thinking sincerely about the self. Certainly, self-development occurs in the context of relationships. But in adults we view thinking about attachment as a quality of self-integration and personal identity that is just as important a representational feature as reflective functioning concepts that stress thinking about the minds of others. It is the internalized secure base in the self that promotes empathy, forgiveness, and relationship reintegration. In an essential way, the internalized secure base creates meaning from within by bringing distressful attachment experiences within the domain of the internal working model of self, which in turn restores representational homeostasis.

On the basis of the foregoing considerations, internalized secure base is coded in AAP story content from descriptions of characters as exploring the self by drawing on the haven of safety strengths in their internal working model of attachment when the attachment system is activated by the picture stimuli. Agency of self is coded only for alone pictures that provide the individual with maximum opportunity to demonstrate internal exploration. Dyadic pictures that portray potential attachment figures do not afford this opportunity. Internalized secure base is most typically evident in responses to those picture stimuli in which the story character is identified by the individual as an adult, commonly the *Bench* and *Cemetery* pictures. It is evident when characters are described as content to use solitude (in contrast to feeling lonely) and "mental actions" to engage in genuine thoughtfulness (clearly expressed without jargon or psychobabble). The topic is personal, with the main character thinking about how a relationship with an attachment figure affects his or her thoughts or feelings. This type of thinking rises above reminiscence or thoughts of another person solely in relation to the self. In reminiscence, memories of activities or the individual are made sentimental (i.e., unearned or barren emotion). Self-reflection emphasizes qualities of the self. The internalized secure base emphasizes the importance of the relationship, self, and other coming together internally to provide courage and sometimes comfort to face an attachment stressor. These qualities are vividly expressed in the following *Cemetery* response, indicated in italics (see also Chapter 6):

> This is his son's trip back to his mother's grave and he stands and contemplates his life with his mother sheds a few. I think maybe the guy has . . . has been doing a lot of *thinking about his mother* and so he just felt the need to go and tell his mother that he loves her and then *he forgives her for all the things she couldn't be.* (What would happen next?) I think he'd go for for a, a little walk . . . and just *let thoughts run through his mind* and let them go, take some deep breaths, and then go **back** to his family—and live in the **present,** instead of the past. (Speaker's emphasis is indicated in bold.)

This picture shows a man standing in front of a tombstone. The story describes how the man visits his hometown and also visits the graveyard where his mother is buried. *He is thinking about the past, how things had been when she was still alive, what she had pointed out to him for his life. He is very centered on the past, remembering many things; at the same time he is gathering courage for the future since he knows that life is transient.* He is keeping to this task for a while, then returns to his apartment *lost in thought.* The next day he leaves his hometown after having visited some of his old friends and some of mother's neighbors. He will visit them again in the years to come when he returns to his own family and his hometown. The importance of his relationship with his mother, and his desire to think about this relationship and create new meanings through repair and forgiveness, take center stage in this response.

Evidence of internalized secure base material in the AAP is independent of the story character's level of distress. The emotional tone in AAP stories varies considerably; some characters are depicted as comfortable, other as distressed, sad, or depressed. Others are described more simply as seeking solitude in order to be alone and think things through (in contrast to being alone and lonely, withdrawing, or trying to escape or avoid others). Consider the range of emotional tones in the following responses to *Window*, indicated in italics:

> The girl just woke up and is looking out of the window, *thinking about what to do today*. It's raining. She's sad because she and her friend had planned a picnic. She has breakfast and calls her friend to come play at her house instead.
>
> This little girl is inside, maybe she's gotten into trouble and she's looking outside wishing she could be outside. Maybe she's on restriction or punishment and maybe she's watching her friends playing outside and, let's see, maybe next time, or after she gets off punishment she can go outside and play. (What is she thinking or feeling?) Uh, she's probably sad that she can't go outside. *She's thinking about what she did to get her in trouble.*

The internalized secure base quality of self does not necessarily lead to satisfactory, resolved, or happy results. What is important is that individuals' internalized sense of safety fosters honest and constructive exploration of a range of events and the attendant emotions. These qualities characterize the following *Bench* response, as indicated by italics:

> A young woman sitting on a bench in a park. Farther back one can see a wall. The woman seems to be very sad or distressed. Perhaps she is just tired and lays her head on her arms. Is she waiting for someone? Perhaps later on the one she has been waiting for is coming. They are going for a walk together in the park and have a nice conversation. But looks rather sad. She has looked for a quiet place where she then, she then can *think about her situation, can consider what has happened, how she can handle the situation. In any case she has been looking for, for the quietness of a, of a different place, not, not her own flat but somewhere outside*. Perhaps a place with which no, no memories are connected. Later on she will perhaps get up and, on a walk, let her attention wander or, or *think*,

> let the thoughts wander a little *but at the moment she prefers to sit on the bench and think.*[1]

Other responses integrate sincere thoughtfulness into a broad cycle of thoughtfulness, as described in the following response to *Cemetery*, highlighted especially by the words in italics. The reader will note that the only event that is clearly evident in this story is the importance of thinking. It is more important to this respondent than describing who the deceased is or any circumstances surrounding the death.

> This guy is visiting a grave of a loved one, someone he loves or cares about. He's just visiting him, just to talking to them. He's probably *thinking about them* for some reason or another. So, afterwards he is probably going to leave, just go home and *think about it some more.* And if it is a loved one that he really cares about a lot because you don't just visit anybody's grave. So he is going to go home and just *think about it even more.*

Haven of Safety

Ainsworth developed the concept of "haven of safety" to describe the attachment figure's role in providing comfort in response to the child's distress (Ainsworth et al., 1978). Haven of safety is coded in the AAP when the main character's actions are a component of a reciprocal, sensitive, and responsive attachment–caregiving relationship. Haven of safety may take two forms in the AAP. In one, the character gives a signal to which the attachment figure responds, or the attachment figure anticipates another character's needs, or there is an integrative reunion following separation between parent and child or husband and wife. In the other, integrated agency involves repairing a relationship, in which the main character apologizes or makes restitution to another person. Sincere reparation—not just going through the motions of saying "sorry"—exposes the self to rejection or anger from others. These feelings must be managed and somewhat overridden by confidence in and protection from attachment figures, who act as safe havens, in order to have the courage to make amends. Over time, this confidence is internalized and fortifies efforts to engage in behaviors that will reintegrate the threatened relationship. The italicized portions of the following examples indicate evidence of haven of safety in AAP responses:

[1] This response was translated to English from German.

Window: A girl, approximately 8 years old, is standing in the apartment and is looking out of the window at the opposite house and the trees. She sees neighbor kids down there playing but can't go out because she is sick. She is standing there in her nightgown. Perhaps she has got the chicken pox and that is why she is not allowed to go out. She is staying there for a while observing the other kids. They are looking up and waving to her and she is always waving down to them. She is a little sad that she too can't be down there. And then, later on, she returns to her bed and reads a book a little and is thinking too bad that she can't go out and is a little sad. The mother is just doing some shopping, that is why *she is feeling very lonely at the moment and is happy when the mother comes back.*

Window: Yes, there is a girl at home, she has the flu and is not allowed to go out because she has a fever. She is standing by the window and is very sad and full of desire and is just looking down there at the children playing and her girlfriend is playing there. She goes back to bed, and falls asleep and dreams about how the others are all playing outside and how she can play along and that she is well again. She wakes up and realizes that it was just a dream and is once again very sad. *Mom is coming and consoled her* and plays with her. They have discovered a gorgeous game that they are playing with each other and then *she is feeling better again.* And in the evening she then goes to sleep.[2]

Corner: Here, a little boy is threatened. He is in the corner holding his hands out because he doesn't want somebody to come to closer to him. He has done something bad and his father wants to punish him. He is anxious and he doesn't know exactly what happened. The father will approach him and will say that he is mad at him, but *it's okay, it doesn't matter what the little boy has done.* And the little boy will go up to him and he won't be nervous any more.

Bench: This little girl, I guess little girl, person was at school and maybe she got in trouble for doing something to another child, maybe being mean or hitting him and she got put on time out. So she's sitting there, she's angry and upset and sad because she can't play. (What might happen next?) *She'll probably apologize to the person or whatever she did* and um hopefully not do it anymore or remember her consequences if she thinks about it again.

---

[2] First two stories were translated to English from German.

Capacity to Act

Capacity to act is defined as the ability of the self to take constructive action and reflects the self's sense of efficacy. It is coded when the central story character is described as engaging in an action, including going to a different location than is portrayed in the picture, thereby successfully managing attachment distress by moving away from the event. At the representational level, taking action keeps the self moving forward; it is a form of problem-solving coping. Agency of self provides ways to confront problems or alternative solutions when thinking about them is not possible, desirable, or perhaps not needed. In addition to the various ways that story characters demonstrate capacity for constructive action, the AAP coding also pays particular attention to acts of self-protection. To protect, ward off, or shield the self from threat is considered productive capacity for action, irrespective of whether these actions are deemed effective in the actual story. The crucial point is that the representational self demonstrates a clear sense of efficacy, in contrast to a sense of helplessness or despair.

In summary, what is important with regard to capacity to act is that it keeps the individual organized when sensitive attachment resources are not available. The following are examples of capacity to act:

> The gravestones are crooked. *The man straightens them* and goes home.
>
> The girl cannot go outside because she is sick. She *goes to bed* and *reads a book* and *watches TV.*
>
> The girl on the bench had a fight with her parents. She sits on the bench for a while and then *goes home.* She doesn't want to speak to her parents, so *she goes directly to her room* without saying hello.
>
> The woman is afraid that she will hurt herself. *She calls 911.*
>
> The man's wife died of cancer. She had been sick for quite a long time. He tells her that he's looking forward to seeing her in heaven and *finds a new wife.*
>
> This child is backed into a corner, um, like he's trying to *protect* himself from being hit maybe by a parent or maybe, maybe by a bully at school.
>
> The boy's brother was teasing him and chased him into the corner. He turns to his brother and *says, "No, stay away."*

Before we leave the topic of agency of self, we draw the reader's attention to the distinction between two types of attachment agency of self. One type pertains to integrated forms of agency (internalized secure base and haven of safety), which serve as the foundation for attachment security. The other type pertains to a functional form of agency (capacity to act), which serves to keep attachment organized but not necessarily evidence of security. We expand on this in later chapters when describing how agency is used to differentiate organized-resolved and unresolved attachment classification groups. The point here is to demonstrate how coding agency of self in the AAP fits with contemporary attachment theory, in particular the conditional behavioral and representational strategies model.

Main (1990) described conditional attachment strategies as biologically based behaviors and psychological processes that permit an individual to achieve the set goal of the attachment behavioral system (i.e., proximity to attachment figures). Primary strategies are fostered when attachment figures detect and respond promptly and sensitively to an individual's attachment signals. Secondary strategies "suppress" or "manipulate" primary strategies when conditions do not permit an individual to gain *direct* access to sensitive and responsive care. These strategies replace primary strategies so that an individual can achieve what George and Solomon call "good enough" protection when the attachment system is aroused (George & Solomon, 2008; Solomon & George, 1996). These strategies modulate the arousal of the attachment system, thereby keeping the individual organized and thus maintaining attachment relationships intact. In persistent, compromised attachment conditions, secondary strategies become an individual's predominant mode of behaving and thinking about attachment (Main, 1990).

For the particular reasons elaborated above, we view haven of safety and internalized secure base as primary forms of agency of self because they subsume (George & Solomon, 1996; Solomon & George, 1996) several representational characteristics associated with integrated attachment. These include evaluations of the self as worthy of care, attachment figures as committed and responsive, and relationships as predominantly desirable and pleasurable. To a significant extent, the integrated forms of agency reflect evaluations of self as confident and capable of thoughtful and constructive actions that ultimately free the individual from worry, anxiety, or fear and in turn generate sincere happiness and joy. By contrast, we view the capacity to act as a secondary, functional form of agency that reflects evaluations of the self as capable of taking steps to remove distress or address problems independent of attachment figures. Under circumstances of persistent attachment figure unavailability, the self's capacity to act camouflages self-evaluations of not being worthy of or needing care, and dissatisfaction with relationships, including feelings of loneliness, sadness, anger, and even despair. Solomon and George recently showed that mothers' memories of engaging in self-protective action in childhood were essential contributors to the mother's ability to provide protection and organized attachment for her own child (Solomon & George, 2006, 2011b).

Of course, the opposite of either primary or secondary forms of agency is the complete absence of agency. This is evidenced when characters are described as taking no action. These characters are vulnerable to succumb to their own distress unless they are "saved" by another person or they create a cheerful, optimistic, or fantasy story endings (e.g., "things will eventually get better," the character "moves on," "in the end they knew they were loved"). Ultimately, without signs of agency, these are "defensive tricks"—thin veneers used to coat the representational incapacity for agency. The following are examples of stories coded as "no agency."

> ***Window:*** This child looks like, uh somebody who maybe, um, I mean her parents aren't home or, uh, maybe they're working and it looks like maybe on a, like a nice day and she's bored, she wants to go outside and play. She's going to stay at home and wait for um her parents or somebody to come home and give her something to do. (What is she thinking or feeling?) Sad, she's sad because she wants to go outside and play and walk around and stuff. (What might happen next?) After her parents come home, *she'll be happy because she has something to do.*
>
> ***Bench:*** This lady looks really sad like maybe she just broke up with somebody or a family member died. She really doesn't have anybody to to help her, to comfort her and she's real sad and she's having a real hard time right now. (What may have led up to this?) Um, a sudden, a tragedy, something real bad that um, um, has affected her emotionally enough to that, um, she has to kind of shy away from the world by covering up her face and closing in her arms. (And what might happen after this?) Um, well, *she'll, she'll get better eventually*. I mean, if something as tragic as what looks like has happened to her, um, you know, it's not easy to get through that but *she'll get better.*

Cemetery: This is a man whose wife died. You can tell he really loved her because he, he misses her. He, uh, he looks, looks sad. Um, he looks like he, uh, it's something happened a while ago, uh . . . a few years ago and he, uh, *he's getting over it* but he still misses his wife. Um, that's, that's it. Maybe he might have had kids, but, no, I don't think he had kids, he didn't have kids. (What may have led up to this?) Um, it was an accident or some sort of disease and she, uh, she, uh, died. (And what might happen next?) He'll uh . . . in a few years, I guess, *he'll move on. It's taken him a little longer to get over this, uh, tragedy.*

Corner: This child is backed into a corner and the way their head's turned is, uh, almost as if in fear or is in fear of whatever is going to happen. What could happen next is that the child could be attacked or abused or something. Or punished . . . the child could be punished. What may have led up to this . . . I'm not really sure. The child could have been unruly. Um, or nothing at all. I mean, if, if the person is, has the mindset to abuse this child, probably wouldn't have, there wouldn't have been anything to provoke it. (What is he thinking and feeling?) Probably anxiety and fear. It's almost as if they almost, they sense what might be happening, um, and there's you know, *the child's face is turned away almost to say this isn't happening, to deny it.*

In summary, it may be said that the concept of conditional forms of agency helps us see that individuals have a range of strategies available to them *depending* on the attachment context. This is equally true for the various forms of agency of self. As we will describe in more detail in the next section (Chapters 6–9), it is the patterns of agency of self expressed in response to the AAP stimuli that differentiates among the organized attachment groups, and the absence of agency of self—combined with the representational failure of the self to find protection and solace in any relationship—that defines unresolved attachment.

CONNECTEDNESS AND SYNCHRONY: REPRESENTATION OF THE SELF IN RELATIONSHIPS

Connectedness

Whereas agency of self was specifically designed to evaluate the attachment internal working model of self, the concept of connectedness was developed to evaluate whether the individual's representation of attachment included other kinds of intimate relationships as extensions of or supplements to attachment relationships. In accordance with ethological theory, over the course of development individuals develop other non-attachment–caregiving relationship systems that make essential contributions to survival and fitness. The two most important forms of these relationships are friendships (social or affiliation behavioral system) and sexual relationships (sexual behavioral system) (Bowlby, 1969/1982; George & Solomon, 2008; Hinde, 1982; Marvin & Britner, 2008).

Connectedness in the AAP assesses the characters' desire and ability to be involved in the full range of relationships that are thought essential to human development. The connectedness dimension is used to differentiate between story responses in which the character is depicted as capable of and desires these connections from responses that block relationships or describe the character as alone and without relationships. Connectedness is only coded for the two alone pictures *Window* and *Bench*. The implicit portrayal of death and abuse in *Cemetery* and *Corner* violate our AAP assumption of coding the possibility of making a connection to others in relationships. And as we show in Chapter 9, connections to individuals who are not alive (i.e., dead) are treated in other ways in the AAP, including evaluations for evidence of attachment disorganization and dysregulation. We do not code connectedness in the responses to dyadic picture because the "connection" is implicit in the stimulus. Connectedness evaluates the individual's spontaneous portrayal of intimate relationships, not the ability to describe a portrayed relationship.

The *Window* and *Bench* scenes evoke a range of different representations of the self's confidence in and satisfaction with individuals in these three forms of intimate relationships—attachment–caregiving dyads, friends peers, and romantic partners. Positive indications of connectedness are coded when the character successfully makes contact with individuals representing these relationships in the response. This includes internalized contact, defined as we have described earlier, by the internalized secure base. The following stories are examples of positive indications of connectedness:

> ***Window:*** The child is standing at the window and it's a sunny day. He says, "I think I'll go outside and play. (What happens next?) He goes and gets his coat and *says, "Mom I'm going out to the backyard. I'm going to go play for a while.*" (Connected to attachment figure)

> ***Window:*** The boy is waiting for his father to come. He goes racing to the door when his father drives up and *they go off to a baseball game.* (Connected to attachment figure)
>
> ***Window:*** Um, she is looking out the window. So, she's clearly like waiting for something. Yeah she is waiting for something like her parents to get home. She wants to play with them, or um, watch TV or something. Take her out shopping (laughter) (What might happen next?) *Her parents* make dinner—um, *take her shopping, buy her a nice pair of shoes.* (Connected to attachment figure)
>
> ***Bench:*** This person looks very sad because it is Saturday afternoon and none of her friends can come out to play and so she went outside anyway because she goes—she enjoys going outside. And she is thinking "Hm, where are all of my friends? I wish they were here so I could play with them." *One of her friends comes along and they go off and play* and are very happy. (Connected to peer)
>
> ***Bench:*** The girl had a fight with her boyfriend and wonders if it would work out if they were married. She *thinks* about what it will be like to be together. *She goes home to tell him* she'll marry him. (Internalized secure base and connected to romantic partner)

Nonconnectedness is coded when the story response is restricted to the character's interactions with people in socially prescribed or stereotypical roles such as teachers, policemen, health care professionals, or neighbors. Nonconnectedness is also coded when access to intimate relationships is unsatisfactory or blocked (e.g., due to anger or rejection). The following are examples of stories that are considered nonconnected:

> ***Window:*** The girl is sad because her parents are at work. She's lonely and wants to play with her friends. *She goes over to her neighbor's house.*
>
> ***Window:*** Now there's a little girl that looks kind of lonely to me. Maybe she's had to stay home from school that day because of a fever or whatever. She looks like she's just wondering what in the world to do all day. (What might happen next?) She sees her *teacher and goes outside to say hi.* (Teachers are not biologically defined attachment figures, even though they may substitute for parents in providing care and comfort for children.)

> ***Bench:*** This person *had an argument with his dad* and is upset and is crying . . . just wants to be alone. (What's going to happen after?) The person will either just keep it in and forget about it or *have it out with his dad*."
>
> ***Bench:*** The girl is sad because *she broke up with her boyfriend*. She's crying. She'll sit on the bench for a while and then go home.
>
> ***Bench:*** That looks like someone who just lost a game for their team or something, it looks like that bench would be in a gym change room or something and um, to me that person looks like someone who's let I don't know herself or someone else or a group of people down, for whatever reason and so she's just trying to, you know take a pause and a break and get her courage back up to, face the world again. She wanders off to *talk to one of her coaches*. (Coaches are not attachment figures.)

Finally, some story responses do not evoke references to any human interaction; in short, positive or failed attempts for connectedness are not an issue. The main character is described as engaged in activities that do not involve others. The character is portrayed as alone by the stimulus picture and remains alone in the story response, as seen in the following examples:

> ***Window:*** She's just making the decision of whether to go out there or not um and find something to do or just wait until the world comes to this person that's standing there looking out. (What happens next?) Yeah that's hard to say which—depends on the individual whether they'll go out.
>
> ***Window:*** Um, this little girl has just gotten up and there's nobody in the house, and she's looking out the window and knows that's, that world isn't real out there because nothing is nothing is as it should be. And she, um, decides to go the kitchen and eat. That's it. (What might happen next?) Um, then she does and she's happy.
>
> ***Bench:*** That looks like an adult to me. Sitting on a bench somewhere. Um, loneliness, rejection, depression, all those things. Maybe she had to leave the house in a hurry. She sits there until she decides to go back home.
>
> ***Bench:*** This person has been, running around a lot, busy, very busy, and, uh, has finally cleared everything away in his home space and made this very sacred space, to create a peaceful world and gath-

ers her body into herself, as well as that space, and just is taking a moment to take. (What might happen next?) Um, then she goes about her rest of her day, feeling much more peaceful.

Bench: Ooh, this is a swimming pool, I think. She's tired, she has done like eighty laps, she is taking a breather, hmm. I don't know, maybe she is crying because she has lost a race. (What might she be thinking or feeling?) Hah, oh, If I had only gone faster. If I had not done the push-ups before, I could have beaten that other chick. And she wouldn't be gloating over me now. (What might happen next?) She'll go home and maybe get some ice cream. Watch *Pride and Prejudice*, curl up with a blanket and fall asleep and say I will beat that chick next time.

Synchrony

Synchrony evaluates the self in dyadic attachment relationships. This dimension is coded only for dyadic picture stimuli. The reader will recall that dyadic pictures were designed to portray characters in potential attachment–caregiving relationships (see Chapter 3). Synchrony assesses the degree to which the story characters are portrayed as involved in contingent, reciprocal, and mutually engaging relationships when attachment is activated. This dimension is designed to assess the representational potential for Bowlby's (1969/1982) concept of the goal-corrected partnership or, more accurately, the representational potential for a goal-corrected partnership. The goal-corrected partnership captures the child's experience of the caregiver in what Bowlby (1951) described as a "warm, intimate, and continuous relationship with his mother (or permanent mother substitute) in which both find satisfaction and enjoyment" (p. 13, as quoted by Bretherton, 1992). The synchronous elements of attachment were defined more specifically by Ainsworth in relation to the constellation of maternal behavior that is the foundation of a child's attachment security: sensitivity, contingency, responsiveness, and completeness (Ainsworth et al., 1978).

Synchrony is evaluated based on the elements of sensitivity, integrated partnership, or mutual enjoyment in the attachment–caregiving relationship. These elements can be demonstrated in descriptions of dyadic interaction or characters' shared thinking about each other. The following are some examples of goal-corrected synchrony:

Departure: I think this couple is at the railway station and, uh, the woman is going home for a trip to visit her parents. There seems to be some tension between the two of them because they're not hugging. I think maybe the *wife's going home to think and sort things out.* (What happened next?) The wife will get on the train and there will be stilted words, goodbye and talk to you soon. The husband will help get the bags on the train and uh she'll ride off and *he'll go home and sit in a quiet room and think about their relationship.*

Departure: This couple looks like they're going on vacation that *they planned together.* Packed lightly it looks like, maybe just away for the weekend, maybe they're waiting in line for their flight and discussing what they're going to do on vacation, anticipating it. Can't wait to get there, to leave home and leave all the hustle and bustle of home to go and relax. (What might happen next?) Mm . . . they could board the plane and lose their luggage, um, have to buy all new clothes wherever they get, or whenever they get to where they're going but still have a good time. It's an experience. (What are they thinking or feeling?) Mmmm . . . I think they're in a good mood, uh, because *they're excited about getting away together, maybe they don't get to spend a lot of time together.*

Bed: Well this looks like bedtime and his mom has just sat down to say goodnight and *this young fellow feels he needs a hug before he goes to sleep. So she slides up a little closer to him and gives him a big hug and strokes his head, his back and then tells him to roll over onto his tummy and she'll give him a bit of a massage and that calms him down and gets him ready for sleep.* She kisses him goodnight and leaves the room.

Bed: The boy has been sent to bed by his mother in the evening. She has read him a story in which there was a monster. And about this monster he has dreamed in the night and has *screamed and tossed and turned in his bed and the mother at once rushed over there, took her boy into her arms, consoled him, is saying to him that all of this isn't true, that everything is just a story and he shouldn't have to worry any longer.* And the boy was really convinced that there a monster were under his bed. And so *she went on to soothe him* and went on talking to him to calm him down until then after a while he finally went to sleep again. *The mother stayed for a while with her son and made up her mind to never again tell him a story with monsters* but only with cars.

Ambulance: Oh boy. Um, well, that looks like a grandparent and a boy or a girl, it's hard to tell. Um and, okay we'll make up a story that grandfather is very ill. One of the grandchildren is over and the grandma, and *they're comforting each other* as they see Grandpa being taken in the ambulance. (What's going to happen?) Oh gee, I think he's going to die, he looks pretty sick.

In many instances, relationship interactions are neither integrated nor maximally goal corrected (i.e., integrative). They lack sensitivity that fosters security, such as responses that are delayed or muted, or thinking about how to get out of a situation rather than being responsive. Positive situations (e.g., a couple going on vacation; mother reading to a child before bedtime) may serve to bring the dyad together, but mutual enjoyment is notably absent. The dyad is described as at least minimally engaged in interaction. These interactions are defined in the AAP as functional. Functional interaction supports attachment organization and, in some instances, is all that is needed to assuage attachment distress. This dimension, therefore, is not evaluated as "good" or "bad" representations of synchrony; rather, it evaluates the individual's potential for sensitivity and integration in relationships.

In some instances, functional synchrony may have the quality of "pseudo" integration; that is, implications that the couple is in a reciprocal relationship but the descriptions fail to describe sincere mutuality. And at best, functional responses capture the fact that another person is "there," even if that person fails to respond to or rejects the attachment need. Just as capacity to act when an individual is alone will keep that individual organized, representations of functional synchrony in dyadic AAP stories demonstrate the ability to keep attachment organized. The following are examples of functional forms of synchrony:

> ***Departure:*** A couple going home for Christmas. What they are each thinking? "Boy, I wish that train would get here." Um, "It's a little chilly out here." What's going to happen next is they are going to jump on the train, take their bags and box of Christmas gifts, and go on to their families. (What are they thinking or feeling?) They're excited to be going for Christmas, to see their families. They got their little package all ready to go, suitcases packed. They're anxious, waiting for the train to show up. They got there early because they didn't want to miss it. (What happens next?) They're going to jump on the train and, and store their bags. And she'll probably sit very close to the Christmas package gift or put it on her lap or something.

Departure: Mmm two people, couple, probably waiting on a turnstile um at a airport, bus station, waiting together. They probably are discussing something, like about what they're about to do or um about them personally. They're about to go off, but seems like they're distant about something, like they disagreed or there's some apprehension there you know. (What might happen next?) They might finish, uh, they might continue to wait on the train, bus, airplane, or whichever, uh. Looks like they're pensive and thinking of, thinking about something but both of them are giving each other the kind of the space. At the same time looks like they know they're communicating because, you know, basically to me looks like they're giving each other the space and time to think of whatever previously just happened.

Bed: Um, this is a mom putting her kid to bed at night and he wants a hug and she's telling him he has to go to bed because this is the fifth hug she's given him (laughs) so she's saying, "Okay now it's time to go to bed" and he wants one more hug. (What are they thinking or feeling?) Um, I think they're both pretty happy, they're both just doing the normal routine of going to bed and he's just thinking that sleep isn't something he wants to do and, but I think they probably love each other. (What might happen next?) She'll leave, that's enough, and go away and he'll go to sleep. (Note how the mother never responds to the boy's attachment signal—he wants a hug.)

Bed: The boy broke his sister's doll and he was sent to bed. He's upset and reaches out for a hug. His mom doesn't want to hug him now. She wants him to understand what he did wrong. He's thinking that he just wants her to hug him and forget about it. She's thinking that he needs to learn a lesson from this so he won't do it again. Afterwards she gives him a hug and leaves.

Ambulance: These people are at a bus station and somebody just got injured so they're watching and they're both kind of nosy and wondering what happened as the ambulance is taking them away. (What are they thinking or feeling?) The boy has never seen an ambulance before and the grandma is explaining how to call an ambulance and what the EMTs do with the injured person. They're both pretty curious and I think they're not really feeling too much, because they don't know the person at all. (What might happen next?) The ambulance will go away and Grandma will explain a little bit more and then they'll just go on their way.

Goal-corrected and functional forms of synchrony demonstrate that an individual's mental representations of attachment have important relationship features. The responses describe some form of reciprocal interaction, even if that interaction is unpleasant (e.g., anger, sadness). There are occasions in the AAP when the story response fails to acknowledge all of the characters depicted in a picture stimulus. For example, only the behavior or thoughts of one of the characters are described; descriptions clearly indicating the presence of the other are omitted. We have found that these types of responses appear to be associated with high attachment stress, such that the individual's representational system cannot acknowledge the presence of "others." In essence, the omitted individual becomes "invisible" at the representational level, even though the character is clearly in view in the picture stimulus. Note the omission of one of the characters in the picture stimulus in the following responses.

> ***Bed:*** The boy is sick and needs a hug. He has a cold and has not been able to get up or go to school for several days. He wonders when he is going to feel better and is worried about getting the homework he missed from school. He lies down and goes back to sleep. (There is no female mother figure in this response even though she is clearly visible in the picture stimulus.)
>
> ***Ambulance:*** The older woman and her grandson are at an art museum. They stopped to look at this painting for a long time. She's thinking about the colors in the painting. He's thinking that he's tired and would like to sit down. They look at the painting for a few more minutes and go and get lunch. (Note that there is no mention of a person on a stretcher in this response, although it is clearly visible in the picture stimulus.)

PERSONAL EXPERIENCE: THE DISSOLUTION OF SELF–OTHER BOUNDARIES

The AAP instructs the individual to make up a story about the character(s) portrayed in the picture stimulus. The task is thereby defined as telling a hypothetical story that should "fit" the stimulus properties of the picture. While individuals may see resemblances in the AAP scenes to their own personal experiences, and briefly and explicitly may comment on these reminiscent qualities either in the beginning or end of their stories, describing autobiographical specific content is a violation of the AAP task and is ordinarily not expressed in the AAP responses. It is a sign that defensive and adaptive stability is being undermined when story content drawn from the individual's personal life is conspicuous in his or her AAP responses; self-references indicate an inability to maintain the boundary between self and not-self.

Several different attachment studies confirm this interpretation. Main defined unresolved attachment in relation to lapses in how personal experience regarding death and abuse is metacognitively managed during the AAI (Main, 1991; see also Chapter 9). George and Solomon found representational blurring of past and present to be especially characteristic of the caregiving interviews of mothers of ambivalent-resistant children and associated with cognitive disconnection defenses (George & Solomon, 2008). The hallmark of cognitive disconnection is confusion and uncertainty (see Chapter 5). George and Solomon also describe forms of mental absorption in personal experience similar to lapses in the AAI as related to caregiving representations of some (although not all) mothers of disorganized children. Buchheim and George (2011) reported that anxiety patients, in contrast to borderline patients and controls, characteristically described in the AAP elements of personal abuse experiences, especially in response to the alone picture stimuli. Even though the hypothetical stories of both anxiety and borderline patients included terrorizing and traumatic themes, the blurring of the hypothetical and personal self was observed significantly less frequently in the borderline patients. In these patients, the occurrence of this form of boundary dissolution in the AAP is associated with conscious flooding of strong feelings of anxiety and fear associated with abuse.

The Minnesota longitudinal study of attachment has reported an association between dissolution of intergenerational boundaries, a form of role reversal that is similar to our concept of boundary dissolution, and abuse. Teens with mothers who were sexually exploited during their own childhoods, and living in homes typified by marital dissatisfaction and drug and alcohol abuse, were observed acting in a solicitous and caregiving spouse-like manner with their mothers (Sroufe, Egeland, Carlson, & Collins, 2005).

Boundary blurring is associated with developmental and psychiatric risk in the family systems and psychopathology literature. For example, Jacobvitz and colleagues report enmeshed family boundaries, which includes some elements of the blurred self–other boundaries conceived from the AAP, as related to depression in girls and ADHD symptoms in boys at age 7 (Jacobvitz, Hazen, Curran, & Hitchens, 2004). Boundary dissolution interferes with agency and is associated with severe problems in personality organization that are associated with frightening experiences, including high-conflict divorce and sexual trauma (e.g., Chopra, 2006; Kerig, 2005; Peris & Emery, 2005). Attachment theory views these types of experiences as threats to attachment and self, situations that are at high risk for failed protection by attachment figures (George & Solomon, 2008; Solomon & George, 1999a, 1999b)

In summary, attachment theory and research suggests that blurring is associated with heightened disconnected stress, anxiety, and dysregulating threats to attachment. We capture representational blurring in the AAP by coding the presence of accounts of personal experiences (i.e., autobiographical material) that interferes with the individual's ability to stay on task and tell a hypothetical story. These violations may appear as a simple comment, such as "This reminds me of when my mother was in the hospital." Sometimes the statements are long descriptions of events embedded in the hypothetical story. And on some occasions, personal experience comprises the individual's only response to the picture stimulus, despite the fact that the interviewer asked the individual to tell a story about the picture character(s). The emotional tone of the personal experience material is not taken in consideration when coding this dimension. The personal experience events described range from nonthreatening or silly descriptions to descriptions of terrifying and disturbing events. Examples of personal experience coded in AAP responses include the following:

> ***Window:*** Oh no. So completely spontaneous I say, *I see myself standing at a window.* A girl that is not allowed to go outside and would want, outside wants and wants to play like the others. But it is not allowed. Instead must do homework. And the girl has no other possibility except to stand in front of the window and to dream that it is playing with others. Phhh, that makes me very sad, so. *I wanted as a child also always to play and I was not allowed. And sometimes when I have told my father about it and he said, "You want to play? Inside when it is dark." And I did not know my way around in the village because I never was allowed to go outside and was afraid outside. And then my brother came and said, "What are you doing here outside? What do you want here? And I have the said, "Papa has said I should play. I do not know where I should go." He then took me with him up to the church and simply ran away. And I have had tremendous fear that I do not find my way home. And then a woman helped me to find home and I rang the bell and wanted back inside because I was afraid. And my father has slammed the door into my nose and said, "You stay outside*

until it is dark. You wanted to play and now you can play." I have never again asked for playing. Yes. Hmhm. I still stand in front of the window today. And how does it then end? It is for me still not finished. I still stand in front of the window. There I cannot, cannot find any end to it in the moment. No. Because it is exactly the point at which I actually stand now. I could go now outside and, and am afraid to go outside. I am as said still standing still in front of the window and dream how it is to be outside. And do not find the courage to go outside. Out of fear. I would like to go outside and do something. To go for a stroll . . . maybe go swimming. But there I do not come up with any end.[3]

Departure: A couple getting ready to go on vacation, preparing to enjoy themselves, not knowing what's going to happen in the future. (What do you think led up to that scene?) I think probably the idea that it's time to go away on a vacation. Let's, you know, let's pack and go and head for the airport and, uh, they're standing at, looks like beside a curb or by a wall. So they're waiting, uh, for either someone to pick them up or to go where ever they're going to go. And I, and I cannot help but think of airline travel right now, I just cannot think of anything else. (What are they thinking or feeling?) *Well I know that my daughter and son-in-law and family went away on vacation and they, just a week ago. And they were looking forward to going, having a good time, family time together. And it was one of the last things they said before they left.* (What do you think might happen next?) Like I said, *based on the last week* I just don't know what's going to happen next. In this picture or anything else.

Bed: Hmm, okay it's a little kid who wants a hug from his mother before he goes to sleep at night. She's telling him bedtime stories and she's tucking in and tell him to go to sleep. (What might have led up to this?) You always give your kids a hug before they go to sleep at night so it's just ritual, routine, bedtime time routine. (Anything else come to mind?) No. *Does remind me of what my son said, though, he says that what he remembers from . . . from my husband's coming in at night and he used to hide under the covers and my husband used to shake the bed trying to find him and he just thought that was th . . . the most special thing* (laughs). This looks like a mother so she wouldn't be quite that vigorous, she does the stories and the hugs (laughs).

[3] The response was translated to English from German.

Ambulance: Well let's see, he called an ambulance, taking someone to the hospital. Little guy, he's worried, Momma or Grandma's telling him it will be all right, I imagine. That's about it. (What do you think led up to that?) He probably was overmedicated and fell a couple of times. *I worry about all my medication now, since they did it to me.* (What are they thinking or feeling?) Well, they're kind of worried, little boy's dad maybe. But, Grandma keeps telling him things are going to be all right. (What do you think might happen next?) Well, they're going to hopefully hurry and get him to the hospital, and Grandmamma and the boy will go there, see that he's going to be okay.

SUMMARY

Agency of self, connectedness, and synchrony comprise the attachment content coding dimensions evaluated in the AAP. These dimensions represent the essence of representational attachment patterns in response to the range of events portrayed by the AAP picture stimuli. We have stated in this volume that the field's traditional dependence on discourse coherence does not completely address the question of attachment coherence. The AAP content coding dimensions we have described here extend our understanding of attachment organization by clarifying variations in their forms of appearance in AAP responses. Agency of self and connectedness reveal specific representational patterns associated with the state of being alone. Synchrony reveals patterns of self and other in attachment–caregiving relationships. The facilitation or inhibition of these dimensions is modulated by defensive processes. Taken together, their integrated and compromised forms, combined with varying expressions of defensive exclusion, foster an appreciation of the complexity of attachment patterns manifested in the AAP. We expand in Chapter 5 and the case examples in Part III on how the content and defensive process in AAP coding elements are combined to understand patterns of attachment.

5

Defensive Processes in the AAP

Despite Bowlby's (1980) major effort to define defense precisely, his model of defensive exclusion has been neglected by attachment writers. For example, there are only six index references to defense in the first edition of the *Handbook of Attachment* (Cassidy & Shaver, 1999) and seven in the second edition (Cassidy & Shaver, 2008). With the exception of discussions of the AAP and George and Solomon's work on child attachment and the parental caregiving system (George & Solomon, 1999, 2008; Solomon & George, 2011a, 2011b; Solomon et al., 1995), the discussion of defense is never operationally defined for application to theory building and assessment; rather, discussions are restricted to summaries or generalizations (e.g., Bretherton, 1985, 2005; Bretherton & Munholland, 2008; Maier et al., 2004).

In this chapter, we first review the general outline of Bowlby's concept of defensive exclusion and the work of others who have elaborated on this concept. This discussion will serve as a preface to the principles of AAP defensive process coding. Following this, subsequent sections of the chapter define defensive exclusion more specifically and provide examples of specific forms of defensive exclusion as they appear in the AAP.

DEFENSIVE EXCLUSION

In explicating the psychoanalytic theory of defense, Freud (1926/1959) drew upon an analogy to the mechanics of energy as understood by 19th-century physics. Bowlby (1969/1982) criticized this concept of defense as reflecting an archaic, mechanistic scientism and for making freewheeling use of vague and imprecise constructs that did not accord well with observable behavior. Despite Bowlby's view that the psychoanalytic explication of defense was off track, he believed that a theory of defense would be invaluable as a bridge between observable behavior and internal mental states. For example, he understood the child's "detachment" to his mother after a prolonged separation from her as the behavioral manifestation of *repressed* affect (Bowlby, 1973). Like Freud before him, Bowlby (1980) based his theory of defense on the popular scientific models of his era. He patterned his thinking on an analogy to human information processing as understood by mid-20th-century psychologists. In a chapter entitled "An Information-Processing Approach to Defense," Bowlby (1980) referred to studies in neurophysiology, cognitive psychology, and information processing as the basis for a new view of and a new language to describe defense.

Just as repression is the key to understanding the psychoanalytic theory of defense, defensive exclusion is the key to understanding the attachment theory of defense. Bowlby observed, "What is pathological is not so much the defensive processes themselves as their scope, intensity and tendency to persist" (1980, p. 35). This statement contains the following considerations:

1. It is customary to use the term *defense* to refer to behavior that exists in ordinary life; that is to say, defense is expected as a part of normal development.
2. The exclusion of distressing attachment information and associated affects is thus an adaptive stratagem in that it preserves the integrity of the internal working model of self.
3. The maintenance of defensive exclusion is adaptive, but only in a limited way because massive and extensive defensive exclusion impedes the recategorization of old memories and restricts the capacity to create new meanings (see Chapter 3).

Thus, with reference to the last point, the process of defensive exclusion is the persistent exclusion of some particular data that should be attended to as signal, but instead is treated as noise. In defining the role of defense in attachment relationships, Bowlby elaborated two general levels of defensive exclusion that he then used to describe adult insecurity in terms of how individuals processed and thought about experience and affect. He proposed that, at one level, perceptual exclusion resulted in the *deactivation* of the attachment system with behavioral and representational consequences that Bowlby termed compulsive self-sufficiency. Deactivation effectively preempts full activation of the attachment system (George & Solomon, 2008) and generally keeps attachment distress from consciousness. At a second level, he suggested that preconscious exclusion leads to stopping the processing of information prior to gaining access to conscious thought. This resulted in the *disconnection* of complete attachment information from awareness. In this case, activation of the attachment system is allowed but accurate interpretation of the meaning of activation disallowed. Bowlby proposed that the two insecure patterns of attachment of compulsive caregiving and anxious attachment resulted from this disconnection of cause and effect. Finally, Bowlby discussed a third form of defensive exclusion that he termed the segregated system. Unlike deactivation and cognitive disconnection, this exclusion mechanism blocks attachment information and affect from consciousness and was conceived as the result of extremely threatening attachment experiences, ones that are intolerable and frightening.

We approach defense and attachment following the perspective that has been defined by George and Solomon's (2008; Solomon et al., 1995) research. Defensive exclusion characterizes all patterns of attachment. As we show in the case examples described in Section III, both attachment security and insecurity are associated with defense. For secure individuals, defense acts as a sorting mechanism—transforming and excluding attachment affect and experience in order to support integration, flexibility, and sincere confidence in the self and attachment figures as agents of care and effectiveness. For insecure individuals, defense takes on more of an exclusionary role, akin to Bowlby's (1980) original thinking. Because deactivating and disconnecting strategies suppress direct expression of attachment memories, feelings, behavior, or thoughts, the concept of defense emphasizes that we must attend to what is substituted in order to differentiate patterns of insecurity. Segregated systems mechanisms exclude attachment affects and memories that threaten to dysregulate attachment representation and behavior. The sections that follow in this chapter discuss how these forms of defense are exhibited in response to the AAP stimuli. Examples of the patterns of defensive strategies that define individual differences between attachment classification groups and among individuals in a particular classification group are presented in Part III. In anticipation of those examples, we provide a brief overview of how defense, combined with information based on the AAP content coding (see Chapter 4), is used to derive an attachment classification group designation at the end of this chapter.

Deactivation

Deactivation is defensive exclusion of attachment-relevant information at the initial perceptual level; attachment distress and the details associated with this distress are never consciously processed (Bowlby, 1980). Deactivation then permits the individual to "not notice" attachment need and to endorse a quality of self-sufficient strength that does not require appealing to attachment figures for comfort or care.

This model of deactivation implies that the attachment system ceases to function and appears to be "turned off." Bretherton (1985) stressed, however, that the process of monitoring attachment need must be continually active, screening access and proximity to the caregiver and the familiarity of the surroundings. The antecedent of deactivation is the attachment figure consistently turning away from distress and need, sending a clear message of instead valuing independence and self-reliance. For this reason, one must recognize that, although the attachment *system* itself is continually active, attachment *behaviors* are only intermittently activated. Therefore, deactivation only appears to turn off attachment by ignoring and transforming attachment events and stimuli so that they are not distressing. This process effectively permits the individual to turn away consistently from attachment need and attachment figures and evaluate themselves as strong and unaffected by life's stressors. Deactivation is a preemptive strategy that maintains the attachment relationship by effectively keeping attachment figures present but not involved, often diverting or transforming indices of attachment need to other developmental domains, such as exploration or, in adults, romance and sexual needs (George & Solomon, 2008; George & West, 2008).

Early on in thinking about attachment, Cassidy and Kobak (1988) attempted to augment Bowlby's (1980) view of deactivation by suggesting that the masking of negative affect serves the same function as avoidant attachment responses; deactivation keeps the caregiver close by avoiding stimuli that have caused rejection and distancing. They further proposed that deactivating individuals deemphasize the importance of giving and receiving care and show information-processing biases that function to control or deny affective distress.

This view is consistent with another early model advanced by Main

(1981) under which the suppression of attachment behaviors actually becomes, in a sense, an attachment behavior itself. That is to say, information relevant to attachment is not excluded but rather comes to be associated with distinct behavioral sequelae characterized by the absence of any externally identifiable attachment behavior. Attachment information is recognized and used to determine behavioral responses. But the very consistency of the behavioral response, the avoidance of any attachment behaviors or affects, betrays a careful attendance to attachment-relevant information.

Evidence of Deactivation in the AAP

Based on the foregoing considerations, we expected that deactivation would be evidenced in individuals' AAP responses by specific story content or themes that exclude thoughts and affects that would activate their attachment systems. We should expect this response because the AAP pictures depict threatening events (illness, solitude, death, etc.), and deactivation works as an attempt to dismiss, divert, or neutralize distressing perceptions and affective reactions triggered by these scenes from consciousness. For example, those who rely on deactivation will make persistent efforts to shift attention away from feelings of distress, sadness, and neediness (similar to avoidance in the Strange Situation or dismissing discourse in the AAI). Deactivation enables the individual to complete the task of telling a story without being distracted by attendant attachment distress.

The following AAP forms of response content are evidence for deactivation:

1. *Shift of attention from emotion-related to stereotypic and role-defined interactions.* This form of deactivation is expressed in two ways.

   a. *Stereotypic and role-defined interactions,* shown by describing established social rules or interactive scripts that specify what constitutes appropriate behavior. For example, themes of age, sex, or role-appropriate behavior (men open doors for women; teenagers are not supposed to act like babies) and social scripts (families gather for weddings; a person visits a family member's grave on the birthday of the deceased or anniversary of the death) are common. These responses have the underlying quality of following an agenda or universally approved set of values that shift attention away from personal involvement.

TABLE 5.1. Examples of Indicators of Deactivation in the AAP

Shifts of attention from emotion

Social roles

A child this age should not need a hug at bedtime.

Grandmother called *911* and the *paramedics* took grandfather to the cardiac unit.

The man came to visit his wife's grave on the *wedding anniversary.*

She packed more suitcases than he did *because women always do.*

The boy is sick and the mother brings him *chicken soup.*

Inattention to attachment distress

The kid sits on the couch and watches *TV.*

Mother turns out the light and the boy goes to *sleep.*

It's been raining all day so she is going to get her book and *read.*

Grandmother tells him that he can play a *video game.*

Authoritarian orientation

Power

The girl's parents are *working a lot in order to get money to buy a big house.*

Prestige: The man is at the cemetery to find the *graves of the United States Presidents.*

He's *stronger* than his little brother.

She's a *fashion model* and is on her break.

Personal strength

The grandmother must be *strong* for the sake of the boy.

He *doesn't have the ability* to tackle this (i.e., not strong)

His *shoulders are straight* and he's *strong enough to take it.*

He is *capable of taking care of himself.*

Authority

His mother sent him to the corner for breaking the vase.

The teacher told him he had to stay in from recess to clear his desk.

The teacher is going to call his parents.

His mother *insisted that he listen and learn how to behave.*

Overemphasis on intellect and achievement

Rational problem solving

She's trying to *figure out* why her friends *ruined her popularity*, and *how she can still go to the dance.*

The had a disagreement and they need clear communication skills in order to figure out if they are going to stay together or separate.

They have their differences and they're going to have to solve them to stay together.

She'll get up off the bench and *go resolve the situation.*

(*continued*)

TABLE 5.1. *(continued)*

Overemphasis on intellect and achievement (*cont.*)

Intellect/achievement

The girl was in a *sports competition*, either *swimming* or *track. They could have done better.* She looks *defeated.*

The boy goes to his room and does his *homework.*

This is a *campus dorm room* and this kid is some kind of *child prodigy who is 8 or 10 years old* putting the polishing touches on her *PhD in neurolinguistic, biochemistry synapse release.*

He's going to grow up and be a *professional basketball player.*

Neutralizing and minimization

He'll take the beating; *he's used to it. It happens all of the time.*

Accept that his dad is gone; it's part of life.

The girl *acts as if she didn't get anything out of it.*

Some small thing led up to it and the adult's reaction is out of proportion. Maybe he just spilled a glass of milk.

Affective tone: Interpersonal relationships

Sexual system

The couple were *just married* and they are on their *honeymoon.*

The man is thinking, "*She's attractive, I'd like to get to know her better.*"

The man's wife died. He knows she'll understand that they'll meet in heaven and in the meantime *he will date other women.*

She's *in love* and *she's going to try to get him to go out with her again.*

Rejection/disobedience

He's been sent to *time out. They want to lecture him* but he doesn't want to hear about it. *He did something wrong, he wasn't paying attention.*

No, go away. I don't want to listen to you.

Mom *pushes him away* and tells him, "No. *You can't sit on my lap.*"

She failed her math test and her parents put her on *house arrest.*

Note. Specific indicators of deactivation are designated in italics.

b. *Complete inattention to attachment distress*, shown by turning attention away from attachment distress and toward activities that completely redirect attention and do not permit distress to enter consciousness such as reading a book, playing computer games, or going to sleep.

2. *Authoritarian orientation.* From the point of view of deactivation, an authoritarian orientation rests on a set of explicit modes of interpersonal relating and cultural values involving strength as a shield from or antidote for distress. This form of deactivation is expressed by references to (a) *power,* such as images of materialism, status, prestige,

and persons known for their achievement or power (rock star, president, doctor, teacher); (b) *personal strength,* which include descriptions of characters in the story who are able to act because of their abilities or their capacity to draw upon physical strength; and (c) *authority,* evidenced by depicting characters in the role of strict authority figures concerned with obedience and punishment.

3. *Emphasis on achievement/intellect.* This form of deactivation leads in two directions. In one direction, the typical ideal of the deactivating person is to be objective, rational, and logical. In the other direction, exploration triumphs over attachment and leads to investment in achievement and rational problem solving. Achievement and intellect allow themes of characters pursing athletic competition and activities associated with education and schooling, all of which bespeak of long periods of attachment "abstinence."

4. *Neutralizing and minimization.* In the manner of storytelling, the deactivating person is often driven to take the charge out of distress elicited by the AAP stimuli. To use a pharmacological metaphor, these maneuvers act as "pain-killing" responses to anesthetize or otherwise strip away negative affect. Accordingly, such affect that creeps into an AAP story is kept on a small emotional scale by quickly evaluating events and emotions as unimportant and even irrelevant. For example, after a parent goes to the hospital, "everyone acts like it's not that big of a deal"; after visiting a parent's grave, the man "acts like nothing really happened" or "he really didn't get anything out of it."

5. *Affective tone: interpersonal relationships.* The deactivating person often copes with attachment distress by appearing armored or distanced from attachment figures. Intimacy needs, when expressed, are restricted to the context of dating and romantic relationships (i.e., activation of the sexual behavioral system in lieu of the attachment system). When avoidance of attachment situations is undermined, a possibility when attachment signals are intense (e.g., the boy's appeal for closeness in the *Bed* picture), deactivation often results in story themes in which one character actively rejects or ignores others. These rejection themes are often accompanied by negative evaluations of the other person as disobedient, manipulative, or deserving of punishment.

Cognitive Disconnection

Cognitive disconnection is associated with conscious awareness of the activation of attachment situations and affect; however, accurate interpretation of the meaning of activation is disallowed (Bowlby, 1980).

Bowlby (1980) proposed that cognitive disconnection is most likely to be supported by exclusion processes and resulting beliefs that "divert the individual's attention away from whoever, or whatever, may be responsible for his reactions" (p. 65). In essence, there is a disconnection of affect, cause, source, and effect. The individual comes to "dwell so insistently on the details of his own reactions and sufferings that he has no time to consider what the interpersonal situation for his reactions may really be" (p. 65). The upshot is confused processing; cues are misidentified and attempts to understand attachment are entangled in irrelevant detail. The antecedent of cognitive disconnection is inconsistency and contradiction in caregiver responsiveness; the individual's childhood experiences were neither marked by clear rejection nor sensitive care (Bowlby, 1980). In these circumstances, the coherence of the individual's internal working model of self necessitates the "chopping up" of attachment experience, as it were, so that the disjunction between attachment needs and the caregiver's responsiveness is avoided (George & Solomon, 2008). It makes sense, then, that attachment experience filtered through cognitive disconnection is associated with anxious attachment. In its most extreme form, individuals may show extreme separation anxiety. Bowlby (1973) proposed that disconnected anxiety was the root of what he termed "pseudo-phobias," that is, phobias that originate from attachment fears rather from specific environmental stimuli such as attachment-based fears that mimic school phobia in children or agoraphobia in adults. Bowlby's assertion has been supported by studies showing phobias and anxiety associated with separation anxiety and ambivalent attachment (Bar-Haim, Dan, Eshel, & Sagi-Schwartz, 2007; Brumariu & Kerns, 2010; de Ruiter & van IJzendoorn, 1992; Peter, BrŸckner, Hand, & Rufer, 2005), for which cognitive disconnection is the main defensive exclusion process (George & Solomon, 2008; Solomon et al., 1995).

Evidence of Cognitive Disconnection in the AAP

What, then, should we expect in the AAP stories of those who rely heavily on cognitive disconnection? The specific indications of this form of defensive exclusion should most of all be found in representations that reflect nonintegrated "pieces" of attachment information. That is to say, the individual's ability to tell a story will be compromised by the inclusion of irrelevant information and affect as well as uncertainty leaving him or her unsettled and continually shifting back and forth. At the extreme, this uncertainty gives rise to the inability of individuals to make up their minds or complete their thoughts when telling of their stories.

TABLE 5.2. Examples of Indicators of Cognitive Disconnection in the AAP

Uncertainty and confusion

Uncertainty

He's *confused* as to what he is supposed to do.

The couple is going on vacation or this is a daughter and a father and the daughter is going back to college after the holidays. (Two plot ideas.)

She is *staring* out the window, *waiting* for her parents to come home.

He gets up and has breakfast or he says goodnight and goes to sleep. (Two endings, and the endings are opposites.)

He doesn't know what happened. He *doesn't understand.*

Affective tone: Disconnected affect in relationships

Anger/feisty

Maybe they were *arguing* or *fighting.*

He was *sassing* his sister, so he ended up in the corner.

They're having a *row.*

The man looks *angry* and *aggressive.*

Glossing

He's just a kid, he'll *grow out of it.*

The woman is very sad, but she'll *get over it.*

He wants a hug and she wants to get this over with and watch TV. *But they are so happy together and love each other so much.*

They'll separate and *soon everything will get better.*

Inability to integrate the conflicting desire for closeness and withdrawal

Entangling

They want to hug but they feeling *awkward.*

Bullies stole his lunch money.

She feels *guilty* because she wasn't home when he got sick.

She's *frustrated* and sad.

Withdraw/withhold

She's sad and *she wants to be all by herself.*

She *holds onto her hand* so that she won't slap him.

He doesn't want to cry in front of his friend.

He has to admit that the event happened and *resign* himself to the situation.

Busy/distracted

She needed to take a walk *so she wouldn't think about it.*

She'll *keep him busy* until his parents come home.

His parents were *too busy to notice.*

He *hums a tune* in the corner to pass time until he can leave.

Note. Specific indicators of cognitive disconnection are designated in italics.

The following AAP forms of response content are evidence for cognitive disconnection:

1. *Uncertainty and confusion regarding people and events.* Uncertainty emerges clearly when the individual's response lacks precision in identifying the characters in the story or the story line is unclear, either because of missing pieces or unfinished plot ideas. Characters are frequently described in terms of the individual's own confused mental state, such as being confused, bored, or in an undefined state (e.g., daydreaming). Often, confusion is expressed in the contradictory quality of representations in which story lines or elements of the story are described in polar opposite ways (e.g., the child is going to bed or getting up in the morning). Missing pieces that lend confusion to the response also include an individual's failure to connect the two parts of an event, dropping the attachment element as if someone just hung up the phone (e.g., "The child went downstairs with . . . and sat on the couch").

2. *Affective tone: Disconnected affect in relationships.* This form of cognitive disconnection is likely to be expressed as disconnected affects, seen especially in the individual's struggle to manage anger. On the one hand, disconnection permits anger, although it may be displaced, diffuse, or overly intense. When this occurs, story themes emphasize anger and feistiness (a diminutive form of anger). On the other hand, because intense anger threatens attachment relationships (Bowlby, 1973) and is difficult to manage and repair once it has surfaced, the individual may make persistent efforts to keep relationships and situations happy. Happiness is a distraction that prevents chronic anger from surfacing. In this way, disconnection is used to purify the responses through glossing, an exclusion technique that skips to the happy ending without addressing the elements of attachment that respond to distress, create repair, or create reciprocal enjoyment.

3. *Inability to integrate the conflicting desire for closeness to attachment figures and withdrawal from them.* Confused by the missing pieces of attachment, including disconnected anger, the disconnected person longs for closeness with attachment figures even though the subjective evaluation of closeness is one that it is often not enjoyable or satisfactory. The basic attachment formula is that physical and psychological closeness ought to lead to the attachment figure detecting attachment signals and providing sensitive care. After all, if one is close, how can an attachment figure miss these signals? Yet the experience of the disconnected individual is that the attachment figure does indeed miss these

signals, and closeness often fails to elicit the desired response. Frustrated but persistent, the disconnected individual vacillates between closeness and passive or angry withdrawal. This is indicated in the AAP response by shifts back and forth between expressions of attachment need and expressions of underlying anger, frustration, and withdrawal. Furthermore, the inability to integrate these elements is to leave the individual in a "holding pattern," as evidenced by themes of staying busy or distracted (e.g., grandmother plays a game with the boy to take his mind off his distress) until decisions about being close can be reached.

Segregated Systems

The concept of segregated systems as a defensive operation is most clearly stated in a series of propositions largely derived from the discussions of Bowlby (1980), Main (1995), George & Solomon (1999, 2008), Solomon et al. (1995), and George et al. (1999). The propositions are:

1. Segregated systems are the product of complete defensive exclusion.
2. Defensive exclusion in its most complete form encodes trauma-related memories and emotions in a separate representational model that is inaccessible to consciousness.
3. Segregated systems are prone to defensive breakdown.
4. Defensive breakdown results in a state of mental dysregulation and attachment disorganization.

Because the concept of segregated systems is a core feature of the AAP and has received relatively cursory attention in the attachment literature, we begin this section with a theoretical discussion of the etiology and functioning of segregated systems in relation to internal working models of attachment and caregiving. This background also provides the reader with a convenient source of clarification of the segregated system concept as it is used in the coding and interpretation of AAP content.

Bowlby (1980) introduced the concept of segregated systems to explain the defenses involved in individuals' attempts to adapt to experiences of loss through death. More recently, this concept has been used to think about attachment trauma, defined as situations that threaten or break attachment relationships, such as abuse or other severe threats to the integrity of self (e.g., rape; Solomon & George, 2000; West & George, 1999). Bowlby proposed that segregated systems were the defensive product under circumstances that required complete defensive exclusion in an attempt to maintain basic integrity. He proposed that the segregated system itself is a representational model of attachment that "contains" traumatic and frightening experience and affect that are necessarily blocked—and thus segregated—from conscious awareness.

As we have seen, behavioral systems such as attachment are organized by mental representational structures conceived in terms of organized working models (Bowlby, 1969/1982; 1973). Thus Bowlby (1980) applied the term *system* in his model of segregated defensive processes to suggest that this traumatic mental representation was separate and self-contained, guided by its own representational rules, postulates, appraisals, and executive control mechanisms. Segregated models are blocked from consciousness; not integrated into behavior or thought; closed to new experience and information about attachment; internally consistent and organized in relation to the goal of the attachment system; and exist in parallel with models that have access to consciousness (i.e., an organized segregated system generally not accessible to short-term memory processing).

As we explicate more fully in Chapter 9, Bowlby (1980) developed this concept to characterize the disorganized states of mind he defined as the foundation of chronic unresolved loss. Main (Main & Goldwyn, 1985/1988/1994; Main & Hesse, 1990; Main & Solomon, 1990) operationally defined the disorganized representational and behavioral states associated with unresolved loss as specific lapses in the monitoring of reasoning analogous to the collapse of organized attachment behavior observed in infants.

Adding this perspective to Bowlby's original thinking, we conceive of the segregated system as the resolution of this collapse. When the pain associated with threatening attachment experience is so great that it potentially undermines the individual's ability to function, mental material related to attachment must literally be "housed" elsewhere, in a form of storage that is segregated and kept, as best as possible, inaccessible to consciousness. As such, segregated systems develop as a form of self-protection in an attempt to block severe and potentially devastating attachment affect from interfering with everyday functioning. The segregated system is thus an adaptive stratagem—adaptive, however, only in a limited and temporary way because it is prone to breaking down under stress.

The short-term benefits of segregated attachment models are outweighed by the risks of the potential long-term maladaptation associated with this extreme form of defensive exclusion. For example Main, and attachment researchers extending her thinking, demonstrated that experiences of threats to the attachment relationship through loss or abuse are associated with dissociative symptoms (e.g., Abrams, Rifkin, & Hesse, 2006; Carlson, 1998; Hesse & Main, 2006; Jacobvitz, Leon, & Hazen, 2006; Liotti, 2004, 2011; Lyons-Ruth & Jacobvitz, 2008; Main & Morgan, 1996).

Bowlby (1980) emphasized that segregated models cannot be blocked from consciousness indefinitely. He described segregated systems exclusion as a brittle and vulnerable defense pattern, prone to fail when attachment is activated and when the individual needs defenses the most; that is, when the individual experiences certain internal or external events that are appraised as threatening. It is precisely when the individual's attachment system is intensely activated that the emergence of segregated feelings is most likely (George & Solomon, 2008; West & George, 1999). Upon the release of segregated material, the individual is prone to dysregulation, a state in which behavior and thought become disorganized and disoriented by either emotional flooding or attempts to prohibit or block these emotions from consciousness (Bowlby, 1980).

In summary, the concept of the segregated system provides a conceptual model that integrates the behavioral and representational features that are now considered hallmarks of disorganization, including the disoriented behavior of disorganized infants on reunion during the Strange Situation (Main & Solomon, 1990), the extreme controlling strategies developed by older children (Main & Cassidy, 1988), dissociative symptomology in adolescents and adults, and caregiver helplessness, rage, and glorification of their children (George & Solomon, 2008, 2011).

It is evident that as indications of dysregulation increase quantitatively and qualitatively in the AAI and AAP, they bespeak severe undermining or collapse of the individual's defensive processes. In this regard, a continuum of operation of defensive processes must be recognized. Viewed broadly, the relative success of defensive processes generally decreases as we progress from organized insecure attachment to disorganization (i.e., dismissing and preoccupied to unresolved). Disorganized attachment represents the failure or breakdown of defensive processes (George & West, 1999; Solomon et al., 1995). Indeed, as Main (1995), paraphrasing Freud, observed, "disorganization is the state to which defense is the alternative" (p. 461). Disorganization marks the failure to accomplish reintegration in the representational world so that progress toward a linear process of completed mourning is blocked. Bowlby (1980) considered dysregulation as fundamental to pathological mourning; that is, the failure to begin or complete mourning (see Chapter 9).

Evidence of Segregated Systems in the AAP

The AAP picture stimuli potentially unleash feelings of fear and vulnerability in those individuals who interpret these attachment situations as physically or psychologically threatening. As in the doll play responses of young children (Solomon et al., 1995), segregated systems are evidenced in the AAP as either forms of overt representational dysregulation or constriction. Dysregulation response themes and imagery unleash the possibility of threat, in addition to feelings of helplessness and isolation that leave the individual in a momentary or more prolonged state of dysregulation due to the breakdown of the organizing deactivating or disconnecting forms of exclusion. Constricting responses block dysregulation, but immobilize the individual. This is a freezing response, a representational form of a behavior response that is used to identify attachment disorganization in infants, and is associated with fear in mammals and in individuals who have experienced unremitting attachment terror (Main & George, 1985; Main & Solomon, 1990; Perry, Pollard, Blakley, Baker, & Vigilante, 1995).

The following AAP forms of response content are evidence for segregated systems:

1. *Dysregulation.* This form of segregated system is expressed as (a) *fear and failed protection*, including images or statements of being frightened or endangered, or elements suggesting abdication of care from attachment figures (e.g., abandonment); (b) *helplessness,* including images of characters as impotent, immobile, or out of control (e.g., drunken, emotional outbursts, acts or threats of violence); (c) *emptiness and isolation*, including images of characters who are completely withdrawn or estranged, notably a state of being that Bowlby described as one of the most terrifying experiences for humans (Bowlby, 1973); and (d) *spectral, dysregulated thinking and obtrusions,* in which boundaries between what is feared and what is real are permanently dissolved (i.e., the wish to be with the dead) or the inexplicable invasion of fears and terror into the story response.

2. *Constricted immobilization.* It must also be recognized that in the face of potential dysregulation, some individuals literally shut down their response to the AAP picture stimulus. Rather than respond, descriptions of extreme emotions and the events surrounding those emotions are blocked. Individuals clearly state that they don't want to respond to a particular picture, and, in some instances, they may give the picture back to the interviewer and ask to go on to the next picture.

TABLE 5.3. Examples of Indicators of Segregated Systems in the AAP

Dysregulation

Fear/danger/failed protection/abdicated care

He's *frightened*. He's *scared* that his father is going to hit him.

She's sad and alone, *curled up in a fetal position*.

The boy had a *nightmare* and he was *scared*.

She enjoys the *feel of fire*.

The girl on the bench just found out that her father isn't her father. She goes home and *stabs him three times in the back*.

His parents *abandoned* him at birth, and now he's at the cemetery trying to find their graves.

Out of control/helpless

He's *backed into a cornered* and *can't escape*.

She was *desperate* and had to leave.

The situation is *hopeless*.

His father was *enraged* and *screamed* at him.

Emptiness/isolation

She feels *alienated*.

The room is *totally barren and empty*.

The police took her to *jail*.

It all just seems so *worthless*.

Spectral/ dysregulated thinking/obtrusions

He's just maybe *having a talk with his dead mother, saying why he hasn't visited or is having some trouble in their life*.

Gravestones predict the future.

She wants to curl up and *disappear*.

The children *look weird, like they are behind glass*.

Constricted immobilization

His dad died. That picture is hard. *I don't like that one. That's enough*.

Whoa. We were smacked when we were in the corner. *Not doing that one*.

I don't want to verbalize that. I really don't want to say something.

I don't want to say. It gives me a headache.

Note. Specific indicators of segregated systems are designated in italics.

ADULT ATTACHMENT CLASSIFICATION USING THE AAP

In order to help the reader integrate the coding material presented in Chapters 4 and 5, we provide a brief description of the classification process. This discussion also sets the stage for the detailed discussion of case examples using the AAP provided in Part III. Classification requires the judge to examine the overall patterns of story content and defensive processing elements in the entire set of responses to the attachment stimuli, administered in the correct order (see Chapter 3). Classification cannot be determined by evaluating only one or a subset of story responses. A summary of the AAP classification decision tree is provided in Figure 5.1. The classification schematic is provided to give an overall sense of how the AAP system works; the material presented in Chapters 4 and 5 is not sufficient to apply to cases without training.

The first step in the classification process is to identify the presence of segregated systems material in the responses. If present, material is next evaluated to determine if there is representational reorganization or containment. Containment or "resolution" means that individuals have drawn upon their internal working models of attachment to integrate or recover from dysregulation. Resolution can occur through the story

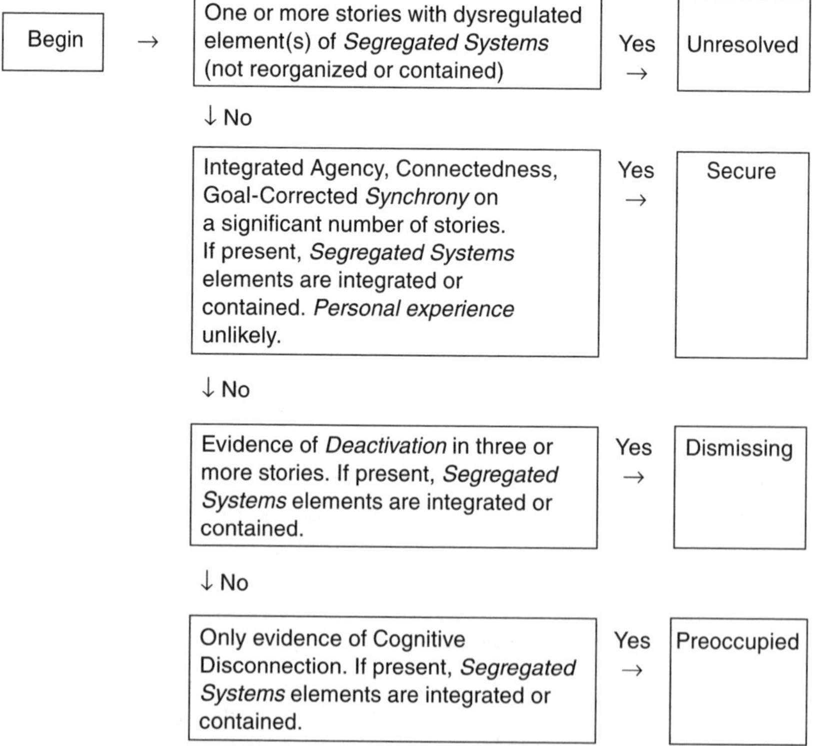

FIGURE 5.1. AAP classification decision tree.

elements coded as agency of the self (internalized secure base, haven of safety, or capacity to act), functional behavior (i.e., activities that address the problem, such as going to the hospital) or descriptions of non-attachment figures providing care or assistance. The failure to reorganize or contain segregated systems material indicates that attachment remains dysregulated and the individual is judged unresolved.

The next step is to evaluate the case for security. The hallmark of security in the AAP is the ability to demonstrate the forms of integrated attachment that constitute attachment relationship coherence. The evaluations of AAP content dimensions are most important for determining security. Security is evidenced by the presence of internalized secure base and haven of safety in alone stories, and sensitivity or goal-corrected synchrony in the dyadic stories. Secure cases typically contain relatively little evidence of defensive processing; when present, defense helps the individual navigate and manage tension or distress. The inclusion of personal experience (i.e., autobiographical information) in secure cases' stories is rare.

If the case is not designated secure, the next step is to evaluate the patterns of defensive processing in order to determine which organized-insecure attachment classification should be designated. Deactivation is the defensive process that defines dismissing attachment. If deactivation predominates in the story responses, the case is judged dismissing. Cognitive disconnection is the defensive process that defines preoccupied attachment. The predominance of cognitive disconnection in the absence of deactivating defenses results in the case being judged preoccupied.

SUMMARY

We began this chapter with an in-depth discussion of the attachment theory approach to defense. Indeed, research has demonstrated that operational definitions of Bowlby's three forms of defensive exclusion—deactivation, cognitive disconnection, and segregated systems—lend themselves to empirical and systematic treatment and are one of the main representational features that differentiate among patterns of attachment (George & Solomon, 2008). We have operationally defined the facets of each of these three forms of defense as they apply to AAP responses and then used the underlying regularity of defensive operations as an aid in classification. In Section III, we present case examples that provide a rich understanding of the adult attachment classification nosology as well as the nuances of each individual's particular representational pattern of attachment.

PART III

Using the AAP

6

Secure Attachment

Bowlby, who approached attachment from the view of a clinician, did not offer a formal definition of secure attachment as a behavioral pattern. Instead, he directed our attention to a set of relatively inflexible and constricted patterns that he claimed defined attachment insecurity (compulsive self-reliance and anxious attachment; Bowlby, 1980). Indeed, it was Ainsworth's methodology for classifying patterns of attachment on which most subsequent empirical and theoretical work in attachment is based (Ainsworth et al., 1978). Ainsworth demonstrated that behavioral phenomena, which at first glance appear heterogeneous, serve the set goal of proximity to a caregiver.

Observations of secure children in infancy through middle childhood have established that attachment security fosters direct expressions and communications of attachment need (i.e., activation of the attachment system), allowing the child to seek proximity to and physical contact with the attachment figure without risk or anxiety (Sroufe et al., 2005; Thompson, 2008). Parents of secure children are sensitive, balanced, and flexible (George & Solomon, 2008). Beginning when children are in the preschool years (typically around age 4), the attachment–caregiving relationship begins to develop the quality of a goal-corrected partnership (Bowlby, 1969/1982). Parents of secure children foster relationship commitment, trust, and enjoyment, and they communicate clearly and effectively (see George & Solomon, 2008, for review).

To be securely attached means that a person is confident that he or she can rely on attachment figures to provide safety, protection, and comfort. Secure attachment is relatively undefended. Secure children do not need to engage in defensive behavioral maneuvers to achieve proximity. As a result, secure children also have relatively defense-free working models of the self as worthy of protection and care and of attachment figures as available and providing care and comfort (Ainsworth et al., 1978; George & Solomon, 2008; Marvin & Britner, 2008; Solomon & George, 2008; Solomon et al., 1995).

Most of the initial work in understanding adult attachment is based on AAI descriptions of "current states of mind" of attachment (Hesse, 2008; Main et al., 1985). The hallmark of secure adult attachment (designated also as "autonomous") is freshness of response and freedom from prescribed and proscribed behaviors when thinking and speaking about attachment. The secure adult exhibits a willingness and ability to recall attachment-related memories and feelings, and to describe these experiences with consistency and clarity. These features of the interview are defined as coherency of discourse about attachment-relevant experiences, particularly with parents, and interview coherency is the "sine qua non" of secure adult states of mind. Coherency in the AAI has a particular meaning because of the central role placed on cooperating with the interviewer-led "conversation" regarding attachment. Indeed, AAI coherence is defined using Grice's maxims of conversational coherence (as cited by Main et al., 1985; Hesse, 2008; see also Chapter 2). What is important in Main's application of conversational rules to the attachment conversation is that a highly coherent transcript is the result of current flexibility and confidence to evaluate attachment. The secure state of mind reveals how the adult simultaneously values and maintains both a clear sense of self and commitment to the importance of attachment relationships.

In summary, to be securely attached ultimately means that attachment relationships are important and that the individual is confident in the present that he or she can expect partners in attachment–caregiving dyads to pay attention to expressions of attachment need and provide safety, protection, and comfort when needed. Following Ainsworth's original studies, individuals with childhood experiences of parental sensitivity tend to carry forward security into adulthood, barring threats to attachment that shift relationships toward insecurity and mistrust, such as major separations and loss (Sroufe et al., 2005; Waters, Merrick, Treboux, Crowell, & Albersheim, 2000). Other individuals "earn" their security through experiences that foster intimate protective and caring relationships, including psychotherapy, that foster thinking, reformulating attachment expectations, and forgiveness. Irrespective of past experience, what secure adults are thought to have in common is behavioral and psychological integration of attachment experience, memories, and affect such that the individual functions in a manner that is consistent with Bowlby's (1969/1982) notion of the attachment–caregiving relationship as a goal-corrected partnership. That is, a secure attachment is a relationship that flexibly integrates the needs and perspectives of both the self and the partner with confidence in the self's ability to seek comfort and protection. Secure adults can classify and recategorize past experience in light of the present (West & Sheldon-Keller, 1994), and are consciously committed to not to repeating the past when attachment figures fostered insecurity and fear.

Because an integrated state of mind and not childhood experiences per se are the essential ingredients of adult representational security, the AAI identified several different secure representational subgroup patterns that are designated following the subgroups of infant security as defined for the Strange Situation (Hesse, 2008). In terms of attachment (aside from coherency), the ability to objectively think about the value and commitment to attachment is the single underlying theme that defines security. Some individuals are initially defensive and restricting as they describe attachment (AAI subgroups F_1 and F_2). Others appear truly autonomous and integrated about their attachment experiences, despite past or current difficulties with attachment figures (AAI subgroup F_3). Others value relationships, but continue to be mentally entangled with attachment difficulties (AAI subgroup F_4) or are somewhat complaining and slightly resentful that they are still trying to please their parents (AAI subgroup F_5).

The Characteristics of Secure Attachment in the AAP

Security in the AAP is evidenced from response patterns that indicate flexible integration with regard to attachment. Unlike the AAI, coherency in cooperating in the discussion of attachment is not relevant to the AAP (see Chapter 2). Following Ainsworth's constructs (Ainsworth et al., 1978), security on the AAP is evidenced by response patterns that demonstrate relative balance between attachment as a haven of safety and attachment as a secure base (see also Waters, 1995). In addition, because secure individuals respond flexibly in different attachment contexts, we may anticipate a range in their expression of distress, including sometimes a lack of attachment need in response to some situations that are generally thought to activate the attachment system. As such, the activated attachment system may not be apparent or seem invisible in some responses. In addition, secure individuals do not necessarily portray attachment figures as available, paying attention, or providing comfort. The responses of secure individuals are, however, realistic; they do not try to present attachment or life in general as perfect or stress free. Viewed broadly, we see in their overall response pattern conspicuous evidence of integrated and goal-corrected mutuality of attachment–caregiving dyads that defines secure attachment.

Because security is defined by flexibility and integration, adults in the secure group evidence the most variation in AAP response patterns of all of the attachment groups. This means that there is quite a range in what would be considered prototypic compared with the AAP records of individuals in the insecure attachment groups. We have selected for this chapter four cases from this range that demonstrate evidence of the prototypic elements of security. The case presentations describe the features of security as evidenced in the AAP record and show how individuals' specific response patterns are related in expected ways to their reported childhood experience with attachment figures. We first present a biographical overview as drawn from the person's responses to the AAI and other information we collected during our research. We next evaluate the case AAP, stepping the reader through first the alone "stories" and then the dyadic "stories" in order to illustrate the person's unique patterns of attachment responses. Finally, we discuss the AAI classification and compare and contrast the AAP and AAI patterns for that case.

SECURE CASE EXAMPLES

Beatrice

Beatrice is a 41-year-old Caucasian, married mother of two teenage children. She completed high school. She was raised with three younger siblings—two sisters and a brother. Her family moved around a lot until she was about 4 years old. They then settled down in the town where she lived for the rest of her childhood. Her father worked in construction and her parents managed an apartment building. Both parents are now dead. Her mother died when she was 17. Her father eventually remarried and died 2 years ago. Beatrice's parents were busy people. She described he mother as not having have much time for her, and Beatrice was made to feel that she was bothersome. "There was a lot to running the apartments. You know, we couldn't bake with her because she couldn't stand the mess. I remember trailing her around in the summertime when she was busy cleaning out apartments and that kind of thing and just wanting to be with her."

Beatrice's mother provided neither a secure base nor haven of safety, and Beatrice recalled feeling rejected by her mother a lot of the time. Her mother was powerful, always giving Beatrice directions. If they had an argument, Beatrice felt "snuffed out." Her mother took care of her physical needs, but was not affectionate. She did not think her mother hugged her as a child, but she recalled being hugged once as a teenager. "And I remember feeling so surprised and uncomfortable because it wasn't anything that, she just didn't do that. She was just an adult who did things for us, and made sure we were fed, got off to school." She recalled that her mother would take care of her when she was sick. Beatrice would sleep downstairs during the day when she was sick instead of upstairs in her bedroom. Her mother would check in every once in a while to see if she was okay.

Beatrice's relationship with her father was a mixture of fun, protection, and frustration. Her father was not a secure base; however, he did sometimes step in and buffer Beatrice from her mother. She recalled that her father taught her and her siblings how to water ski. He also came out to support her sports competitions.

Beatrice said that she was frustrated by the fact that her father never spoke about his emotions. He conveyed compliments and pride through others. Her father was prone to getting angry when he was upset. She described a time when she stepped on a piece of glass when doing chores and her father got mad. "Of course, that was something I didn't understand. Mom explained that he was upset and he didn't know what to do with it so he was angry. Anger seemed to be the only emotion that was shown in our family."

Punishment in Beatrice's household was by spanking. Her father "was the ultimate in punishment. If we got into serious trouble, we would go to him and he would give us a spanking and that was always a very, a very fearful time for all of us." She thought her parents' emotional tone was sometimes abusive. "We were called stupid a lot and, you know, there was very little praise. There was a lot more criticism than there was praise."

Beatrice remembers separations from her parents as being trips to visit her grandparents. She enjoyed those trips immensely and said she did not miss her parents. She also did not remember affection or hugging upon returning home.

Beatrice experienced several losses as a child. Her maternal grandfather died when she was 4; her paternal grandfather died when she was a young teenager. The most debilitating loss was her mother's death in a car accident when Beatrice was 17 years old. Beatrice had picked her mother up one evening from work and a drunk driver struck her mother, who was sitting in the passenger seat. The rescue team was not able to open her mother's side of the car and asked Beatrice to go over and comfort her mother. "So I went over and put my arms around her and she just told me to go away. She had a number of broken bones at that point. She died later that night."

Beatrice described the guilt that she felt for many years about her mother's death. She believed it was her fault and attributed her problems with chronic depression to the accident. She sought therapy when she noticed inappropriate bouts of anger with her children and said therapy had helped come to terms with her mother's death: "I decided that it really wasn't my fault."

Beatrice's father had a series of heart attacks over several years and died 1 year before Beatrice's interviews with us. She didn't see changes in her relationship with her father between childhood and the time he died. She felt he continued to have a very "tight rein." But she was also committed to making changes in their relationship, despite the heart attacks.

Beatrice was judged secure on the AAP. The attachment content in her response revealed strong indications of sensitivity and attachment goal-corrected partnerships in almost every story. Her responses were balanced and demonstrated how defensive exclusion supported rather than undermined flexibility and thoughtful integration. Beatrice demonstrated a range of deactivating capacities, including shifting distress to achievement themes (shifting attention to exploration themes), shutting off attachment feeling, and the feelings of negative evaluations and rejection that we explained earlier are defined in the AAP coding system associated with deactivating defenses. Her responses also revealed a range of cognitive disconnection themes, including uncertainty and confusion, busy distraction, and entangling anger. The only time she became dysregulated during the AAP was, understandably, during her response to the loss stimulus. Her response to loss evidenced the most integrated and thoughtful reorganization and relationship repair that we have ever seen in the AAP. Although Beatrice continues to struggle periodically with depression, there was no evidence in the AAP that she considered loss or her experiences of parental failures as traumatic.

Alone Stories

Beatrice's alone responses provided a complex picture of agency of self and connectedness. Story themes ranged from attachment–caregiving relationships to achievement and competence. The defensive exclusion in her responses generally served representational integration, reorganization, and personal and relationship flexibility.

> ***Window:*** Well, I think this little girl might have some sort of an illness, she can't go outside, something like ahh chickenpox, something like that, so she's standing at the window, it's a nice day out, she wants to go outside and be with her friends. Ahh, well she asks her mom if she could read her a story, but Mum's too busy. So she just goes back to the window—rests her hands on it, on the window sill and, and puts her head down on her hands and just watches. (Anything else?) Hmm, no.

Unlike the majority of the other secure responses exemplified in this chapter, Beatrice's response to *Window* demonstrated how the inability to be connected in relationships was the initiator for attachment distress for her. The girl's attachment system is activated by the fact that connection to her friends was not possible due to illness. The girl attempted to get her mother's help in deactivating her distress (read a story). She does not seek comfort but rather her mother's instrumental help in shifting attention away from her longing to be with friends. Her mother was disconnected from paying attention to the girl and too busy to pay attention (busy/distracted—cognitive disconnection). The story demonstrated how attachment distress could not be remedied in any relationships because access to individuals in both the attachment and affiliative system domains were blocked. The girl was left to tend to herself, which she accomplishes with a minimal capacity to act (changing her posture when she returns to the window).

> ***Bench:*** Well, this looks like a gal who's been in a volleyball tournament and she's just played many games and she's very tired, and the last game was a close one and they lost, so she's sitting on a bench to sit and regroup, think about the game and, and try and reorganize her thoughts and get her body and her mind pumped up again to go off and play again (What do you think might happen next?) Well, I think then she'll go and have a bite to eat, present herself at the appropriate time and, and have the energy she needs to play the next game, and play it well (Anything else?) No. (Okay.)

Faced with failed achievement (deactivation) and a negative evaluation of self (losing the game—deactivation), the girl is tired (cognitive disconnection) and uncertain about her ability. She capitalizes on the solitude provided on the bench "to think about the game and . . . reorganize her thoughts." The girl's internalized secure base fosters action (eats, plays the next game) and competence (plays well).

> *Cemetery:* Well, this is his son's trip back—to his mother's grave, and he just kind of stands and contemplates his life with his mother—sheds a few tears. (What do you think led up to that scene?) I think maybe the guy has, has been doing a lot of thinking about his mother and so he just felt the need to go and and tell his mother that he loves her and then he forgives her for all the things she couldn't be. (What would happen next?) I think he'd go for a little walk and just let thoughts run through his mind and let them go, take some deep breaths, and then go back to his family and live in the present, instead of the past. (Okay, something more?) No.

This story demonstrates the interrelationship between Beatrice's representation of secure base and haven of safety, and the importance of these elements in attachment relationships. The man's internalized secure base is the impetus for going to the cemetery in the first place (has been doing a lot of thinking about his mother). He demonstrates the use of dysregulated moments of spectral and spiritual connection at the grave site (segregated system) to repair their relationship. He felt the need to go tell his mother that he loves her and then he forgives her for all the things that she couldn't be (haven of safety–repair). The man's thoughtful consideration of his relationship with his mother continued after he left the gravesite (just let thoughts run through his mind). But the repair permitted transformation and reorganization of their relationship. Drawing from attachment theory, the man's mourning was now complete (Bowlby, 1980). We see, then, that the man can change his perspective to the present and focus on connections in living attachment relationships.

> *Corner:* Uhm, I think this little fellow and his brother were playing house, and this guy had been doing something wrong, so the brother who was pretending to be the dad sent him to the corner and ahh the father was trying to explain, he shouldn't be doing this and he shouldn't be doing that and the little boy put up his hand said, "Uh! I don't want to hear this anymore, go away, leave me alone," and so the pretend father goes away and does whatever he's

he was doing before, and the little boy in the corner puts his hands in his pockets and leans back and watches his pretend father with resentful eyes. And then pretty soon he starts to daydream and he's thinking about something else and he starts to whistle, hum a little bit, and pretend father sees what he's doing and tells him, well you might as well come out of the corner I see it's not doing you any good anymore. And then they go off, go outside and play in the backyard for a while.

Themes of caregiving sensitivity and haven of safety were embedded in this complex story of sibling pretend play. Beatrice's first response to the stimulus is to soften the blow, so to speak, by disconnecting and contextualizing in play the affective intensity she experienced as the result of a parent's authority and negative evaluation (dad sent him to the corner; been doing something wrong—deactivation). The boy similarly deactivated and rejected the father (go away, leave me alone). Once in the corner, the boy disconnects his distress. He becomes entangled and angry (resentful—cognitive disconnection) and distracted himself (whistle, hum—disconnection). Unlike her descriptions of her own relationship with her father, Beatrice transformed parental power into sensitivity. The father's caregiving system was activated by the boy's behavior in the corner. He forgave the boy (haven of safety). Defensive exclusion of attachment experience and affect were integrated, and the children were now free to engage in new activities. They go outside and play in the backyard (capacity to act).

Dyadic Stories

Each of Beatrice's dyadic stories demonstrated goal-corrected synchrony, suggesting that when attachment figures are accessible she expects their relationships to be sensitive or mutually enjoyable.

> ***Departure:*** I think this couple is at the railway station, and the woman's going home for a trip to visit her parents and there's some tension between the two of them because they're not hugging. So I think the wife's going home to think and sort things out. (What happened next?) I think that the wife will get on the train and there'll be stilted words, goodbye and talk to you soon, and the husband will help get the bags on the train and she'll ride off and he'll go home and sit in a quiet room and think about their relationship (Anything more?) No.

Preoccupied with tension, this couple's relationship became disconnected. The separation provides each of them with the opportunity of solitude to think. In this story, Beatrice's integrated synchrony in this couple relationship was essentially mutual forms of the internalized secure base observed in response to being alone. Beatrice demonstrated in this response how the social roles that define behavior (a man helps the woman with her bags—deactivation) can help support the thinking process. As Ainsworth observed, attachment security endures over time and space (Ainsworth et al., 1978).

> ***Bed:*** Well, this looks like bedtime and Mum has just sat down to say goodnight and this young fellow feels he needs a hug before he goes to sleep, so she slides up a little closer to him and gives him a big hug and strokes his head, his back and then tells him to roll over onto his tummy and she'll give him a bit of a massage, and that calms him down and gets him ready for sleep, and she kisses him goodnight and leaves the room.

The boy needed a bedtime hug. Beatrice identified that attachment signal immediately and described the mother's sensitive response without hesitation. The boy went to sleep. Sleep, coded deactivation, was not in the spirit of defensive exclusion in the context of this story. Rather, deactivation permitted the boy to turn his attention away from his need for his mother, which is the natural result of caregiving sensitivity.

> ***Ambulance:*** Hmm. Well, I think the family has gone to visit Grandma and Grandpa, and while they're there, one of the parents becomes ill, and so the child is going to stay with Grandma while the other parent goes with the one who's sick to the hospital, and Grandma is going to explain what happened, reassure the child that everything's going to be okay and that the parent is going to be fine and will come home. And they go off together and they do some baking together, to help take the child's mind off their parent. (What do you think might happen next?) Well, I think that baking the cookies will be so much fun that the child would forget about the parent for a while and then Grandma and the child would sit down and have tea and cookies and maybe by then the other parent would be home to help reassure the child that the other parent's going to be okay. Hmm . . . I think that then the parent will take the child on her knee and give him a big hug and soothe him.

This story described instrumental care and comfort for a hierarchy of attachment figures. Beatrice differentiates between primary and secondary caregivers and described how the coordinated efforts of multiple generations in a family can together protect and comfort a child. The source of attachment distress was a parent's illness. The parent dyad in this story functions as a unit; the other parent accompanied the sick parent to the hospital. In the meantime, the grandmother provided the child with the functional care to keep the child safe and organized, including explaining the situation, reassuring and distracting the child from the parent's situation (baking together to help take the child's mind off their parent—cognitive disconnection). It is not until the primary attachment figure—implied to be the mother—returns from the hospital, however, that the child receives real comfort: "The parent will take the child on her knee and give him a big hug and soothe him." In Beatrice's mind, comforting is reserved for primary attachment figures and grandparental second-generation attachment figures play an important role in supporting synchrony. And again we see how organizing defenses support attachment integration and comfort as opposed to undermining it.

Summary

Beatrice was judged secure-autonomous on the AAI (F_3). She clearly "earned" her security through carefully thinking about her childhood insecurity and disappointments with her parents. Although guilty and depressed in response to her mother's death, psychotherapy appears to have helped Beatrice develop a state of mind that values attachment relationships and forgiveness. She had lost her mother at a young age, but thought she had time for change in her relationship with her father. "I feel cheated. It's not fair to lose two parents at a young age. I may be 40 but I still feel young. It just doesn't seem fair." When asked to think about her childhood she concluded, "I think I've learned the importance of relationships. I'd have to put that on the top of my list."

Beatrice's AAP consistently revealed elements of every form of security and integration we could evaluate using the AAP coding system. Her responses described both children's attachment needs and sensitivity and anticipation that are associated with secure caregiving (George & Solomon, 2008). Her stories were sophisticated, especially developing sensitive caregiving in the context of pretend family play (*Corner*) and creating a hierarchy of instrumental and sensitive family-based care in the family unit described in *Ambulance*. Her AAP clearly echoes her own statements about commitment and the importance of attachment-caregiving relationships.

Susanna

Susanna is 25 years old. She is Caucasian, single, and college-educated. She has three siblings—a younger brother and two younger sisters. Her father worked as a computer professional. Her mother did not work outside the home. Her family moved frequently while she was growing up because of her father's job and she lived in many different North American towns and cities.

Susanna described being close to her parents as a child and says she always felt loved and cared for. She has vivid secure base memories. Her parents were actively involved in supporting her exploration, problem solving, and competence. She fondly recalled when she and her mother practiced swimming lessons, made Halloween costumes despite her mother's lack of expertise as a seamstress, and going out to breakfast together. She appreciated her mother's dedicated help with projects that were beyond her developmental reach, such as organizing a letter-writing campaign to save an old house in their community: "She didn't tell me that it wasn't a big deal."

She described her father as cheerful and fun. She recalled being excited when he took her to the store to select the decorations for a dollhouse he had made especially for her. Although her memories with her father typically included her siblings as well, there were elements in her descriptions that her father had a special connection to her. The fact that her father valued her opinion was important to her, such as a time when she convinced him to let her and her brother try out some challenging athletic activities that he initially thought were beyond their capabilities. Susanna also appreciated her father's patience in answering the questions fueled by her endless curiosity.

Susanna's memories of her parents as a haven of safety were mixed. Her tone when describing attachment situations was emotionally subdued, and her memories of comfort tended to be eclipsed by the details of instrumental parent care. Susanna seemed disappointed that practical safety was accompanied with comfort. For example, one of the only details that Susanna remembered regarding a serious illness that kept her housebound for several weeks was that her mother cancelled the other kids' swimming lessons to stay home with her. In another example, Susann described a big gash on her face that the result of falling off her tricycle, "And I remember going up to my mom and, you know, not wanting her to touch it but at the same time wanting her to take care of it. I think well her first priority was, was calming me down, not necessarily taking care of the wound. You know, it was also done, but the first priority was making sure that I was calm and not screaming."

Her memories of relationship conflict are subdued: "My dad was going to throw a surprise party, so it was my job to keep [Mother] out of the house that day. And I told her she needed to go to the store or something. And she didn't want to go and we had a big deal, it had to happen. And then she found out why. And that night, um, she put me to bed and we just talked for a long time. After she'd been annoyed with me (laughs)." Although she can now consider this event with a sense of humor and recalled how Mother repaired the situation, the quality of Susanna's description of the repair remained subdued. When describing other memories, Susanna sometimes abruptly disconnected feelings potentially related to emotional distress. She recalled a time, for example, when her brother's teasing made her so mad that she retreated to her room. "Which I was never in my room as a kid. I was always out. But I remember staying in my room like almost all day. I remember everyone couldn't figure out why I was up there, what had gone on, but . . ."

Susanna's descriptions of childhood separations from her parents demonstrated knowledge of parental commitment but managing separation distress with muted emotions. She and her brother began to visit her grandparents several times a year beginning in middle childhood. "You know, it was a special trip. It didn't feel like I was not going to see them again. It wasn't anything like that. I knew it was going to be over. It wasn't a big deal. They made sure that I, that we knew when we would see them again. So it was very clear, but it wasn't really a big deal." Her father's extended absences to work away from home, which started around the age of 5, were more difficult than visits to her grandparents. "I don't know how long it was exactly . . . it seemed forever. But even after that the relationship seemed a little distant." She says she wanted to talk to him every night when he was home and remembered getting upset if that wasn't possible.

There was no evidence of threat, loss, or abuse in Susanna's childhood. At the time of the interview, Susanna evaluated her current relationships with her parents with overall positive regard, although we continued to hear in her description of the present the quality of subdued emotional tone that characterized her descriptions of childhood events. She described now feeling close to her parents, a closeness that she evaluated as a reintegration with her parents following a period of adolescent conflict she attributed to personality clashes. She has reconnected with her mother and says they talk frequently. "I can connect to her on, on the mother–daughter level that I consider mature, normal." She doesn't talk as much with her father, but says her relationship with him "has become more equal, our opinions are shared." Her views of her current relationship problems were difficulties with peers, not parents. She proposed that her problems in making peer connections were due to the family's frequent moves during her childhood: "I never felt like we'd stick around."

Susanna was judged secure on the AAP. Her responses to the picture stimuli demonstrated that relationships, especially attachment relationships, are important; every response portrayed interaction in intimate relationships. Attachment figures were present in her stories, and Susanna even created attachment figure characters in stories for which no attachment figures was visibly portrayed in the stimulus picture. Portrayal of self and attachment figures as integrated and goal-corrected was the most prominent content feature in Susanna's stories. The responses also demonstrated that Susanna evaluated her capacity to take constructive action as connected with integrated attachment (i.e., attachment–caregiving as goal-corrected relationships). Story elements associated with attachment security were linked with Susanna's capacity to act in alone stories and constructive functional action in dyadic stories.

Susanna's main organizing defense was deactivation. Transforming attachment distress by interpreting events based on social rules or neutralizing the emotional content in the response permitted Susanna to face her attachment situations and feelings rather than ignore or become completely dysregulated by them. Deactivation did not fully protect Susanna from distress, however. Her stories sometimes revealed negative evaluations of self and feelings of rejection. These are common representational indices in the AAP that emerge when deactivating defenses have not successfully disabled distressing affect and anxiety. Susanna also demonstrated another response pattern that we often observe as associated with deactivating defenses. This pattern is to tell stories in which attachment distress is shifted to the affiliative system. Although Susanna evaluated peers as currently more distressing than parents during her interview, her AAP response pattern demonstrates how Susanna deactivates attachment distress by shifting her attention from the attachment system to the affiliative system.

Cognitive disconnection was also evidenced as an organizing defense in Susanna's AAP. Susanna revealed a range of cognitive disconnection indices, including confusion, worry, and sometimes anger. Her responses indicated also that she managed attachment distress in some situations by withdrawal and emotional withholding.

Overall, Susanna's AAP transcript demonstrated how deactivating and disconnecting organizing defenses supported her fundamental security, the ability to experience and think about attachment relationships and her own attachment distress so as to reintegrate and maintain connections in relationships.

Alone Stories

Susanna's alone responses at first focus on affiliative system problems and shift to attachment problems at the end of the AAP sequence. The characters in the *Window* and *Bench* cannot make connections in the peer relationships, and we see that attachment figures and adults in roles of authority are represented as not helpful.

> ***Window:*** Um . . . I think she's maybe . . . um . . . maybe she's sad, looking out the window. Looks like she wants to be out there. But she can't for some reason. Maybe she's sick or something. (What do you think led up to the scene?) Um . . . um, I think she was doing something inside and then heard other kids playing outside or something drew her attention to the window. (And what do you think might happen next?) She might ask her parents if she can go outside. I think for some reason she can't. (Anything else?) No.

The girl's affiliative system is activated by the sound of kids playing. But an attachment problem prevents her from joining them—she is sick. The girl asks her parents if she can go outside (capacity to act → successful connectedness, attachment system). This attachment connection, however, does not remedy the fact that a connection to peers is not possible (blocked connection, affiliative system).

> ***Bench:*** He looks very unhappy. I think he looks like a kid who maybe got in trouble. Did something he shouldn't, um, so now he's in a time-out. Or some other form of punishment negative evaluation, so he looks very unhappy about being there. (What do you think led up to the scene?) Um . . . maybe he got into a fight with another kid, maybe he hit somebody, and um, he's probably in a schoolyard and his teacher sent him over here. (What is he thinking or feeling?) Um, he's probably thinking that it's totally unfair. (And what do you think might happen next?) Um . . . I think he'll be allowed to get up and he'll probably feel like getting back at the person who told on him, whoever got him in trouble, but he won't because he just got off of being in trouble. (Anything else?) No.

Attachment distress is now exclusively directed to the affiliative system. The kid gets in trouble for fighting and the teacher punishes him with time-out. Her anger at her peers brings out negative feelings of self, to the extent that Susanna sees herself as punished by people who are in roles of authority and who enforce rules. There is no evidence of agency of self or connectedness. Instead of confronting anger, the kid withholds his emotions (cognitive disconnection).

Susanna's responses to the last two alone stimuli demonstrate how deactivating defenses are used to moderate her emotional reactions so that she can think about events (internalized secure base), take initiative for constructive action (capacity to act), and ultimately reintegrate self and relationships.

> ***Cemetery:*** Looks like he's visiting an older relative, a parent or grandparent, someone close to him. (What do you think led up to the scene?) Um, maybe it's the anniversary of their death so he came for the day to be with them. So he probably just does this trip regularly. (What is he thinking or feeling?) He's probably remembering the person, the relationship they had, things they had done together in their life, and he might be a little sad but I think he's come to terms with them. (What do you think might happen next?) I think when he leaves that he'll probably go home. I think maybe in terms of giving some time to this person. (Anything else?) No.

Confronted with loss, the idea of attachment figure death momentarily unnerves Susanna. Stating that one "visits the deceased" or "came to be with them" in the AAP is an indication of dysregulation that indicates a spectral merging between living and dead. Susanna is also confused by the stimulus (disconnection), only vaguely identifying the deceased as an attachment figure (parent or grandparent). The element of the anniversary of the death is a deactivating element that helps regulate emotion by placing it in the context of a socially designated time and place. Similarly, emotionality is deactivated by regularization ("he . . . does this trip regularly"). However, the spectral dysregulation of attachment must be contained in order for Susanna to maintain an organized state of mind. We do not code the connectedness dimension in the *Cemetery* response because of the reality that a living person cannot make a physical connection with a dead person. Proximity to the deceased can only be representational or spiritual. With emotions now subdued and the context of this spectral connection specified, the man can remember their life together. This togetherness, which is synonym for mutuality, permits him to come to terms with the loss. The internalized secure base leads to the capacity for constructive action. The man goes home.

> ***Corner:*** (What's going on in that picture?) Looks like maybe he's pushing someone away or wants to keep them away. Um . . . for some reason he wants to be by himself. Maybe someone's mad at him and he doesn't want to get in trouble so he's trying to stay away or maybe he's sad about something and wants to be alone. (What do you think led up to the scene?) Um . . . probably one of his parents noticed that something was wrong and trying to talk to him and he wasn't ready for it. (And what is he thinking or feeling?) I think he's probably confused, which is probably why he's looking for some time alone, to sort out what he's feeling. (What do you think might happen next?) I think his parent is going to uh . . . sit down with him in the other room and try to talk to him about what's going on and help him out. (Anything else?) No.

The threat portrayed in this stimulus immediately activates self-protective rejection (deactivates attachment to protect the self). While pushing his attachment figures away, the boy feels his anger is wrong and becomes confused by his heightened emotional state (cognitive disconnection). He withdraws (cognitive disconnection). This defensive maneuver establishes the solitude he needs to sort this out (internalized secure base). He can then accept his parents' attempts to help him out. Susanna's current capacity for personal integration and balance fosters her connection with her parents that helps her accept their instrumental support.

Dyadic Stories

The themes of Susanna's responses to the dyadic stimuli all portray attachment figures as present and accessible. Security is again sometimes portrayed in subdued interactive and emotional contexts.

> ***Departure:*** Um, looks like a woman getting ready to leave. And I think the man is not going with her. He's walking up to say goodbye. (And what do you think led up to the scene?) Um, I think probably, they're probably close and he came to the train station to drop her off. (And what are they thinking or feeling?) Um . . . they're feeling sad for her to be leaving. But I think she's coming back, so um . . . I probably think they're worried or . . . (And what do you think

> might happen next?) She'll probably get on her train and be thinking about what's coming up wherever she's going, she's doing, and, um, I think he'll probably drive home thinking about her. (Anything else?) No.

Susanna interprets the scene as a separation goodbye. Her attention focuses predominantly on descriptions of the characters' internal states, and Susanna provides only skimpy background details. The sadness surrounding this separation is heightened by worry, which in the AAP is evidence of confusion and uncertainty (cognitive disconnection). There are defensive deactivation indicators in this story. As in *Corner*, Susanna's confrontation with heightened emotional states serves as the catalyst addressing confusion with integrated attachment without the need to tone down the intensity of the situation. The man thinks about the woman, which is evidence in the dyadic stories of a form of synchrony that is analogous to the internalized secure base elements in Susanna's alone stories. Thinking about the relationship demonstrates the importance of the attachment relationship and helps to restore balance during the separation.

> ***Bed:*** Um, looks like maybe the child is reaching to his mom for a hug. For some reason she doesn't look too ready to reach right now. Maybe she's trying to have a serious discussion about something that's going on. Maybe he's trying to avoid it or trying to . . . trying to make her feel like it's okay if I give him a hug. (What do you think led up to the scene?) Um, he probably did something that day that he wasn't supposed to and she chose this time at bedtime when they were together and had some time to sit down together. I think that she'll, when she feels like she's made her point she'll probably give him a hug and reassure him. (What are they thinking or feeling?) I think he feels scared that his mom might reject him because of the way he's been. But I think she feels um . . . feels like she needs to make a point to help him out. (Anything else?) No.

The attachment and caregiving systems are portrayed as having conflicting goals. In Susanna's story, the boy wants a bedtime hug (attachment signal). The mother wants to have a serious discussion and deactivates the boy's signal by focusing on her caregiving agenda—discussion of the boy's misbehavior (negative evaluation). This story element is defined as evidence of deactivating defenses because diversion to behavior management has been shown to be a common correlate of caregiving rejection (George & Solomon, 2008). Unable to avoid the situation (the boy's attempt to reject the mother's agenda) brings Susanna face to face with negative self-evaluations (more deactivation) and confusion (cognitive disconnection). Her deactivating defenses have not successfully excluded or transformed the threat of maternal rejection and becomes momentarily frightened (dysregulated segregated system).

Secure relationships are not perfect. Susanna's response to the *Bed* stimulus demonstrates that she expects to be rejected when parents interpret her behavior as inappropriate, and these feelings elicit strong attachment insecurity. She knows the relationship will eventually be repaired—the mother eventually responds to the boy's attachment need—however, Susanna continues to be confused as to why parental rejection is so frightening.

> ***Ambulance:*** Um . . . it looks like a grandmother and the grandson are watching someone be taken away, probably one of his parents was sick or injured and so he's probably very worried and she probably is worried too but she needs to look brave for him to reassure him that it will be okay. (What do you think led up to the scene?) Um, probably some sort of accident happened and I think maybe the boy called his grandmother and she came over to be with him. (And what do you think might happen next?) Um . . . she'll probably talk to him about what happened and what's going to happen. She'll probably take him to the hospital to visit his parents. (Anything else?) No.

This story portrays attachment figures as vulnerable and a surrogate attachment figure as an acceptable temporary substitute that keeps attachment organized until contact with attachment figures can be reestablished. The grandmother provides instrumental care—she provides reassurance and information. This form of care, however, does not meet the level of synchrony we evaluate in the AAP as evidence of an integrated and comforting relationship. Susanna's response to physical threat once again emphasizes deactivating its intensity. She portrays the grandmother as needing to be brave (deactivation) in order to be able to care for the boy. We also note that, although not formally integrated into the AAP coding system, the pattern of events in the story plot is one typically found in the stories of children whose secure attachment is organized by deactivating defenses (Solomon, George, & Melamed, 2007; Yamakawa & Takahashi, 2007). The boy called the grandmother to come over and be with him, a form of instrumental agency in which the child takes the initiative to seek attachment figure care. The threat of physical vulnerability is deactivated and relatively unimportant to Susanna. In comparison to separation (*Departure*) and parental rejection (*Bed*), attachment comfort is not required and an integrated reunion with parents (i.e., more than a functional visit) is not needed.

Summary

Susanna's AAI classification was a form of security that is described as "somewhat distanced or restricting of attachment" (F_2). The main feature of her AAI-based security was Susanna's confidence in and value of her relationships with her parents, combined with her thoughtfulness. Susanna's AAI convincingly demonstrated that she was comfortable with her parents, and she described her childhood experiences vividly and with genuine fondness. Her memories emphasized her parents as a secure base and evidenced deficiencies in parental haven of safety (i.e., emotional comfort). Susanna believed that they made conscious efforts to be caring and involved in ways that they did not experience as children and that her experiences as a child made her a caring and trusting person.

Susanna's AAP and AAI demonstrated consistent themes. Confidence in parental caregiving was most evident in her AAP responses to situations in which Susanna envisioned the self alone and in need of attachment care. Susanna's AAP also echoed attachment relationships that were not always satisfying and problems with peers. The deactivating defenses Susanna evidenced in her AAP responses were consistent with the distance and emotional restriction shown during the AAI.

Several features of Susanna's AAP were not clearly evident in her AAI. One was her strong association between representations of integrated agency of self and her confidence in her ability to take constructive action. Both her thoughtful consideration of attachment (internalized secure base) and successful care by attachment figures (haven of safety) fortified her capacity to act. The AAP elucidated the degree to which parental rejection potentially dysregulated her, whereas she denied feelings of rejection in the AAI. The range of attachment situations portrayed in the AAP also helped us understand Susanna's evaluation of different kinds of attachment situations. Being alone and separation (including the separation of loss) were interpreted as very stressful and eliciting the need for relationship reintegration; rejection blocked integration; and threats of physical illness were manageable with basic care.

Fran

Fran, 31 years old, is a college-educated, African American single mother of two young children. Her father worked for a utility company, and her mother held several administrative assistant positions. Although both parents worked, her family was poor. Her parents divorced when she was 3. Her father lived nearby after the divorce. She lived with her mother and maternal grandmother until she was 12 years old, with regular overnight visitations with her father. She unexpectedly moved in with her father when she was 12, which no one explained to her. Fran lived with her father and two younger half-siblings for 6 years. She moved back to her mother's house for 1 year and moved out on her own when she was 19.

Fran described her relationship with mother as emotional. She thought they were close and said she felt loved. She remembered her mother hugging and kissing her and making her feel loved. She remembered her mother holding and comforting her when she cried when she returned home after a visit with her father. She said her mother loved her so much that she would do anything to make Fran happy, for example buying her a bedspread in her favorite color. Sometimes their closeness felt like they were sisters. She felt she could tell her mother anything while she was growing up and she liked the singing duet act that they performed together at family gatherings. Other times she said she felt more like her mother's doll than her daughter and she would run away from her mother when she began primping and tugging at her to make sure she looked just right.

Neither of Fran's parents acted as a secure base or haven of safety. Despite reported feelings of being close to her mother, Fran notably described her as absent. She could not remember any events that her mother was present when Fran needed her. Once when Fran was very sick, she remembered being confined indoors for many days. She stayed by herself when her grandmother left for work and until her mother returned home several hours later. She recalled how hard it was on her because she did not feel well. Fran's viewed her mother's failure to go on school field trips as another indicator of her mother's absence in their relationship. She remembered only one occasion in elementary school when her mother made an effort to come along on an overnight camping trip "because she knew how much this affected me. She wanted to show me that she could be there, so she did." Although Fran interpreted this event as one time her mother showed her that her feelings were important, she noted that her mother left before nightfall and returned the next day only to pick her up.

Fran described her mother and grandmother as strict; they spanked and reacted harshly when she and the other children in the family misbehaved. She remembers one day when she and her cousin got in serious trouble when they played outside after dark. They were so frightened when they returned home that they hid in the house. Her grandmother spanked them with switches and then they got in trouble again with Fran's mother and her aunt. "Three times for that one, it was my fault." She remembered during a family gathering when her mother "grabbed my leg and dug her nails in it and gave me this look like you're not supposed to" in response to Fran's comment that she thought an adult family member was acting foolish. "Immediately I knew that I wasn't supposed to say that, that is was disrespectful."

As a young child, Fran thought her father was magical and full of fun, taking her to the amusement park and on helicopter rides. So moving in with him as a young teenager was at first exciting. After living with him, she realized that he, too, was an absent parent. "He was just never there." She described her father during that time as stern and noncommunicating, and she remembered not understanding why he was so rigid. She was confused by his refusal to let her try on fashion clothing and his tendency to shout at her rather than explaining a situation. She did not think her father was interested in her as an individual, but rather viewed her as his personal source of achievement. "He chose all my classes for me. That's when I realized, he wasn't there. I assumed he'd be like my mother would be, 'What are you going to do?' I realized I didn't know this man."

Fran described her teen years as increasingly difficult because her father could be mean. He seemed to have no regard for her as a person. He would not let her see her mother. He made her pick up a snake even though she was terrified of snakes. She resented his rigid conformity. She said she finally "went crazy" and got herself into all kinds of trouble with curfew, drugs, and sex. She remembered one night that her father locked her out of the house when she returned home. The message was clear—she returned to live with her mother. "I was relieved and confused. I knew what was going on, why it happened, but it seemed really severe and out there. But I was happy to finally be away from him, to be honest."

Fran's separations as a child were visitation with her father until he had her move in with him in at age 12. She didn't see her mother during that time, which was distressing but out of her control. Fran's final childhood separation was moving out of her mother's house at 19. Her mother and grandmother were critical of her lifestyle and wanted to change her. "So I moved out. And that was traumatic, actually."

Several of Fran's family members died, beginning when she was a teenager. Her first loss was a close uncle. She says that she was numb when it happened; that it was like a dream and that she could not face this loss until several years later. Her maternal grandmother died 8 years ago from complications during a routine hospital procedure. Fran said she balanced her memories of her grandmother's strictness by remembering the good things her grandmother said to her before she died that she could use to examine her life. Another uncle died unexpectedly 5 years ago. He had been a part of her life when she lived with her father, and Fran says she took the news pretty hard. More difficult, however, was witnessing her father's pain, something she'd never seen before. Her uncle's death had since been a catalyst of change for her because she saw how it changed her father.

Fran discussed how she has concentrated in her adulthood on redefining her relationships with her parents. She sees her mother daily and is grateful for her mother's help with her education. She says she is trying now to teach her mother more about who she is as an individual, "show my mother what my limits are and try to have her have some respect for my boundaries." Redefining her relationship with her father has been more of a struggle. She felt they reconnected to a point where she could at least talk to him. She talks to her father with some regularity, although not as frequently as she talks with her mother. "I have to keep him at bay. I have to stay on guard with him. So when he starts doing all of his controlling kinds of manipulative kinds of negative talk, I say, 'You don't mean that.' "

Fran was judged secure on the AAP. Her responses demonstrate a mixture of integrated thoughtful agency and attachment–caregiving sensitivity—internalized secure base and synchrony. As is characteristic of most secure AAPs, the integrated elements that evidence security were not observed in every story; however, their pattern was characteristic of her overall responses. We also saw a connection in some responses between integrated relationships and positive action—how Fran's representation of attachment was linked to her capacity to take constructive action.

Fran's main organizing defense was cognitive disconnection. The splintering effect of cognitive disconnection was confused for Fran and often made access to attachment information and affect while telling attachment stories blurry or oblique. Cognitive disconnection also heightened her emotionality when attachment was activated, and Fran still struggles with entangling attachment feelings such as anger, embarrassment, and shame. Her integrated dimensions rebalance her affect, but do not necessarily result in the clarity that she still seeks in understanding the details of her attachment experience.

Evidence of defensive deactivation and attachment dysregulation were rare. Organized mainly by cognitive disconnection defenses, Fran did not seem to need to cool off attachment distress nor was she likely to become overwhelmed by it.

Alone Stories

The alone stories suggest that Fran's secure representation of attachment is maintained by thoughtful consideration of attachment events (internalized secure base) combined with her capacity to take action. The characters must face attachment events on their own. Attachment figures are noticeably absent from her stories. As a result there was no real evidence of Fran's desire or ability to connect to others when distressed. She faced attachment stress alone and drew upon her own resources.

> ***Window:*** Um, this kid is probably sick and um, in the house and would like to go out. I think she's probably sad and um, what happened before, is she probably was laying down and decided to get up and look at what she could be doing outside. (What will happen next?) Um, she'll probably go back and lay down. (Anything else?) No.

Fran's first response to the AAP task is functional but passive. There is no evidence of the desire to be connected in relationship or defensive exclusion. The girl begins the scene sick and alone and ends the same way. The girl's distress is moderated by lying down. Her agency at least takes her away from the distress of not being able to go outside, but does little for the girl's sickness—the main attachment event in this story.

> ***Bench:*** This lady's depressed. Before this she probably was walking around. This must be a lake or something and she probably was just walking around, looking at the water, thinking about what was going on and she decided to sit down and she's probably crying, very depressed and crying. (What will happen next?) I don't know. She may be contemplating jumping in but hopefully she'll allow this time to meditate and get through whatever her problem is and you

know, figure out some way to deal with it. (Anything else?) No, that's it.

The intensity of aloneness in *Bench* confuses and dysregulates Fran. Cognitive disconnection (uncertainty and depression) obscures Fran's ability to specify the contextual details that account for the lady's distress. Fran depicts the bench as a possible place of solitude that provides the lady a context in which to think, even though the nearby lake tempts the lady with suicide ("jumping in"—segregated system). We have found that extreme dysregulating images such as this one in *Bench* is an indicator for attachment trauma, in this case suggesting that Fran's desperation in response to being alone is related to physical or psychological abuse (see Chapter 9). Confidence in the lady's ability to think through this problem (the internalized secure base) reorganizes and rebalances succumbing to depression and fear, although Fran's ability to describe productive agency (i.e., clear capacity to act) is obscured.

> ***Cemetery:*** Okay, this is a guy who is at a cemetery. Um, before this he probably was walking through looking for the gravesite of someone. I assume it's a relative. Um, I guess he's feeling sad, introspective. Maybe not so sad but just thinking about you know, whoever this person is, or death something like that. And um, I think after this he'll probably go away walk, you know, toward his car and go home. (Anything else?) No.

The man at the cemetery deliberately engaged with the theme of death ("looking for the gravesite"). Fran's attention focused on his internal processes (internalized secure base), yet once again cognitive disconnection interfered with her ability to specify other important features of this attachment event. Fran was not able to specify the man's relationship with the deceased (e.g., a relative). Facing the theme of loss head on, however, the man thought about the intensity of this experience. We noted too that, unlike Fran's *Bench* response, the man demonstrated at the end of the story the clear capacity to take constructive action following thinking, one of the hallmark patterns of security in alone stories ("walk toward his car and go home").

> ***Corner:*** I don't like that picture. This looks like a kid who probably is being abused or possibly hit by maybe a parent or a sibling or something. And um, he uh, doesn't want it to happen and is sort of pushing it away. Um, probably before this there must have been

> some sort of argument or maybe he was being scolded or something and um, he ran in to a corner. Um, I think he's feeling probably scared, afraid, and um, sad, embarrassed or something. Ashamed. And, after this, I don't know, I'm hoping that he you know, whoever this is will look at this scene and decide to stop it or turn around and walk away. So, I'm hoping that's what'll happen. I don't know, though, with his hands up it looks like possibly he might get hit. After this um, I think he'll probably feel sad, go to his room.

Fran's attachment system became dysregulated by fears of abuse and disconnected entangling emotions that she is still not able to integrate and understand (ashamed, scolded, embarrassed). At the height of the drama in this story, the best the character can do is try to disconnect from these feelings by hoping that the perpetrator will stop or leave. Themes of abuse are common in the *Corner* story; indeed, as we noted when describing the development of the picture stimuli, the *Corner* picture was added to the stimulus set for this reason. Combined with the suicide theme in Fran's bench story, however, it seems even more likely that Fran's attachment experiences of harsh parents is interpreted as some form of abuse. We noted, though, that Fran disconnected and obscured the identity of the perpetrator, even though the boy gets hit, suggesting that Fran continues to be troubled by the realization attachment figures could be so cruel. The boy's response to the threat of abuse provided evidence of Fran's representation of self as capable of taking action. We saw for the first time in the AAP how deactivation was used for self-protection—the boy tries to push it away (rejection). And in the end, even though the boy was probably hit, he demonstrated the capacity to remove himself from the situation, reorganizing attachment dysregulation by finding safety alone in his room.

Dyadic Stories

The attachment–caregiving responses in Fran's dyadic stories portray adults as confused and caregiving responses as interrupted and defused by false positive emotion. Only the surrogate caregiver in Ambulance was capable of providing comfort and security.

> ***Departure:*** This is a picture of . . . two people waiting for a bus or a train uncertain and um, needing to engage with each other. I think that um, I think that before this, they probably were standing apart from each other sort of just waiting and, um, probably the

guy decided to come and engage in a conversation with the woman. And what I think, oh, how they're feeling? I take it from their hands being in their pockets that, um, they're not necessarily happy, that they might be feeling some sort of sad emotion or introspective type of emotion about why they're leaving or where they're going or what they're doing. And um, what I think will happen next is that a train will come and they'll get in the train and they'll leave. (Anything else?) No.

Fran's first response to a dyadic stimulus was emotion laden and disconnected. It was difficult to determine what this couple is doing or why. *Departure* is the second stimulus in the AAP series, and the stimulus evoked the same quality of passivity evidenced in Fran's response to *Window*. The story theme for *Departure* was waiting, a form of disconnection that renders attachment events as almost endlessly bewildering. Waiting means one must stay in place until something happens—the individual is uncertain, and attachment and caregiving cues become confusing and potentially misunderstood. Waiting slows down one's capacity to remedy negative affect or solve problems. In the end, the only outcome that Fran developed was the couple's capacity to go forward—they get on the train. They were able to do something to move away from the center of their distress. Without other forms of constructive action, the distress lingers and follows them onto the train.

Bed: This is a picture of a mom and a son, it looks like, and it's probably time for the little boy to go to bed. Probably before this the parent was reading a book or telling a bedtime story and, um, it's time for the baby to go to bed and so he wants to embrace his mom for a hug goodnight. I think that, um, I think that they're both feeling really good and you know, a loving connection. I think after this, the boy will go to sleep (deactivation) and the mom will leave. (Anything else?) No.

Fran interprets as a context in which the son's attachment system is activated by the night time separation. Unlike other response, Fran's description of the boy's attachment signal is unambiguous—"he wants to embrace his mom for a hug goodnight." The mother's sensitive response was clearly missing from the story. This type of response typically occurs in the AAP when attachment figures have camouflaged their caregiving insensitivity (i.e., inability to provide sensitive comfort) with illusions of closeness and affection. Fran's response disconnects the mother's response by failing to include it in the story and focuses on themes of love and connectedness in their relationship as a defensive smoke screen that obscures underlying disappointment. In the end, the boy goes to sleep—defensive deactivation that cools down potential realization that his mother's love is an illusion.

> ***Ambulance:*** This picture looks like it's a grandma and probably a little boy. And, um, possibly someone in the neighborhood got sick and the ambulance came to pick them up and the little boy is feeling really sad. Before this he must have heard the ambulance or something and decided to come and see what was going on and became sad and the grandmother must have seen him sitting there and decided to come and kind of console him. And um, he uh, I think he's feeling sad and the grandmother's feeling concerned. I think after this the ambulance will pull away and the two will probably engage in some more conversation and maybe go eat some milk and cookies or something. (Anything else?) No, that's it.

The central element of Fran's response to *Ambulance* was her description of a caring attachment–caregiving relationship—the grandmother noticed the boy's sadness and consoled him. This feature was not evident in any of the other dyadic stories. The consoling theme was clear, and not transformed or obscured by defensive processes. We noticed, however, that the boy's distress was not connected to specific attachment–caregiving relationships in the boy's family. Aside from the grandmother's response, the story was impersonal. The sick character was a person from the neighborhood and someone not likely to be close to the boy. The relationship was not important enough to pursue and the ending was seemingly nice, but superficial.

Summary

Fran's AAI classification was "secure with some preoccupation with the past" (F_4). Fran's parents were insensitive despite the fact that she camouflaged their insensitivity to her childhood attachment needs with false memories of love and closeness (for mother) and fun (for father). Her experiences growing up were entangling, inconsistent, and often emotionally overwhelming. Both of her parents could be mean, although there was nothing in her AAI to suggest that Fran was abused. Her memories of childhood were vivid and often, although not always, thoughtful. Fran could literally "disconnect" (e.g., stop mid-thought) and seemingly jump over details when the descriptions were becoming too intense to handle. Fran appears to have earned her security subsequent to her adolescent rebellion and moving out on her own. The defining feature of her adult attachment security is her reintegration in current parent relationships and how hard she is working to establish a balance that probably was not present in her childhood.

The disconnecting defenses that were evident in Fran's AAP provided even more insight into Fran's mental representation of attachment. Her smoke screens were more evident in the AAP than the AAI, such as covering up her disappointment in caregiver insensitivity with illusions of love in the *Bed* story. The AAP provided a clearer snapshot of the strengths that Fran has developed on her path to earned security. Some responses demonstrate how truly difficult this is for her, based on observations of how attachment distress can only sometimes be faced with passive actions and minimal functional care. The AAP also suggested that her parents' harshness with her, described as strict in the AAI, were more dysregulating than she acknowledged during the interview. The trauma indicator evident in the *Bench* response demonstrated how horrible and frightening parental anger and physical punishment really was for Fran, as suggested by the combination of the *Bench* and *Corner* themes. Two of the alone responses, however, clearly demonstrated how Fran has developed strong integrated agency—the internalized secure base and capacity for action—that is likely her main source of stability as she works on her relationship to parents now as an adult.

Seti

Seti is a 21-year-old college student. He is single and has no children, and is the only child of Indonesian and American parents. Seti's father owns an airport transport business; his mother is a scientist. He spent his childhood in the same urban neighborhood and now lives in a nearby city.

Seti described himself as close to his parents as a child and remembers always wanting to be with them. He described his mother as caring, entertaining, and nurturing, and his memories suggested that she provided him with a haven of safety and secure base. He thought it was "great that his mother was so protective" of him. He recalled that she stayed at preschool as long as he needed if he was upset when she dropped him off. He remembered fond times together, such as his mother picking him up from kindergarten and going home and playing with blocks. When he was older, she cheered him on when he played games at the local arcade. His mother helped him with his homework every night. "When I was a little older, we had history tests and she would just read to me 'cause I would have trouble sometimes, but . . . yeah, she'd just, uh, read to me. She also helped me a lot with math homework, like adding, multiplication, I remember we just started adding . . . so we went off and she helped me like with multiplication and division and everything."

He similarly remembered his father as caring, entertaining, and helpful, also as providing him with a secure base and a haven of safety. He recalled his father as being devoted to fostering Seti's interests. His father was enthusiastic when Seti expressed interest in learning how to play basketball. He took Seti to the local playground courts and they played regularly as he grew up. His father was involved with Seti's care. His mother worked, so Seti woke up early to be with her. But his father stayed and played with him in the morning before taking him to his afternoon kindergarten class. "I was always, like, really scared to go to go to school. I can't think of why, I guess I just was, I didn't want to be left alone without my parents. So he was very helpful, when he'd just, like, you know, walk me up there and just wait till I got comfortable and he'd leave and he'd say, 'I'll be out here, so if you need me, just come out.' And then eventually I'd just get comfortable and then he'd just leave."

As Seti thought more about his fear of separation from his parents, he proposed that this was due to losing them on two occasions at amusement parks. The first incident occurred when he was preschool-age. He actually did not remember the incident, but his parents told him about it. The second incident occurred several years later. He recalled, "I went on like the high ride, and then I got lost. Then I just went to tell someone working there, I'm lost. So I went to the, I don't know, there's some kind of the main center or something, I just waited there. And eventually my parents found me. I remember I still wanted to play. So they said, okay, and I guess they just kept a tighter watch."

Seti viewed these experiences as fortifying his trust in his attachment figures and his personal confidence: "Even though I had so much fear of being alone, I kind of view myself as really confident now. I don't know, just after, other than being lost, like they'd always find me. Even when I feared being alone, being left or abandoned or something, it never happened, so . . . I guess that contributed to knowing that someone would always be there for me, just contributed to my self-esteem. My confidence."

Seti's paternal grandmother and maternal aunt died when he was a child. He had only met them on a few occasions and did not think their deaths influenced him in any way.

Currently, Seti was satisfied with his relationship with his parents. He developed a passion for golf in adolescence, and Seti and his father now enjoyed playing golf together. He visited home a lot of weekends. "I guess it's always been on my terms, but even more so because when I want to be with them, I can, and when I just want to do whatever I want to do, I do that." We noted, too, that his discussion of current relationships with his parents had the quality of self-centered assuredness that characterizes young people in the post-teen stage developmentalists term "emerging adulthood" (Arnett, 2006).

Seti was judged secure on the AAP. His overall response pattern revealed integrated agency, capacity to act, and relationship synchrony. The tone of his responses covered a wider range than demonstrated in our other secure cases. Seti could be confident, tense, and playful. The strongest tension was associated with threat of separation and loss, evidenced by feelings of danger, isolation, and helplessness. The residue of his own experiences of getting lost as a child was prominent in his AAP stories.

Seti's main organizing defense was deactivation. Signs of deactivation appeared in the three responses related to the potential threat of being lost: loss in *Bench*, nighttime parent separation in *Bed*, and being trapped in *Corner*. For Seti, deactivation neutralized tension and/or supported thinking and mastering his fear through achievement.

Seti's responses also had a consistent undercurrent of cognitive disconnection. This was mostly evident in discourse-style forms of confusion (e.g., I don't know). Seti also demonstrated some preoccupation and entangling, and anger.

Seti's responses included stress indicators that are somewhat unusual for secure individuals. His first response brought personal experience into his story, evaluated in the AAP as indications of blurring the self with the hypothetical character. Later during the task, he interrupted his story with a shift in attention that we call a "rule of life." Individuals use a rule of life to explain a situation and shifts attention away from the specific to the general in order to preempt or interrupt affective experience.

Alone Stories

Evidence of the internalized secure base and capacity to act were the main themes of security in Seti's alone stories. Attachment figures were never portrayed as a haven of safety and, with the exception of connection to family in the *Cemetery* story, Seti's responses demonstrated little connectedness and a tendency to deal with or minimize his problems (*Corner*). His stories demonstrated that being alone was stressful and frightening. The tension of the alone self was evidenced in *Window*, and feelings of loss, isolation, and helplessness were confronted in *Bench* and finally mastered in *Corner.*

> ***Window:*** It seems to be a little girl looking outside her window, this could be her house and she could be just thinking what she wants to do for the day. I know sometimes I would just stare out the window and just stare, and she could be thinking, and next she would, I guess, do whatever she was thinking, maybe. (Anything else?) Um, hmm, I would guess that maybe it would be maybe a weekend and she's just thinking. I don't know, sometimes I do my best thinking just staring out, especially out of a window so big. Yeah.

Internalized secure-base thinking is the central feature of this response. A girl at home on the weekend is thinking about what to do. There is little evidence of defense in the story itself, although here is a hint of what we might interpret as nervous disconnection ("I guess"—uncertainty). Seti's stress in response to the girl's aloneness is indicated by telling about his own personal experience while developing the story. This blurring of self and other suggested to us that Seti may not be as nonchalant about being alone at the window as the story line implies.

> ***Bench:*** This looks like someone I guess maybe a woman sulking on a bench. Something, either she is really tired, or something bad must have happened to her and she is thinking. She is just pondering whatever has happened to her and she is just sitting there just thinking about the consequences of what happened to her and what she should do next so, she is not really sure what she wants to do next, that's what she is trying to figure out. (And what led up to it?) Um, well, I guess it could have been some news she heard or yeah. Could have been devastating like, the loss of a loved one and it saddens her and she's contemplating the effects it has on her, so I guess if that is the case she would uh, go to, go back home later and mourn, I guess. (Anything else?) No.

The alone self in this response elicited feelings of being preoccupied and entangled in relationships. The woman was sulking (cognitive disconnection). Seti's emotional heightening and confusion (tired, or something bad happened) about fear (loss of a loved one—segregated system) emerged as the story progressed. Finally, at the end of a descriptive string of disconnected feelings, Seti described addressing attachment distress in terms of the internalized secure base. The long description of thinking that followed demonstrates how defensive exclusion can support balance and integration (not really sure what to do next–disconnection; that's what she's trying to figure out—deactivation). Once contained and balanced, Seti was able to describe the woman's dysregulated state and she now has the capacity to take action. She mourns at home. Once again, we saw the hallmark association between two forms of agency that is more prevalent in secure individuals than individuals in any of the other attachment groups. This is the juxtaposition of the internalized secure based and capacity to act.

> *Cemetery:* There is a man in a cemetery with a, he's particularly fixated on one tombstone and I am assuming that it could be, uh, someone. The tombstone would represent someone that he was very close to, probably the mother or father. Uh, the man is, I guess, he is an older gentleman, certainly not a kid, and he's just paying his respects. This could be some kind of, it could even be his wife. This could be an anniversary of the person who died or it could be a birthday or some special occasion where he is just trying to pay his respects and he is just thinking or reminiscing in his own mind of that person. Seems I guess very sad but just trying to think back to good memories. (And what might happen next?) Um, I would imagine that he would stay there for a while, but when it is all over I guess he'd go back home to maybe his family or what's left of his family and, um, try to get back to life.

The internalized secure base was again the central theme of this story. Seti seemed struck by the intensity of the stimulus (he's particularly fixated) and disconnects. Disconnection obscures his capacity to specify the identity of the deceased attachment figure or why the man was at the cemetery. The man's thinking about the deceased person, however, demonstrated the importance of this relationship, disconnected and heightened a bit by elements of sentimentality (special occasion, reminiscence, good memories). Once again, the internalized secure base theme was followed by the capacity to act, which led the man to reconnect with living attachment figures (what's left of his family).

> *Corner:* This actually looks like a kid who's, uh, wants to mime. He's got, his hands are up in that manner and he's trapped in a box.

> He is practicing his miming techniques. I guess I guess he is showing this to someone, maybe his parents, and it seems fun for him. I guess his parents, I don't know if they support it but, it seems funny to me, to pantomime. (And what might happen next?) Either his parents are going to applaud him and laugh or they are going to tell him to knock it off. Yeah. But I think it's all in good fun, nothing serious. (Anything else?) No.

The picture of a cornered boy potentially dysregulated Seti's attachment system. "Trapped in a box," the boy was isolated and helpless (segregated system). The agency evident in Seti's other alone stories was absent in this response, and Seti managed attachment dysregulation only with defensive exclusion. Potential dysregulating affect was disconnected. The threat was contextualized as pretense (mime) and given a positive spin ("it's all in good fun"—glossing). We also noted that selecting the character to be in the role of a mime literally disconnected speech from action. Communication when one is a mime depends on exaggerated mimicry of behavioral and facial action; that is, the mime disconnects and exaggerates communication cues. The threat theme was also managed with deactivation. The character was described as practicing his technique (achievement) and the situation is not serious (neutralize). Although dysregulation was now effectively blocked, Seti remained confused about the involvement of attachment figures. Were the parents supportive or annoyed? In the end, his own feelings were contained (i.e., reorganized), but he remained confused about attachment figures.

Dyadic Stories

Goal-corrected synchrony was the main theme in Seti's dyadic stories. Seti's representation of attachment figures was generally one of mutuality and sensitivity. However, his *Bed* response demonstrated his concern with failed synchrony in response to separation.

> ***Departure:*** Uh, it appears to be a man and a woman, they could be married, and they have some baggage right next to them. I would think that they would be on their way to some type of vacation. Maybe they could be at the airport. Actually, it could be just one of them going on vacation and, uh, the other one just wishing good luck and saying their goodbyes. So, I guess next the one going on vacation, I guess it kind of looks like the woman's going on vacation because there is more baggage near her. But they are just wishing each other goodbye and she'll be on her way.

This adult attachment–caregiving dyad was initially a bit unsettled and disconnected (wishing, I guess). Once Seti settles on the story, however, he developed the synchrony of mutual goodbyes ("wishing each other goodbye").

> ***Bed:*** This seems to be a mother and a child. Um, her child, that is. They are laying on the bed and, uh, it looks like the child is somewhat young, probably around the age of 5 or less. And it's time for this kid to sleep and, uh, I guess he doesn't want to sleep without his mother. Sometimes kids grow very attached and, uh, they feel like they don't want their parents to leave especially at nighttime when it's all dark, so. But eventually his mother does leave and the kid gets over it and he goes to sleep. (Anything else?) No.

Seti's story of mother–child separation is defensive and there is no evidence of a synchronous goal-corrected partnership. He launched into the story with surprising clarity, as compared with the disconnected beginnings of his other AAP responses. The identities of this dyad was specified, as well as their posture, the child's age, and the time of day. The tension of the imminent separation increases and cognitive disconnection defenses interfered with Seti's ability to complete the response. His uncertainty interrupted what would have been a natural description of the boy's signal to his mother; he instead jumped to a description of the boy's angst about the separation ("he doesn't want to sleep without his mother"). Seti's failure to ascribe meaning to the boy's outstretched arms in this scene was striking in that it is one of the most common elements of most individuals' AAP responses. Disconnected and emotionally heightened, Seti's obliquely acknowledged an attachment signal without actually describing it. Instead, he recited a "rule of life" statement about children at bedtime that interestingly includes all of the attachment elements that Bowlby (1973) defines as natural clues of danger—separation, darkness, being alone. Seti described the situation intellectually, but he was not able to ascribe it to the character. Without a clear signal, the mother's response and the boy's implied distress are disconnected. The mother left the room and the child got over it (disconnected glossing). As with Fran's *Bed* response, the illusion and confusion of ambiguous attachment signal and response were deactivated by sleep, and cognitive disconnection blocked integration of the mother–child relationship when threatened by nighttime separation.

> ***Ambulance:*** Um, there is, this seems to be a I guess a mother and a child. Staring out their window and they see an ambulance where

> somebody's being carried out. This could have been due to some kind of car accident they witnessed. I doubt that the actual incident has to do with the mother and the child. Because they are, I guess, they are not there with them. With the one who's hurt and I guess they just. They are just watching it happen and, uh, I guess they are amazed that it seems to be that the mother is trying to console the child after seeing such something, I guess. It could have been something horrific and, uh, the ambulance is taking the person or possibly just the body away to the hospital and, uh, yeah. (Anything else?) No.

Seti's uncertainty about attachment figures' sensitivity to the separation portrayed in *Bed* was countered in this response. The adult figure in this story was clearly identified as the mother, who successfully provided comfort in response to the tension (disconnection—uncertainty) and fear (segregated systems—amazement, horrific, a body connoting someone has died) the child experiences when life events were shocking and horrific. This mother–child relationship is a synchronous integrated goal-corrected partnership.

Summary

Seti's secure AAI classification had elements of being "somewhat distanced or restricting of attachment" (F_2). He believed that he had a pretty nice life as a child, and most of his belief appeared to be sincere with regard to parents as a secure base for exploration. His childhood haven of safety memories included a mixture of parental presence, care, and inconsistency.

Seti's AAP response pattern, that of integrated and personal agency combined with goal-corrected synchrony, is evidence of his confidence and sturdy security. The AAP also revealed the restricting or distancing elements of attachment through his use of deactivating defenses. Consistent with Seti's AAI evaluations, there is no evidence in the AAP that his parents devalued their relationship, evaluated him negatively, or rejected him. Rather, his attachment tension is clearly centered on the threat of separation, which is evident in a bedtime scenario in the AAP and not confined to worries about getting lost, as he suggested in the AAI. The AAP shows that these childhood separations continue to haunt him, which belies the sturdy self Seti described in the AAI. He remains somewhat overwhelmed and confused about these experiences and his attachment figure's responsiveness.

CONCLUSION

Published investigations in the field of attachment generally support the conclusion that secure attachment is biologically "natural" and the most developmentally adaptive; researchers have been concerned with the conditions that support or hamper its development. The results of meta-analytic studies indicate that secure attachment is overrepresented, with upward of 55% of individuals classified as secure (Bakermans-Kranenburg & van IJzendoorn, 2009). The upshot of this finding for the present discussion is this: Because the goal of integration appears to foster individual differences in secure attachment organization, we must therefore accept that it is impossible and incorrect to define only one "optimal" type of secure attachment. Instead, we need to accept, as has been empirically demonstrated, that there is a range of workable secure organizations. The four cases presented in this chapter represent different contexts in the development of integrated attachment. In their AAP records, the patterns of their story content dimensions all emphasized the importance of attachment relationships. To varying degrees, characters showed agency of self in the form of internalized secure base and haven of safety, and they engage in synchronous, goal-corrected partnerships. It was their shifting position with respect to a basic reference point, defensive exclusion, that defined the differences in their security. From the relatively undefended AAP records of Beatrice and Susanna to the increasing appearance of deactivation (Seti) and cognitive disconnection (Fran) in the AAP records of the other two, we observed a range of defensive operations. Of any kind of defense, however, we may ask, to what extent and how well does it serve an integrative purpose? Seen this way, it is not self-contradictory to speak of defensiveness in the service of genuine attachment integration. In this instance, the individual's basic adaptive and defensive position support attempts to integrate attachment experience, memories, and affect. There are different kinds of effective integration and tolerable defensiveness in secure attachment contexts, expressing themselves accordingly in AAP stories.

From the consideration of Fran and Beatrice, it would also seem unwarranted to expect that secure attachment derives solely from a history of empathic responsiveness of the caregiver to the child's attachment behavior. Against actual attachment-related experiences, we must also allow for the self-generation of new meanings out of the ramifications of the individual's attachment experiences, thereby transforming them and gaining the expansion of the agency of self. Despite compromised attachment histories, Fran and Beatrice were able to inwardly work on the connectedness of their past and present attachment experiences and creatively transform their internal working model of self. The creation of new meaning in both their cases was a transformative experience that extended their sense of agency of self. They were, in other words, able to bootstrap themselves from within.

7

Dismissing Attachment

Minimization, normalization, and neutralization form a deactivation defensive strategy that typifies the dismissing individual. A general emphasis on deactivation inevitably disrupts the integration of attachment experiences and the feelings that accompany them. Although defense by deactivation is an integration-disruptive solution, it does, however, work to purify otherwise negative aspects of the dismissing individual's past caregiving experiences and the self; painful attachment realities and feelings of distress are denied. Then, in addition to accomplishing this purification of their attachment experiences, deactivation supports persistent efforts, through minimization and reversal in idealization, to present their past attachment experiences as normal and supportive. In these respects, dismissing individuals succeed in defensively mastering the breakthrough of attachment distress and are relatively effective in modulating the arousal of their attachment systems, thereby keeping them organized and connected in relationships.

When we focus our attention on dismissing individuals' past attachment experiences, we cannot help but be compelled by their representational use of deactivation to rearrange and transform these less-than-optimal experiences. The childhood prototype of dismissing attachment in adulthood is avoidance characterized by the child's ability to unemotionally turn away from or ignore the attachment figure during reunion in the Strange Situation (Ainsworth et al., 1978; Cassidy et al., 1987–1992; Main & Cassidy, 1988). Avoidant infants also use toys and objects in a weak attempt to redirect their attachment needs to the exploratory system (Ainsworth et al., 1978).

Infant observations in the home, however, indicated that avoidant infants were often upset and not as independent and sturdy as they appeared to be in the laboratory playroom. Avoidant infants were observed to be less settled, communicative, and responsive than secure infants. They cried more, were more upset when their mothers left the room when at home, were less likely to respond positively to being held, did not settle in, and were more likely to retreat when seeking contact (Ainsworth et al., 1978). Ainsworth et al. (1978) observed that avoidant infants were indeed outwardly anxious, and it is noteworthy that they expressed the most anger at home of infants in any of the organized attachment groups, which is in direct contrast to their seemingly non-angry cool laboratory behavior. Other researchers have described avoidant child–parent attachment as characterized by inhibition of interpersonal closeness (including aversion to physical contact), communication, and emotionality (Britner, Marvin, & Pianta, 2005; Isabella & Belsky, 1991; Moss & St-Laurent, 2001; Pederson & Moran, 1995; Solomon, George, & Silverman, 1990; Weinfield, Sroufe, Egeland, & Carlson, 2008).

Deactivating defenses are the foundation of avoidant children's prototypic response to reunion in the Strange Situation and their parents' approach to caregiving (George & Solomon, 2008; Solomon et al., 1995). The avoidant strategy develops in a relationship of mutual rejection of attachment and caregiving (Ainsworth et al., 1978; Solomon et al., 1990) in which parents emphasize "distanced care" and redirect children's attachment needs away from them (George & Solomon, 2008; Solomon & George, 1996). Caregiving distance shifts attention from intimacy, reduces the probability of conflict, and redefines children's needs for closeness and comfort to what these parents deem as the child's basic functional needs (George & Solomon, 2008; Solomon & George, 2008). Basic functional needs typically include physical safety and socialization, especially the emphasis of these parents on the importance of manners, behavior management and intervening in misbehavior, and achievement as a means of getting ahead in life. Parents and children maintain a facade of connectedness that focuses on interaction through objects (e.g., toys) and activities (e.g., field trips, vacations). They monitor children from afar and often give major caregiving responsibilities to parent substitutes, such as nannies or babysitters.

Ainsworth et al. (1978) noted with regard to avoidance, "there seems to be more basic conflict between the kind of comfort and reassurance that they want and are prompted to see, and the fear or at least an avoidance of just that" (p. 131). According to Main (1990), a strategy of avoidance and distance offers the best possibility for the child to satisfy the goal of the attachment system (physical and psychological proximity to attachment figures) when parents are not flexible and cannot provide closeness. Avoidant children respond to their distanced parents with attempts to immobilize attachment and remove attachment distress from conscious awareness. This defensive "switching off" of attachment feelings allows the child to remain near enough to the attachment figure to seek contact if needed, although the threshold of expressed need is higher than that of the secure child. These immobilizing attempts, however, are somewhat ineffective. Deactivation does not completely manage heightened arousal and anger, as evidenced by the behavioral insecurity, separation anxiety and the sadness, hurt, and negative images of self that are associated with relationship distance and rejection (Ainsworth et al., 1978; Dallaire & Weinraub, 2005; Lutz & Hock, 1995; Solomon et al., 1995; Sroufe et al., 2005). And under severe circumstances, deactivation is subject to collapse (see Chapters 5 and 9).

In adulthood, dismissing attachment is evidenced by current states of mind that appear to be cut off from or devalue the importance of attachment experience. In the context of the AAI, responses to questions requiring dismissing individuals to describe their attachment experiences are marked by restricted, unreflective thinking about difficulties related to these experiences (Hesse, 2008; Main et al., 1985). Their thinking about attachment events consists of unrealistically edited or idealized versions of caregiving experiences. As applied to these past experiences, the overarching formulae are simple: It did not happen or it was not painful. Deactivating denial is completed by idealizing reversal; for example, painful childhood experiences with attachment figures are transformed into positive accounts, unsupported by memories. Within the AAI, it appears that dismissing individuals strive for normalcy by editing out attachment events and/or distress from their generalized views of relationships and the self. Unlike the childhood manifestations of the analogous avoidant age groups described above, dismissing adults appear during interview responses to attachment to be better able to prevent affective leakages of attachment and separation anxieties.

The dismissing pattern that has been described is that encountered when deactivation serves as the predominant defensive process used to insulate the individual from the emotional charge of attachment relationships (George & West, 1999; Solomon et al., 1995). It is important to recognize that "dismissal" of attachment through deactivating distress carries no implication that the distress is integrated, only that defensive processes are enlisted to prevent distress from affecting the individual's current consciousness. The inability of dismissing individuals to face the feelings of anger and sadness that accompany disappointments in the relationship with their caregivers leads to detachment from any kind of deep attachment feeling. Their portrayal of themselves as detached, independent, and strong covers a soft-hearted center full of perpetual feelings of longing, sadness, and anger.

There are three common subgroups of dismissing attachment in the AAI (Hesse, 2008; Main, 1995). The first subgroup of dismissing adults (Ds_1) idealizes attachment, prettying-up and sentimentalizing their past. This denial may be carried beyond the point of normalizing past attachment experiences by claims of failure to remember them at all. A second subgroup of dismissing adults (Ds_2) devalue or derogate the importance of attachment relationships in their lives, cultivating instead personal mastery of the surrounding world wherein achievement, self-reliance, and strength figure prominently. Our study of attachment suggests that this derogatory posture is probably better understood in the context of Bowlby's model of pathological mourning than as a normative form of dismissing attachment and we expand on this discussion in Chapter 9. A third and final subgroup of dismissing adults (Ds_3), with the help of strong defensive deactivation, are able to tolerate the awareness of many negative aspects of their lives, including rejection and problems with closeness in parental relationships. It is not unawareness of these attachment problems that distinguishes them but rather their inability to integrate and think about how these experiences influence who they are as adults and their current attachment relationships.

THE CHARACTERISTICS OF DISMISSING ATTACHMENT IN THE AAP

Dismissing attachment in the AAP is evidenced by an individual's reliance on deactivating defense to manage their responses to the attachment stimuli. The indications of a strong deactivating emphasis were described in detail in Chapter 5. Only a few general points will be made here.

The AAP pictures portray major activating elements such that threatening events are easily perceived in the stimuli. We designed the stimuli as attachment activators, a design that is supported by recent fMRI brain activation studies of the AAP (Buchheim, Erk, et al., 2006;

see Chapter 10). Dismissing individuals are then in the position of having to make persistent efforts, through deactivation, to shift attention away from events and feelings that arouse their attachment systems. They strive to develop story lines that deny or shift attention away from the existence of distress; instead, themes that emphasize relationships guided by stereotypical social roles, materialism, authority, or personal achievement are evident. Attachment themes may be displaced to the affiliative (peer) or exploratory system. Sustained deactivation may not always be possible, and distress and painful feelings may well up within the dismissing individual. In such circumstances, the individual will attempt to neutralize or minimize these subjective difficulties. Also, themes of distress are often accompanied by negative evaluations of characters (e.g., the character's distress is the product of undesirable qualities or their actions deserve punishment or rejection by others). Finally, and because of their beliefs about the unproductiveness of attachment, dismissing individuals rarely seek help from attachment figures and are forced to fall back on taking action themselves. The internal attachment resources (e.g., internalized secure base, haven of safety) and attachment figures as external resources that are optimal in reestablishing attachment equilibrium are notably lacking in dismissing AAPs. However, dismissing individuals are characteristically able to portray the self as taking action (e.g., capacity to act; agency) or seeking relationships with attachment figures or others so as to obtain functional care (e.g., connectedness to non-attachment figures, especially friends, and functional synchrony).

The following section describes two cases judged dismissing on the AAP. These cases represent the scope of how deactivation can transform or reduce potential distress. We show how these dismissing response patterns are related in expected ways to their attachment experiences.

DISMISSING CASE EXAMPLES

Daniel

Daniel is 20-year-old college student. He is Caucasian, single, and has no children. He has three siblings—an older brother by 3 years, and a younger brother and sister. Daniel was raised on the farm near a small town. His father was a farmer, and worked in health care at the local hospital and at a local store. His parents owned and managed several rental homes in the area.

Daniel described his childhood relationship with his parents as "really good," and his parents as loving and caring. Childhood was portrayed as fun. Daniel's descriptions of his family life, however, lacked vivid detail. Descriptions of memories of parent interaction were predominantly generic, and Daniel described combined experiences that included his siblings. His memories were rarely personal. The activities he described were situations of "functional togetherness" (George & Solomon, 2008); that is, situations that served to organize attachment and caregiving by maintaining an illusion of security. These situations often focused on basic care, such as Daniel's parents putting a Band-Aid on a scrape or taking him to the doctor. Functional activities were sometimes pleasant and enjoyable, such as hiking together, a trip to an amusement park, or his parents attending a school academic awards ceremony. Daniel's functional interactions with his parents, however, lacked the integrated goal-corrected elements of secure attachment as associated with parent–child mutual enjoyment, synchrony, and emotional attunement.

Daniel's mother did not work outside the home, so she was involved in her children's daily care. Daniel recalled enjoying his mother rocking him and his siblings to sleep when they were little and, when older, listening to her bedtime stories. He was proud of the fact that his mother made sure their lunches were waiting in the school office if forgotten in the morning. His fondest memories were times when his mother played games with him and his siblings. "She would turn everything into a game . . . just make up a game when we had to wait for Dad to come home for dinner wait in the van. We'd play for hours." He recalled that his mother also generated ideas for activities when he and his older brother were bored from hanging around the house: "She'd tell us to go out and build a fort or work in the garden."

Daniel described how he enjoyed spending time with his father on the farm. He remembered riding around on the farm machinery and sitting on his father's lap so he could drive. He spoke of enjoying times when his father spontaneously took his sons out for the day to car shows. "He'd buy us motorcycles or get us started on some new crazy thing. He'd spoil us."

Both of Daniel's parents were involved in their children's daily routines. They tucked the children into bed at night, and on Saturday mornings, "we would run into Mom and Dad's room, jump on their bed, and watch morning cartoons with them."

Daniel's childhood memories emphasized attachment relationships as fostering exploration and learning over attachment. Daniel chose the word "learning" to describe his childhood experiences with his parents: "I don't know how to put it, like learning educational kind of thing, that sums it up." He discussed at length how his mother's stories helped him learn the alphabet and school lessons and how his mother helped her children with their nightly homework. He appreciated how his father taught him the practical things associated with farming. One of his most vivid childhood memories with his father was when his father taught him how to repair a tractor. "We had to rip it all apart and play with the gears and stuff and he taught me how gears worked and, the little and big and the different ratios and stuff, and we fixed it. It all made sense. It was just these big machines that looked too complicated, but once you took off the top and looked inside they really aren't that bad. It was very practical."

Daniel's discussion of his childhood attachment events evaded attachment feelings. He played down upset and endorsed the benefit of his difficulties. He would "suck it up" when he was upset, and upsets did not last long. He said that he sometimes went to his mother to get one of her "magical Band-Aids that would make it all better." As with his other memories, these attachment memories tended to be generic rather than personal. He interpreted illness an opportunity for him and his siblings to "take it for all it was worth," which he equated to his parents bringing them chicken soup. Staying home sick from school was an opportunity to read and watch TV. Parental care equated to them bringing him chicken soup, and he never mentioned parental comfort.

His parents managed misbehavior by spanking, sometimes with a wooden spoon. He remembered getting in trouble a lot when he and brother were young but never described any specific events. What he recalled the most about these situations was his older brother's tough attitude; his brother refused to cry when spanked. He also stressed that knew that he was in big trouble when his father got involved in their punishment and that his father's spankings really hurt.

Daniel remembered two frightening attachment experiences. His description of these experiences demonstrated how deactivating strategies transform serious threat by shifting attention away from the breach in the attachment relationship to a positive outcome. One memory was when Daniel got lost at a car show when he was 5 years old. His discussion failed to acknowledge how frightening it must have been to be lost and any tendency he might have had to express this to his father was deflected by his father's casual reunion. "I went to the stand and said, 'I can't find my dad.' So they took me to a place and said it's okay and they gave me pop and I got to play games and stuff." [Daniel's older cousin picked him up when he heard Daniel's name announced over the intercom.] "They said, is this your kid, and he's like yeah, I'm like his cousin.

So it was fun and then I got a shoulder ride for the rest of the day. Dad was cool with it. He was just said, 'Where'd you go?' "

The second memory was a time when his brother put him in the deep end of a swimming pool. He admitted to being afraid of water as an adult but could not describe any other details about this childhood event (e.g., how old he was, where his parents were at the time, his parents' reaction). His fear was deactivated and transformed into an experience that he evaluated as a contributor to his personal strength as an individual. He also stated that he does not like to jump into a pool but "once I'm in I can swim for miles." Daniel concluded, "I'm not scared to try new things now because of in the past I think that being forced to, like, with Dad he'd always teach us new things or go on adventures with us and, Mom would always have, we'd always have fun kind of thing." This statement suggested Daniel probably had other scary childhood experiences besides the two mentioned and was forced by his parents to carry on.

Daniel's memories of peer experiences (the affiliative system) eclipsed his attachment–caregiving memories. He ascribed his feelings of childhood rejection to his peer group, a problem that he addressed intellectually instead of emotionally. "Once with a group of friends it was different. There was three of us in the group but always two of them that were closer. Triangle theory. At the start I was kind of like, 'oh man, this sucks,' but later on I don't know, it really wasn't that bad because there was a lot of people too."

Daniel described having other attachment figures during his childhood, in addition to his parents. They were adults who led his teen church youth group rather than other adult family members, such as grandparents, aunts, or uncles. His parents held the church youth group at their home every Friday night. "I'd go to the big people and they babied me. I had fun with them because I was the little guy."

When asked to describe experiences of loss, affiliative system losses were more prominent in Daniel's mind than attachment relationship losses. He described a long succession of deaths in high school and the school's script for handling each death. The loss of a college friend a year and a half ago was described as his most difficult loss. He emphasized the inconvenience of the loss because it occurred during the academic finals period and any thinking about the importance of this interpersonal relationship was deactivated and deflected. "It was more nerve-wracking because it happened right in the middle of finals. I had to finish finals and I found out the morning before my last final. I wrote a big essay for half an hour and then I just kind of got up and left and went home. That one was hard. He was a good friend. He was always open to talk to people. We'd have a lot of talks about how things were going. And so it was just a loss of a friend. It made me realize that you don't know when your time is up and you got to live each and you got to be ready to die today. You got to live each day for what it's worth and treasure the little things in life."

Losses of family members seemed to be less prominent or important to Daniels. Just over a year prior to his interview, Daniel's grandfather died several years after a stroke. He felt that his grandfather was inaccessible prior to his death, in part because of his psychological deterioration. In addition, Daniel's father wouldn't let the children visit his grandfather while in the hospital because his father wanted their last memories of their grandfather to be positive memories from childhood. His family had a big party for his grandfather's funeral. "His funeral was more of a celebration. It wasn't dramatic or sad. It was kind of fun."

Daniel did not think there were any changes in his relationship with his parents between childhood and the present. He said that he had never been angry or rebellious against his parents and he was satisfied with their current relationship. "It's pretty much been a secure kind of steady thing the whole time."

Daniel was judged dismissing on the AAP. His response demonstrated evidence of pervasive deactivating defenses that reshaped and depersonalized attachment events and emotions. Deactivation typically appeared in the story themes as related to intellectual activities, personal strength, and the importance of social rules of conduct. Attachment figures were rarely present in Daniel's stories. Rather, Daniel represented a self with the capacity to act in the absence of attachment figures or integrated internalized agency (i.e., no internalized secure base). Attachment distress in the alone stories was transformed to themes of play and fun. The story themes also evidenced how deactivating defenses shifted attachment toward relationships and interaction organized by other behavioral systems. The exploratory system eclipsed attachment needs, and attachment themes were displaced to the affiliative system. The stories revealed, however, how Daniel struggled to manage anger, fear, and the pain of loss, and how defensive deactivation processes managed these emotions so that Daniel's representation of attachment remained organized.

Alone Stories

There were many elements of deactivation in Daniel's responses to the alone stimuli. He generally interpreted attachment events as intellectual and exploratory pursuits, also defused by a glossy veneer of playful fun.

It is only through these maneuvers that the characters in Daniel's stories were capable of demonstrating the capacity to act (i.e., functional agency). Daniel's responses, however, suggested that underlying feelings of anger, negative self-evaluation by parents, and worry about loss challenged his ability to maintain his cool veneer.

> ***Window:*** Ah, I think it just snowed outside and, this is a little kid hoping that school's canceled for the day and after this she might run outside and play in the snow, build snow angels. (Anything else?) She's inside and it's warm. (laughing) No.

Daniel momentarily disconnected from the stimulus (uncertainty, hoping) but immediately deactivated attachment so as to continue his story. He described a kid who, released from by social rules from school-based exploration, was free to play. Any attachment distress she felt by being alone was neutralized by images of the warm indoors. Daniel deflected his attention from the aloneness represented by the stimulus picture by building a story line that demonstrated how the capacity to act fosters activities that keep attachment distress at bay.

> ***Bench:*** Um, hm, I think, for that one it looks like he's sleeping maybe he's fallen asleep on the front porch kind of thing. He's hiding from a water fight. (A water fight?) Don't squirt me, no. (So what might have led up to this?) Um, could be that he was playing, maybe he, it could be that he did something bad too and he's having like a time-out kind of thing. Um, depending how you look at it, I don't know I think he's, I think of having a nap actually, what first comes to mind. After watching the sun go down on the front porch sitting having a nap. (What might happen next?) Um, he'll get up and go to bed.

The intensity of the *Bench* stimulus was more difficult for Daniel to manage, as evidenced by introducing two different story responses. Although he managed the attachment distress in both stories, the themes of these stories are quite different. Daniel's first response was a disconnected awareness of the fear (hiding) generated by anger (water fight). He quickly deactivated his fear; the character was already sleeping and impervious to emotional distress before Daniel described the other elements of the story.

When prompted to say more about this scene, a new deactivation emerged. Daniel momentarily entertained punishment as a story line, although he quickly dismissed the possibility of this story. Punishment themes are coded in the AAP as associated with the negative evaluation of self and others engendered by the distance and lack of real intimacy in avoidant and dismissing attachment relationships. As we have already noted, attachment relationship distance is often maintained by emphasizing themes of misbehavior and behavior management. Violations of intimacy and security are transformed into violations of the rules of social conduct that must be controlled and sometimes punished (George & Solomon, 2008; Solomon et al., 1995). Punishment threatens the attachment bond, no matter how necessary, and the bond is not repaired when the focus is on transgression over attachment. Relationship anger must be neutralized and displaced. Cool disciplinary techniques for which no repair is deemed necessary (e.g., time-out) are preferred to expressing anger or repairing punishment with interpersonal closeness. This process results in a cycle of distance and rejection—unmitigated behavior management strategies promote feelings of rejection and negative self-concept that then perpetuates the cycle of distance in the relationship.

> *Cemetery:* Um this one, I think, ah visiting a grave (laughing) how observant. Um, going to see, making it personal it would be like after Grandpa was buried going out to see his grave. Kind of thing. But it's not a sad time. (What might he be thinking or feeling?) I think he'd be thinking of past experiences with him. What he's learned from the person. What, like, life lessons he's learned. He might also be going through an issue now, and, um, by going to the grave remembering like thinking what would he have done if he were in this issue kind of thing. And, yeah. (What might happen next?) Next. He would . . . get in his car and drive away. I don't know, he's going to leave, he's not going to stay there forever.

Daniel deliberately made his response personal by connecting the gravestone in the stimulus picture to his own grandfather's grave. The character's emotional tone is completely deactivated, however; potential feelings of distress from the loss are transformed into the intellectual pursuit of life lessons. The man's mental activity was self-centered and focused on the past, which bypassed the quality of thinking about the relationship that the AAP coding system would evaluate as the internalized secure base. Daniel once again depicted his capacity to take action when attachment is activated, but his behavior is not based on integrated security. The character got in his car and drove away much as Daniel has set aside his own grandfather's death.

> ***Corner:*** No, don't squirt me. That one is, um, yeah no that one is actually it's kind of playful. In the corner is the idea, but it's not a negative thing I don't think. That one's very much, yeah. Actually, I think of hide and go seek, because when I was little I had this philosophy that if I didn't see the person then they couldn't see me (laughing) so I'd hide in places like the corner when I was a little little kid. (And what might he be thinking or feeling?) Thinking or feeling? Ah he'd be well it would be a game kind of thing, and it would be fun for him. Ah, he would be really quiet, he wouldn't be trying to say anything or moving at all. (And what might happen next?) Well obviously, it's not a good hiding spot. So he's going to get found.

Daniel's response to the *Corner* stimulus was essentially a reenactment of his *Bench* story. He deactivated attachment fear by rejecting it and contextualizing events in fun. The theme of using rejection as a form of self-agency is strong in Daniel's reaction to attachment distress in the alone stories. Daniel was not rattled by the *Corner* stimulus like he was by the *Bench* stimulus. He even deliberately interrupted the story to explain how potential threat was not necessarily interpreted as negative and described his philosophy of hiding. Rejection and fun were attempts to make attachment fears invisible, although he admitted that these strategies are not necessarily successful. Immobilization in this story does not work and the boy was eventually found, suggesting that Daniel does have to face his distress on occasion, as revealed in other responses as anger, fear, and strong feelings of deserving punishment and negative evaluation by others.

Dyadic Stories

Not surprisingly, Daniel's predominant response to stimuli depicting attachment dyads is also to deactivate potential attachment distress. In these stories, we see how attachment was shifted to the affiliative system (i.e., peers). We see also how characters' functional interactions create a false sense of security and love. The *Ambulance* response showed how vulnerable Daniel was to loss of peer relationships loss rather than family-related death.

> ***Departure:*** Um, automatically I thought of hitchhikers (laughing), which is kind of weird. Standing on the side of the road waiting for a ride waiting to go somewhere. But I don't think it's like a bad

> thing, I think it's fun, I think they're traveling and they're having a good time and they're seeing new places and they're going on a grand adventure kind of thing. That's helping them out. It's like an experience that they're never forget kind of thing. (So what might happen next?) Um, they might get a ride, they might walk for a bit, but they're going to come across some new place that's going to be exciting, a new adventure. They're young, they're not too old, they're like, well mid 20s early 30s.

This story turns away from themes of potential attachment synchrony and mutuality by shifting to themes of peers (affiliative system) and traveling (exploratory system). The activities of these young adults were contextualized by North American social stereotype of young people on a hitchhiking adventure (deactivation through stereotyping).

> ***Bed:*** Oh, okay. This little boy's getting tucked in bed by Mom. Kind of thing. Getting ready for a goodnight hug. Um, she'll, next she'll tell a story to him until he falls asleep. (What might they be thinking or feeling?) It would be love, and caring kind of atmosphere, between the two of them. It's very secure. (What might happen next?) Ah she'd, tell the story until he falls asleep.

A mother putting her child to bed is a common response to the *Bed* stimulus. Daniel's would be story of love and care is a sham, however. The boy's outstretched arms are interpreted generically as the dyad "getting ready for a hug." Daniel maintained illusions of security, despite the fact that his story theme deflects attachment to the mother telling the boy a story and the mother never acknowledges or responds to the boy's signal. Mother–child deactivation is mutual: The boy responded reciprocally to the mother's deactivation (telling a story) with deactivation (he goes to sleep).

> ***Ambulance:*** Okay, this one is, um, automatically I think of death. Somebody's died and the ambulance attendant taking him away. The family are there there's Grandma kind of thing, maybe someone's grandma. I can't personally relate to it, though. Like I'd be more looking at it I could see it as a friend. But more specifically it would be like one friend whose mom died, that's who I think of right away. And, watching as they take her out. (What might they be thinking or feeling?) It would be a tremendous loss. Tremendous loss. Pain. What would happen next would be the family would

come together and there would be lots of different people there to support but still they'd feel tremendous loss and pain.

The *Ambulance* stimulus immediately dysregulated the feelings of distress and pain Daniel associates with loss. Although he seemed to know to tell a story about a family death, he explained that he could not relate to that theme and told a story rather of loss of a friend (the affiliative system). Once again, Daniel's attachment distress is displaced to affiliative relationships over the importance over family. At the end of the story, Daniel's description of events became generic. Social rules that guide behavior and decorum at these times cooled down the personalized intensity of loss. As Daniel explained, the survivors were supposed to "feel tremendous loss and pain," acknowledging exactly the feelings that Daniel's sturdy deactivating defenses were keeping at bay.

Daniel's AAI was judged to be in the dismissing subgroup most cut off from conscious evaluation of attachment (Ds_1). The main qualities of his AAI classification were parental idealization and his inability to recall the details of specific attachment events. He avoided the emotional components for those events he did describe, such as when he was lost, when his brother threw him in the pool, and his grandfather's death. We saw distress in the AAI as fun and personal strength in both the AAI and the AAP. As is typical behavior for avoidant children, both Daniel's AAP and AAI demonstrated how the representational attention to the exploratory system deflected attention to attachment. In attachment intervention, this error is termed a "miscue" (Hoffman, Marvin, Cooper, & Powell, 2006; Marvin, Cooper, Hoffman, & Powell, 2002), which in Daniel's case substitutes cues of exploration for attachment need.

Daniel's AAP also demonstrated the extent to which attachment is deflected to the affiliative domain. Daniel discussed peer relationships in the AAI, but it was even clearer in his AAP that peer relationships are elevated to be more prominent and important than parental attachments. The AAP also elicited Daniel's feelings that were not evident in the AAI, feelings of rejection, anger, and negative self-evaluation as deserving punishment. Feelings of fear and pain that were minimized in the AAI were prominent in his AAP, as was the extent to which deactivating defenses characterized how Daniel attempted to block these feelings from conscious awareness.

Contrary to his sturdy dismissing stance in the AAI, Daniel's AAP suggested that his attempts to dismiss and hide from attachment distress were fallible. His AAP stories demonstrated that, at some basic level, his disguise of rejection, negative self-evaluation, and fear, like the boy in *Corner*, was at risk for malfunction and discovery. He was unable to permit himself to address the importance of these emotions and the role of attachment figures and loss in his life. Defensive deactivation organizes and maintains his insecurity and hinders the reintegrative processes he needs to achieve real security. But importantly, Daniel's deactivation of attachment affect and experience help him stay in attachment relationships.

Debora

Debora is 37 years old and Caucasian. She is divorced and has two elementary-school-age children. She has an older brother and younger sister. Debora was born in the United States, but her father's government job took the family to Latin America when she was a child. Her mother stayed home during this time and, with the assistance of household maids, took care of the children. Debora was 5 years old when her family returned to North America. Her father decided to make a career shift and her parents then both worked outside the home while also attending college. Debora's mother worked part-time until she was 8. The family moved again when Debora was a young teenager and her father took an academic position. Her parents divorced when she was 15 years old, but her father had been living part-time in an adjacent state for quite a while prior to their divorce.

Debora remembered "always feeling close" to her parents. She described her early childhood as "comfortable and warm" and she fondly recalled the loving atmosphere of living in South America.

Her potential secure-base memories focused on superficial relationship connections and family activities. She remembered feeling connected to her mother and she described pleasant activities with her. Debora described these times as "peaceful" and how these events typically involved her mother providing the children with delicious food and drink. Debora described her mother as loving, recalling how she scratched Debora's back as fell asleep at bedtime or watched TV. Her mother's actual presence in these memories would best be described as pleasantly distant. Elements of synchrony and interpersonal involvement were absent from Debora's memories. For example, she recalled how her mother sat on the blanket at the beach while her children played in the water. She recalled how her mother set up the Christmas tree and decorations while the children were sleeping. They would come out on Christmas morning and "it would all be just magic."

Debora described her relationship with her father as distant, which she attributed in part to the fact that he traveled quite a bit for his work. She felt, however, that he was mentally distant even when he was physically present. Debora interpreted her father's psychological absence by drawing from her knowledge of gender stereotypes. "We'd go to my mom for things we needed. It was okay for the husband to be out of it. They had their work outside of the home and that was okay then." Their interactions were dictated by her father's preferences and had little to do with her interests. He enjoyed sports and supported Debora's sport activities, even though she personally did not care much for sports. She also described her father as kind and generous. She remembered him splashing around in the water with his kids and reading stories at Christmas time.

Debora had no memories of parental comfort. At best, they provided for her physical care. Debora suggested that her closest connections with her mother were when she was sick. She hated elementary school, so her mother let her stay home sick a lot. Debora said that she took advantage of this time home to catch up on reading, homework, or just stay in bed. Her mother's presence, aside from the fact that her mother stayed home from work on these days, was mentioned only as an aside. "I would get treated in bed and she would bring me lunch or breakfast or dinner."

Debora described longing for emotional care. She said she felt rejected by both parents as a child, although she did not think they realized this because their lives were so busy. Debora lamented her mother's shift to full-time employment: "There was a babysitter that would take care of us. She was a good baby sitter that wasn't—she wasn't there to make snack after and all of this food stuff I guess that's what mothers do." She felt that her father's rejection was accentuated by the fact that he closed himself off in his office to study.

Debora's childhood emotional needs were never met. Debora described becoming upset a lot as a young child and remembered her mother being publicly embarrassed by her tantrums. She screamed at bedtime each night and her parents shut the bedroom door so she "would cry it out and go to sleep." She said that her tantrums diminished to whining as she grew older, recalling whining at her mother's feet while her mother was studying when Debora was 5. Her mother's response was to shoo her away, saying, "Stop your whiner, you're going to break your whiner."

Debora described terrible fights with her brother throughout childhood. She claims that he was verbally abusive and that her only recourse was to fight back physically. But he was bigger and stronger than she was, and she was frightened of him. She said her parents did not know how to deal with the fighting and tried to "erase it" by sending them to their rooms.

By age 7 Debora tried to be stoic, and it seemed that her yearning for parental care was transferred from attachment figures to medical professionals. This was clearly evident in her description of being hospitalized. She described waking up unable to walk on her seventh birthday and, embarrassed to reveal her injury to her family, tried to conceal it. Clearly injured, her parents took her to the doctor. Debora narrated the hospital scene carefully, including describing the surgery that was required to remove a small, sharp object from her knee. Yet her narration never mentioned her parents' involvement. Rather she stated, "I loved being in the hospital. I'm doing everything to try to get back into the hospital so I was there for 2 weeks. I just loved the attention, the idea that you can ring the bell at 3 in the morning and they'd bring you ginger ale, that there were always nurses coming and checking on you and poking you. At one point they were concerned that my parents were abusing me as a child because I was so calm. Once I fell on a rock and cut my head. I remember them rushing me to the hospital and just really concerned and worried. The doctors took them out to investigate if this had been some kind of abuse issue because I was just happy as a clam because I'm back again. So I was thrilled to get to the emergency room anytime I could get there. I got there and I was cut here and I remember once just feigning an injury playing with my crutches and pretending that I couldn't walk to the point where my parents took me to the hospital."

Despite enjoying being in the hospital, Debora still craved her parents' attention and the vehemence of her parents' rejection. She remembered a dramatic scene in middle childhood when her father was working on a school project. "I remember saying something like, if I don't get some attention, I'm going to kill myself. And instead of the reaction which I hoped was 'Oh honey, come here, let me you know,' he said, 'Would you be quiet so I can get my work done.' I was just shocked because in my life they never hit me and suddenly he's after me. I ran into my room, I closed the door and locked myself in and like wow (laughing), this is really not the reaction I was expecting."

By the time Debora was in middle school, she had internalized her parents' rebuff and tried when possible to take care of herself. Debora described her parents as aloof and that they expected her to manage situations on her own. For example, she remembered being so frightened by a bully that she stayed home from school until she felt she could manage the situation herself. She recalled the events of several 2-week summer visits to her grandmother, during which she endured what she called her grandmother's volatile temper and humiliating tirades. "I think my parents' idea was just that she's just that way and you have to just watch yourself when you are around her." When caught stealing out of student lockers in high school, her father was so angry that he wouldn't talk to her. Threatened with school expulsion if she was caught with the other teens involved, she took matters into her own hands. "I pretended like I didn't know them. I walked down the hall. I didn't have friends for the rest of that year."

Debora's only real havens of safety were her aunt and uncle. She visited them every year and said she felt close to them like parents. "I just remember them always being present and they were really helpful."

Debora remembered separations from her parents as being pretty normal. She and her siblings had lots of babysitters. She stopped visiting her volatile grandmother when she realized that "she attacked my sense of self in a way that was really damaging." She described her parents' divorce as her most difficult separation. The announcement that they were divorcing was abrupt. Debora remembered being really angry with her father and yelling at him for several years after the divorce when he visited her. She says that she became her parents' confidante and, by her later teen years, she knew more than she cared to know about their marriage and new relationships.

Debora's first loss was her great-grandmother's death when Debora was 18. More recently (in her 30s), her grandfather and her aunt also died. She has never been to a funeral. She says that she feels bad for the people who died, but has little else to say about the experience.

Debora was judged dismissing on the AAP. The attachment content in her stories demonstrated representations of the self's capacity to act when alone but no evidence of internalized security. Alone stories were devoid of attachment figures and the themes of these stories shifted attention from attachment to peers (i.e., affiliative system). Her stories demonstrated a desire for connectedness in attachment and other relationships that was never achieved. Attachment dyads were never described in synchronous goal-corrected relationships in her dyadic stories—attachment relationships were neither sensitive nor capable of mutual enjoyment.

Debora's deactivating strategies were mainly evidenced by themes of personal strength, rejection, social roles, and negative evaluation of self. There were also undercurrents of defensive cognitive disconnection in Debora's stories, which demonstrated an undercurrent of confusion, ambivalence, and entanglement. Debora risked intense emotional arousal several times during the interview, as evidenced by literally disconnecting and breaking off descriptions of events or feelings. The AAP demonstrated that she could become momentarily overwhelmed and frightened by loss. Deactivation emerged as the main organizing defense that fosters the agency she needs to keep these feelings under control and move forward.

Interestingly, although deactivated, Debora was unable to maintain self–other boundaries for the entire AAP. Anxious, her *Corner* response is interrupted with descriptions of her son's experience, deflecting her attention temporarily from her own feelings.

Alone Stories

Debora's stories revealed a profound sense of aloneness. The majority of the alone stories suggest that Debora was generally unable to acknowledge problems with attachment figures and her feelings tended to be deflected to affiliative system problems. She could not portray connection to others when alone. Her one story that included an attachment figure character revealed hidden feelings of emptiness and loss. Debora managed her aloneness with deactivation, and deactivation was present in each of her alone responses. It appeared that deactivation served to deflect Debora's attention away from feelings of anger and preoccupation. This deflection managed distress to the extent that Debora could portray characters as capable of taking the action needed to solve problems in the absence of assistance from others.

> ***Window:*** She is looking outside. It looks like something might be stuck in the tree, I don't know maybe that is just the tree. Um, it looks like she just wants to go outside and play. Um, and maybe she is by herself in the house, and maybe she can't go outside. So, she is not able to go outside and play, but she wants to. Um, or she might be shy and not want to go outside, but, then she might decide that she wants to do, just get up the courage to go outside and open the door, go outside and play with, see if the people outside want to play with her. (What do you think led up to the scene?) Um, perhaps she was watching TV or playing in her room. Or it could even be in the morning and she might have just have gotten up a little while ago. (What do you think she is thinking or feeling?) I think she is trying to decide whether she wants to go outside or not. She is, something seems to be holding her back. (What might happen next?) Um, I think that she will get up the courage to go out there.

The character's (note that the character was not named) attachment system was activated by her desire to go outside. The story implied that connection to peers will assuage her tension, yet her desire for such a connection was never clearly achieved. This suggested that Debra cannot envision herself in meaningful relationships or interactions with others. The first elements of Debora's response evidenced arousal and defensive disconnection; she cannot settle on the story events. The character is described as entangled ("she might be shy") to such an extent that she becomes confused by contradictory feelings ("go outside or not"). We noted then that Debora had to interrupt her storytelling, a form of cognitive disconnection that indicates the need to abruptly break away from the growing intensity of the situation to prevent becoming overwhelmed. Debora also revealed that relevant information about attachment was being withheld ("something seems to be holding her back"). Deactivation was Debora's resolution to this mixture of confusion and heightened emotion, and once deactivated by an appeal to personal strength ("courage"), the character had the agency needed to take constructive action (opens the door and goes outside).

> ***Bench:*** It looks like maybe a teenage girl. Or a little bit older girl. Um, she is crying from sadness about something. It looks like she is in a public place on a bench. (What do you think led up to the scene?) She broke up with her boyfriend (laughs). (And what is going to happen next?) She will get over it (laughs). She might be sad for a while.

The *Bench* story described the sadness of a peer relationship breakup. The relationship connection is severed. The girl retreated to a bench in a public place. This is interpreted in the AAP as contextualizing attachment to follow the social rules that dictate emotional control over intense emotion in public. Once deactivated, Debora disconnected from the situation by glossing over the importance of the relationship ("she will get over it"). Debora's representation of attachment in the context of a severed relationship shows no evidence of the capacity for personal agency or repaired connectedness.

> ***Cemetery:*** Um, he is looking at the tombstone. It looks like a very unkempt, not well-kept cemetery. And maybe this is, maybe he hasn't come for some time. And this gravestone has toppled over. So it might be somebody who is a relative that died a couple of years ago. Maybe his father, who died a long time ago. And he hasn't had contact, I mean you know, maybe the father died and he didn't, um,

have contact with him. (What is the character thinking or feeling?) Probably feeling sad, or a little bit ambivalent. Like here I am, all these years we didn't have contact. And then you died I felt a hole. Here your grave is all uncared for. I feel, I think he feels ambivalent, but a little bit like he should try to do something for that, for the grave in the future so that it is better kept. (What do you think might happen next?) I think he will find out what he can do to help maintain the grave.

The character (again not clearly identified) came to his father's grave after many years of distance when his father was alive. Debora's overarching approach to this stimulus was to interpret the scene through the lens of deactivation. The superficial theme of the story centers on the unkempt grave. The problem of loss becomes the question of how to fix the external difficulties ("he should try to do something . . . for the grave in the future") produced by the enduring distance in their attachment–caregiving relationship. Deactivation, however, was not successful in managing the character's sadness, and disconnected relationship ambivalence heightened and surrounded the character's awareness of the loss. Organized defensive control became dysregulated and, in a spectral state as if his father is present, the man blurted out the emptiness left behind ("then you died I felt a hole") from their deteriorated relationship ("Here your grave is all uncared for"). Longing for a proper relationship, attachment was reorganized by the personal agency needed to at least maintain the superficial elements of their relationship ("he will find out what he can do to help maintain the grave"). The relationship in real life can never be regained when someone dies. However, Debora demonstrated her ability go forward without having to think about that relationship very deeply.

Corner: I don't want to play anymore. Stop throwing that ball at me. Maybe it is an older sibling or sister that is being difficult. Or a friend perhaps, saying stop, stop! The child, the antagonist is not stopping. He is just doesn't understand the word no. What is going to happen next is that the boy will get out of the line of fire and find an adult to come help. I have tried all of my words and they are not working (laughs). (What do you think the character is thinking or feeling?) He is probably thinking I am so sick of playing with this friend who doesn't seem to understand the word no. Every time we play we have the same problem (laughs). It is very autobiographical, not for me, but for my son (laughs). He has got a friend like that.

The theme of this story is the unsatisfying cycle of rejection and distance in relationships, once again focused on problems in the affiliative rather than the attachment domain. In this response, Debora's agency was represented as rejection. Pushing others away and telling them to stop are actions are self-protective actions ("I don't want to play anymore"; "stop throwing that ball at me"; "stop, stop!"). Rejection is also an attempt to block awareness of the intensity of distress. Debora, however, was also confused, as evidenced by her inability to specify the actual source of peer conflict and her inability to understand why the friend does not understand her clear signals. We noted that the story implied that adults could be a haven of safety for peer conflict, but Debora was not able to specify who those adults might be. So in actuality, the adults were not really available and peers wouldn't listen. Deactivating defenses maintain moving forward, but are not successful in fixing the situation or modulating the intensity of distress peers create.

Dyadic Stories

Debora's dyadic story themes describe failed synchrony, interrupted and misinterpreted attachment signals, and functional activities that shifted family members' attention away from themes of intimacy. We note that Debora was relatively unable to deactivate attachment distress in response to the dyadic stimuli. She had more difficulty interpreting these scenes than the alone stimuli, and cognitive disconnecting defenses typically resulted in confusion about relationships and events in response to these stimuli where potential attachment figures were visibly present.

> ***Departure:*** They have their hands in their pockets. Maybe they have had a little bit of a . . . One of them is going to be going away. Maybe the woman because she is next to all of the luggage. And since they have their hands in their pockets it doesn't look like they're not wanting to touch each other. So maybe, you know, this is a goodbye forever. (Laughs) Um, but, what led up to it. Maybe they are ending their relationship, they are going to their car, she is going on a plane. (What do you think the characters are thinking or feeling?) Um, probably a little bit of sadness. Maybe what happens next is that he drives off and she goes off on the plane.

The *Departure* described a permanent relationship breakup. There was no illusion or attempt at synchrony or togetherness. The tension portrayed by the position of the characters' hands immediately captured

Debora's attention, but she quickly disconnected the thoughts generated by their posture ("Maybe they have had a little bit of a . . ." [breaks off thought]). This defensive maneuver suggested that she was confused and could become overwhelmed by the nature of this couple's problem and did not wish to address it. The remainder of the story described the couple's departure—a functional goodbye that was defined as having no capacity for repair ("a goodbye forever").

> *Bed:* She has got slippers on, so it is either nighttime or morning. Um, maybe it is in the morning and there is a little voice good morning mommy, come give me a hug. What led up to it, the little boy had a bad dream. Maybe it's not the morning, maybe it is the middle of the night. And maybe afterwards she is going to comfort him.

Debora was confused by this stimulus. Cognitive disconnecting defenses were revealed by Debora's inability to stay with a theme and the choppiness of the story line. The child's signal and the mother's attachment reply are disconnected by events and time. She is first confused as to the context ("nighttime or morning"). Settling on morning, she described the boy's "little" attachment signal to his mother, asking for a hug. Not able to describe the mother's response, Debora suddenly shifted the theme to a nighttime bad dream. She interrupted her description of potential immediate comfort with a discussion that explains her confusion (cognitive disconnection). Even though the mother's comfort emerges as the final event in the story, the AAP story reveals how the misinterpretation of signals and context prevents this dyad from achieving attachment synchrony.

> *Ambulance:* It looks like that is a grandmother with the boy. It could be a girl, too. They are watching as Grandfather is taken in the ambulance. He is very sick, the neighbor, if he is still alive. Maybe he is dead, because you don't really see. It looks like he is covered. If he were dead they would be much, look like they would have a different kind of body position. Maybe the person is being taken to the hospital and maybe it has happened before. So, it's not, so they are not as surprised at having this person go into the hospital. They are just watching out the window. Somebody they don't know. Because if they knew the person, you would think that they would go out there with them. So maybe they are just watching from their apartment window, while the person next door is going to the hospital. And it is kind of sad, but since it is not someone

> that is that close to them. What is going to happen next, they will probably talk about some stuff, someone had to go to the hospital. Maybe go talk to the other people left in the house next door.

The *Ambulance* story described a grandmother and her grandchild watching from their apartment window as an unknown neighbor is taken to the hospital. Debora immediately deactivated and distanced the family characters from the emergency. The character on the stretcher is first identified as the grandfather, but his identity smoothly shifted without clarification to become an unknown neighbor (i.e., demoted identity, deactivation). Debra is momentarily dysregulated by the intensity of this scene. Thoughts of death frightened and confused her, and she disconnected her thoughts in the same abrupt manner that we have observed in other stories ("Maybe he is dead, because you don't really see" [breaks off thought]). The remaining elements deactivate the situation into a series of functional events. This has happened before, so the dyad is not surprised (neutralize). Synchrony and comfort are not necessary because nobody is upset and the grandmother and boy engage in functional behavior ("talk to the other people left in the house").

Debora was judged dismissing with restricted feeling on the AAI (Ds_3). There was clear evidence of lack of closeness with and rejection by attachment figures during the interview. She seemed to have little or no insight as to the source of her continued longing for attention from her parents both during childhood and now in adulthood. Her feelings of hurt, failed intimacy, fear, and rejection were often rationalized. Her father's distance was sometimes contextualized in male gender roles. Her parents' inability to address sibling conflict was ascribed to their youth, as they were only in their 20s when the children were born. Yet her memories of her parents' rejection and distance did not undermine her general endorsement of her childhood as warm and comfortable.

Debora's AAP revealed a level of confusion and preoccupation with attachment that Debora kept under control in her AAI. The AAP *Departure* story revealed her continuing inability to think about her parents' divorce and how she continued to be confused by the circumstances surrounding their announcement that the relationship was breaking up. She described in her AAI how her current relationship with her father was irritating. The *Cemetery* story in the AAP suggested that her view of this relationship goes beyond her statements of angry annoyance. She clearly felt she has lost this relationship with her father, as if he had died. She described in the AAI how her father is always correcting and trying to change how she runs her life and takes care of her children. Her

AAP *Cemetery* story demonstrated how truly debilitating her father's criticism has been and her commitment nevertheless to trying to find a way to maintain a superficial relationship with him. The AAP *Bed* story reveals how confused Debora still is about her relationship with her mother. The intensity of their failed synchrony in the *Bed* story gives more meaning to Debora's statement in the AAI about her mother's care. "We're still working on the mothering thing . . . she'll tend to want to take care of too much and then I sort of let her because I want to be the daughter." Debora struggled between still wanting her mother's comfort, as in *Bed*, and "needing to be the responsible adult."

In the AAI, Debora attributed her adult personality to her parents' inability to face and resolve conflict. This theme was evidenced clearly in the *Corner* story, both by describing a recurring story and her inability to specify attachment figures as a haven of safety. Her current representation of self in attachment, however, seems to go beyond her parents' failure to manage her childhood sibling conflict. The AAP evaluation demonstrated the pervasive influence of parental rejection in the context of confusing and difficult family life events. Throughout the AAP, we saw that Debora's preferred mode of operation, in spite of her continued longings, was to be responsible, take action, and distance herself from attachment intimacy and emotional arousal. We also saw how quickly and consistently her superficial strength could become undermined by disconnected currents of confusion and preoccupation. The AAP demonstrated the degree to which individuals who are plagued by restriction of feeling in dismissing relationships are really quite confused by their attachment relationships. Deactivation turns Debora's attention away from confusion, cools down her emotional response, and, like Daniel, keeps her involved in attachment relationships.

CONCLUSION

According to the attachment rationale of dismissing attachment, we have observed the following dynamic configuration in the cases of Daniel and Debora: Painful attachment conditions in which their attachment figures were unwilling to respond to or satisfy their attachment needs resulted in the attempt to "switch off" the attachment system through defensive processes that deactivate from conscious attachment-related desire and affect. On the side of the denied, therefore, we have seen in their AAP records how they avoided or ignored direct expressions of attachment in their story lines. Only brief and abortive breakthroughs of attachment distress occurred in their stories, and from these they quickly retreated into defense by deactivation. Perhaps because of their beliefs in the unproductiveness of attachment, story characters were portrayed as having to fall back on taking action themselves. What was notably absent in their stories was evidence of internal and external resources (internalized secure base and haven of safety) that are optimal in reestablishing the attachment equilibrium required for security.

Also noteworthy in the AAP stories of dismissing individuals is the deemphasis on attachment relationships. It seems that persons who rely heavily on defense by deactivation direct their desire for connectedness to affiliation and sexual relationships. For example, in Debora's *Bench* story problems occur in a romantic relationship with a boyfriend. In extreme form, dismissing individuals stories are devoid of relationships altogether: the girl in Daniel's *Window* story is described as involved in her own activity.

The unproductiveness of attachment relationships for dismissing individuals is clearly evidence in the evaluations of synchrony. Descriptions of sensitive, reciprocal interactions are typically absent in their dyadic stories. This was indeed characteristic of Daniel's and Debora's *Bed* stories, in which there were no indications of sensitive and timely responsiveness from the attachment figure.

Finally, a generalized emphasis on deactivation means that successive modifications and recategorization of old affective categories cannot occur (see Chapters 2 and 5). Despite the costs that interfere with the development of fully flexible goal-corrected partnerships, dismissing relationships are organized, and all of the deactivation operations make it possible for them to mute their attachment distress and maintain connectedness in their relationships. In this respect, we may encounter some instability rather than failure of deactivation in their AAP records, with sufficient resiliency to effect fairly good recovery from the breakthrough of attachment distress.

8

Preoccupied Attachment

Cognitive disconnection underscores the relentless uncertainty and ambivalence that pervades the preoccupied individual's (cf. Ainsworth et al.'s [1978] ambivalent pattern for children) state of mind with regard to attachment. As described in Chapter 5, underlying the process of cognitive disconnection is the separation of attachment experience and the accompanying feelings from their sources of arousal and distress. Cognitive disconnection can be so disruptive that individuals with a preoccupied state of mind are completely unable to integrate attachment experience, memory, and affect. Instead, they continually "worry the wound," turning again and again to the details of their attachment experience or how they are feeling in a futile effort to achieve felt security and an integrated self.

According to Bowlby (1973, 1980), the childhood experiences of preoccupied adults were marked by confusion and contradiction, which in turn generated strong feelings of anxiety and ambivalence. If the experience of dismissing individuals was consistent caregiver rejection of attachment signals, then we may say that the experience of preoccupied individuals was inconsistent caregiver responsiveness to attachment signals. The childhood prototype of preoccupied adult attachment is ambivalent resistance, characterized on reunion in the Strange Situation by strong separation protest juxtaposed with the inability to be soothed and comforted by the attachment figure. Unlike the smooth turning away observed in avoidant infants, Ainsworth et al. (1978) noted that the behavior of ambivalent-resistant infants is a contradictory mixture of contact seeking and resistance. Some infants are passive; others are angry, sometimes to the point of throwing a temper tantrum; still others redirect their attachment behavior to the stranger. In childhood, this group is characterized in the Strange Situation by exaggerated separation protest (i.e., exaggerated for their age group), intimacy, and immaturity that is often displayed as coy or cute "notice me" behavior (Cassidy et al., 1987–1992; Main & Cassidy, 1988). The ambivalent quality of older children's responses to the attachment figure is often evident in jerky or uncomfortable cycles of proximity seeking and movement away from the parent (Main & Cassidy, 1988). Unlike the attempts to divert attention to the exploratory system observed in avoidant infants and children, children in this group appear to be so thoroughly upset by attachment distress that it undermines their ability to explore and play, especially in infancy. Attempts to play often seem frantic or incoherent because their attention darts among objects or play themes (Pederson & Moran, 1995; Solomon et al., 1995).

Observations of ambivalent-resistant infants in the home confirmed the contradictory behavior patterns observed in the laboratory. Ambivalent-resistant infants were conflicted about close physical contact with their attachment figures. Ainsworth et al.'s (1978) observations also showed that the infants' worry about their mothers' availability inhibited secure-base behavior (exploration). They described also how mothers' attempts to engage their babies in exploration activated attachment distress, resulting in their anxious need for reassurance. It is noteworthy that ambivalent-resistant babies were neither as angry at home as they were in the laboratory nor as angry as avoidant infants observed at home. Other researchers have described the ambivalent-resistant children and their parents as characterized by dependency (sometimes to the extent of appearing helpless); exaggerated needs for personal closeness; lack of personal agency (i.e., not competent, cannot explore); impatience; unnecessary calling attention to the self; emotion regulation problems (especially anxiety and depression); intense and unpredictable emotional fluctuation (e.g., conflict–harmony, attuned–nonattuned); and confused signaling (e.g., parents engaged in resentful intimacy or tickling while disciplining the child; Britner et al., 2005; Cassidy & Berlin, 1994; Moss & St-Laurent, 2001; Pederson & Moran, 1995; Solomon et al., 1990; Sroufe et al., 2005; Weinfield et al., 2008).

Disconnecting defenses are the foundation of the ambivalent-resistant relationship (George & Solomon, 2008; Solomon et al., 1995). Cognitive disconnection exclusion patterns develop in a relationship in which a complex mixture of ambiguity and outright rejection heightens worry about caregiver accessibility and sensitivity, which in turn intensifies anxiety and chronic need (Bowlby, 1973; George & Solomon, 2008).[1] Ainsworth et al. (1978) suggested that the anxiety in ambivalent-resistant relationships "lies in the discrepancy between what they want and what they expect to receive" (p. 131). When organized by disconnecting defenses, a strategy of maintaining physical closeness in order to achieve care and protection is preferable to distance and separation (Main, 1990).

The core of this pattern is the wish to restore positive affect, an outcome posited by researchers as central to maintaining emotional regulation and mental health (Tronick, 1989). Intimacy and physical closeness is the almost unilateral path associated with positive affect in these dyads. In this regard, George and Solomon (2008) described how the parents of ambivalent-resistant children emphasized in their caregiving descriptions how much they enjoy cuddling with their children as well as their efforts to nurture intimacy so as to circumvent distress and anger. They described being confused by distress and anger that leaked into their relationship in spite of their efforts. Unlike the mothers of avoidant children, cognitive disconnection did not transform affect and memory to prevent their awareness of the emotions they were working so hard to cover up. Confused by their simultaneous awareness of negative and positive affect and experiences with their child, they expressed the importance of turning away from the relationship because being a parent had become a burden (George & Solomon, 2008). Turning away, however, felt like a separation to these mothers, and the frustration of

[1] The terms used to describe attachment processes are important in that they provide us with insight into the meaning of different attachment-based mechanisms. We differentiate in our work between the terms "heightened" and "hyperactivation" of attachment. Some attachment theorists define the processes in the ambivalent-resistant/preoccupied attachment group as hyperactivation, also often paired with the term "hypervigilant." The prefix "hyper" means to be above normal, beyond that which is thought to be minimally healthy. The use of the prefix "hyper" as associated with ambivalent-resistant/preoccupied attachment originated in studies that only focused on three attachment groups. In comparison with flexibility (secure) or deactivation (avoidant/dismissing), describing the underlying processes of this group as hyperactivation may have seemed appropriate (e.g., Kobak & Madsen, 2008). We have described in this book and other papers, however, how deactivation and cognitive disconnection are organizing defenses. As such, cognitive disconnection supports the goal and function of the attachment system. We reserve the terms hyperactivation and hypervigilance to describe the processes associated with fear that dysregulates and disorganizes attachment (Solomon & George, 2011a, Chapter 9).

maintaining closeness became a source of worry and guilt about their accessibility and availability to their child.

Preoccupied adult attachment is the group conceived as analogous to the ambivalent-resistant child attachment. These adults cannot free themselves from a preoccupying enmeshment with past attachment relationships and, while attachment topics are open for discussion, these individuals are entangled in worrisome and annoying rumination. Bowlby (1973) posited that the experience of extended unpredictable and highly conflicting interaction and emotions contributes to the development of multiple confusing and incompatible models of self and other. The preoccupied adult pattern, therefore, belies a marked lack of unity in the underlying representation of attachment experience and affect. Cognitive disconnection interferes with the capacity to integrate or deactivate the positive and negative spectrum of emotions normally associated with attachment closeness and disappointment. This fosters preoccupation with affect over experience, especially negative affect that is associated with chronic sadness, depression, worry, and anxiety (George & Solomon, 2008; West & George, 2002).

Consequently, preoccupied individuals must literally disconnect from attachment or they are at risk of becoming overwhelmed and frightened. The disconnection is incomplete, however, and leaves the individual unsettled and continually shifting back and forth between positive and negative emotions and evaluations of attachment. We would expect, and do indeed find, that attachment distress and intimacy needs often appear to others as a unilateral self-focus in relationships.

We interpret the lengthy AAI descriptions (violating the quantity maxim), wandering tangentially off topic (violating the relation maxim), and a plethora of run-on, entangled, and vague thoughts (violating the manner maxim; Main, 1995) of the preoccupied individual in terms of disconnected defenses. This incoherent quality of preoccupied AAIs is different from the incoherence exhibited in the AAIs of dismissing adults. The preoccupied AAI transcript is laden with contradictory elements and unneeded detail. Despite the detail, it has the quality of a mental void. Preoccupied individuals fall into two AAI subgroups: One subgroup is notably passive (E_1), while the other subgroup continues to be angry with parents (E_2) (Hesse, 2008; Main, 1995).

We have argued that defensive exclusion by cognitive disconnection is the unifying construct that explains the thinking patterns of these two somewhat different AAI preoccupied subgroups (George & West, 2004). In the passive pattern, disconnection keeps the individual distracted from the wish for continuing overinvolvement with attachment.

Although distracted, the passive individual remains entangled in attachment relationships because disconnection disrupts integration. Disconnection is less effective in sorting out negative emotion in the angry pattern. The person's confusion is punctuated by one or more strong, interruptive angry descriptions of attachment figure injustice. Some preoccupied individuals may also adopt a pseudo-intellectual facade during the interview in an attempt to portray to themselves and others that they have achieved a grounded, integrated understanding of unsatisfying attachment experiences.

THE CHARACTERISTICS OF PREOCCUPIED ATTACHMENT IN THE AAP

When defense by cognitive disconnection is pervasive and rigid, preoccupied individuals find it impossible, either from deficiencies in external experience, internal organizational capacities, or both, to integrate conflicting and opposing representations of self, attachment figures, and relationships. Cognitive disconnection creates confusion at many levels in the AAP responses of preoccupied individuals. The prototypic indications of defense by cognitive disconnection are most of all found in conspicuous uncertainty and contradiction. Disconnection fractures integration, and negative emotions well up in their stories, especially entangling emotions such as anger, frustration, and guilt. Unable to tolerate the intensity of sadness, unhappiness, and loneliness in their stories, they will often strive to disconnect and shift away from negativity to describe situations with syrupy sentimentality, nostalgia, or develop a sugarcoating story ending (see *glossing*, Chapter 5) in the absence of evidence of attachment sensitivity and mutuality (i.e., internalized secure base, haven of safety, goal-corrected synchrony, see Chapter 4). Some individuals circumvent distress by literally disconnecting from their tension and abruptly stop speaking midsentence.

Confusion also creates the need to pay attention to small stimulus details that presumably would provide clarity where clarity is lacking. Preoccupied individuals are at risk of becoming consumed with the details of the stimulus drawing. The details are carefully analyzed to get the information needed to complete the storytelling task, including information about the characters' emotions. Under the dominating influence of cognitive disconnection, the prototypic approach of preoccupied individuals to the AAP task is to split attachment information into multiple images or storylines. Story themes often take two opposing directions in which one situation is evaluated as good, the other as bad; or story characters are described in terms of positive and negative characteristics (the first story is happy, the second sad). In the final analysis, uncertainty is evidenced when the individual is unable to make decisions about the story line or events, when they second-guess their ability to tell a story, or when there is evidence that they are mentally preoccupied with affect. Although common, disconnection does not always result in fractured (i.e., lack of clarity about a single theme) or opposing themes. It is not unusual for story lines to only focus on pleasant events or affect, especially in response to *Bed*, which potentially portrays parent–child intimacy (disconnected negative affect is momentarily out of conscious awareness).

The AAPs of preoccupied individuals demonstrate a diminished sense of agency of self. When faced with attachment distress alone, self-agency is extended and strengthened in secure and dismissing individuals by representational integration or deactivation transformation, respectively. Although preoccupied individuals may on occasion integrate or deactivate attachment distress, disconnection fractures their capacity to think or take constructive action. Characters in the alone stories do not enter and actively explore their internal working models of attachment (no internalized secure base). They do not consistently use attachment relationships for support or exploration (no haven of safety and no secure base). The self characters are portrayed as incapable or only minimally capable of removing the self from the source of the attachment distress. For example, the character in *Bench* may simply *get up*; this action only minimally regulates attachment distress because the individual has not demonstrated the capacity to productively move away from its source.

The ability to portray integrated attachment–caregiving relationships or connectedness to others in meaningful relationships is undermined by the preoccupied individual's representational confusion and polarization. While positive emotional appraisals in stories can (e.g., happy, sentimental) generate representations of satisfying relationships themes, this is more difficult for preoccupied individuals to describe when emotions are appraised as negative. Satisfying relationship themes are more likely in response to dyadic than alone stimuli. The overarching representation of the self character in response to the alone stimuli is the loneliness of facing distress in the absence of connectedness to other human beings. If connectedness is described, specification of other characters in the story is typically blurred (e.g., someone, person), which is an indication of lingering tension. Characters are typically portrayed as engaged in functional synchrony; mutuality is interrupted or not possible because of an acknowledged problem in the relationship (e.g., the child in *Bed* must signal the mother several times before she responds). When story themes describe characters as distressed, it is difficult for preoccupied individuals to develop stories that displace attachment distress away from the self and seek solace in an attachment relationship, or any other relationship, because they often perceive people as the source of negative affect.

It is important to note, however, that in this sea of confusion and contradiction, preoccupied individuals can sometimes describe thoughtful agency (internalized secure base), successful and satisfactory connectedness to attachment figures, or genuine sensitivity and mutual enjoyment in the attachment–caregiving relationship. We are reminded that the childhood experiences of preoccupied individuals were not pervasively marked by attachment figure rejection, but rather by an ambiguous constellation of caregiver comfort, rejection, interrupted care, and passivity (Ainsworth et al., 1978; Cassidy & Berlin, 1994; George & Solomon, 1999, 2008). In short, these individuals did on occasion have their attachment needs met.

In what follows, we consider the AAIs and AAP responses of two preoccupied individuals. Their responses are good examples of how reliance on cognitive disconnection splits, confuses, and heightens attachment distress and dissatisfaction to the extent that preoccupied individuals are distressed but also have developed a murky or sentimental smoke screen that helps keep them in attachment relationships in spite of their distress. We also show how these preoccupied response patterns are related in expected ways to the attachment experiences recounted in their AAIs.

PREOCCUPIED CASE EXAMPLES

Paige

Paige is a 57-year-old Caucasian mother with two adult children. She and her first husband divorced when her children were young, and Paige raised them as a single parent. She was the youngest of five children and always felt that she was the "tagalong" child because all of her brothers and sisters were quite a bit older. The family moved frequently because her father purchased and renovated farms. The family would live in a home for only a year or two before they sold the property and moved on. Her mother was educated to be a teacher, although she did not work outside the home. Paige's paternal grandmother lived with their family until her death when Paige was 5. Paige's parents lived into their 80s and died within the last decade. Paige has remarried.

Paige's descriptions of family life suggested little interaction between Paige and her parents, allowing that she had to be clever to capture her parents' attention. She remembered reading at the dinner table because there were no conversations. Paige was dissatisfied with the pervasive message at home that expressing emotions was unacceptable. "There was a tradition in my family, pretend that emotions did not exist if possible. If they happened to appear, you got rid of them as soon as possible." This memory is countered, however, by the fact that her parents argued a lot and there was also a lot of parent shouting and fighting with her siblings.

Paige described her mother as a sweet woman, and she respected and admired her mother's public generosity and community involvement. She was impressed that her mother always knew the right thing to say. Yet her mother's savvy also frustrated Paige. For example, Paige said she tried hard to give her mother birthday gifts that would "make her more excited. She'd be polite and say thank you. And it would really hurt when I found out that she never used the gift." Her descriptions of their relationship dwelled on her mother's emotional void; her mother did not like emotions—she was neither happy nor angry, she neither laughed nor cried. Paige was critical of what she called her mother's dishonesty; she said could never trust her mother. Her mother expected family members to pretend that all was "nice and beautiful, regardless of what we were really feeling." Paige wanted emotional communication, but her mother would only discuss events. There were "no deep sharing of feelings, she was very uncomfortable hearing my feelings. I wanted her to know what my life was even if she disapproved of it."

Paige emphasized that she felt closer to and trusted her father because, although he was moody, she believed his emotions were at least genuine. Sometimes he was fun. He father liked to laugh and hug. He did fun activities with his children, such as skating or playing ball in the backyard. Paige could not recall being involved in these activities, though, because she was too young to play. She remembered watching from the sidelines. Sometimes she felt he could be totally unreasonable. For example, on one occasion, he insisted that she help him with chores, but he really didn't need her and she sat around with nothing to do. Paige thought he was too authoritarian and critical of her mother and her siblings, but glad that she had her father's approval. Sometimes he was very angry. "I think he even slapped my face for something and that was okay with me. At least I knew where he stood . . . I'm sure my mother felt like slapping me and didn't, and that was less acceptable to me." But

Paige was simultaneously grumpy about the fact that her father would never apologize.

Neither of Paige's parents provided her with a safe haven or secure base. Frightened by thunderstorms, she remembered running to her father during storms, but she has no memory of how he responded. "I must have learned somewhere along the way don't bother telling Dad if you're afraid." She said that her older sister was upset when her parents fought and assumed Paige was upset as well. When she was a young child, her sister would take Paige outdoors and read to her to get away from their fights. As soon as she was old enough to read alone, Paige used to read to "hide" from their fighting. When she was really upset, she rocked "furiously" in her rocking chair. Paige never told her parents when she was upset, and her parents never noticed. She said that her mother would talk with her when she had personal upsets (e.g., problems with friends), but Paige viewed these talks as long, unhelpful lectures.

When asked about hurt or illness, Paige only recalled bits and pieces of these events. Her memories suggested that her parents' responses were passive or they minimally managed these situations. "I fell down our basement stairs once, but I don't remember it. I remember being told about falling down and having a crack on my head, but I don't remember the . . . I suppose Mother would be the one who would be around when I did . . . I never asked." Her family did not like sickness. "I learned not to be sick, like it was never rewarded. If something happened that wasn't supposed to happen, you got over it as fast as possible." She remembered once needing to have her appendix out. "I remember having to prove that I was really sick because you would just hope it would be better tomorrow, so I don't imagine being rushed to the hospital." She considered her parents' response to her hospitalization as minimal. "Nobody was reading to me for hours or fussing over me. That was not part of our family culture."

Paige circumvented acknowledging separation distress. She identified her hospitalization as a major separation but did not associate this separation with distress for her parents. Rather, she said she did not like the hospital because she was afraid of the possibility of needing surgery. The issue of surgery had never come up in their family because there were never conversations about illness. To Paige, surgery was a frightening unknown. She was not separated from her parents again until high school, when she worked away from home for a summer. To Paige, being physically separated from her parents was not an issue; however, the degree of psychological separation she felt was huge. She discussed at length how she always had felt psychologically removed from her family.

She said she never had identified with her family; she was not like the rest of them. But she was also confused about why she felt this way.

It was striking that Paige's first response to loss was not to describe death, but to discuss loss of trust—presumably the loss of trust in her mother. In terms of deaths, the earliest death was the loss of her grandmother when Paige was 5. She complained that there was no closure regarding her grandmother's death. Her parents told her that she couldn't see her grandmother anymore and her mother decided Paige was too young to attend the funeral. She had to spend the day with a neighbor whom she "hated." In Paige's eyes, her grandmother had just disappeared, and her death was a "total mystery." She groused that she had wanted a photograph of the funeral or to visit the grave, but that her family's lack of sentimentality prevented this.

One of Paige's older brothers was declared missing in action during a war when Paige was still a young child. She said that she was struck at the sight of her father crying, tears that she attributed to regret from having fought so much with her brother when he was alive.

Paige's parents died when she was a middle-age adult. She stated, "You had time to grieve one and then a few years later the other, to get as comfortable as you ever get with an ending." She said that she didn't visit their graves for several years because it was the memorial service and not the grave that was important to her. She worked hard to get what she called "closure" about their deaths because she was not supported in getting closure in childhood. Paige described how she got closure around death when her own father died. She gave her children the choice of attending her father's funeral, in direct response to her own mother blocking access to her grandmother's funeral. For Paige, then, closure was defined by the actions related to the events surrounding the loss, not the emotions; however, her description was marked with some sentimentality.

When asked to discuss abuse or trauma, Paige's response shifted from childhood to her own experiences as a parent. She immediately responded that she was disappointed by the birth for her first child: "I was gypped because I didn't have any pain." Later in the discussion, Paige described what she considered traumatic in her own childhood. Her discussion eventually circled back to the incident when her father slapped her. At this point in the discussion, she called his action a "physical assault"—a descriptive tone that was quite different than her description of this event earlier in the interview. Her description, however, did not have the quality of being assaulted. "He probably just did it once. And I don't remember crying, I just remember being surprised." She said her parents' regular fighting was traumatic as well; the fights had been going on forever without ending or resolution. She spent her childhood "waiting for the next one to happen, sort of, when one happened probably puzzled like I don't understand what happened and I don't know when it might happen again, but sort of probably resigned to it."

As an adult, Paige indicated that she had demanded changes in the family culture around emotions and death. Most of all, she wanted honest communication with her mother. She said that she insisted on honesty with her mother, even though her insistence had made her mother uncomfortable and other family members told her to back off. She wanted a "friendship" relationship with her mother that was not threatened by disagreement or disapproval. She had achieved equal emotional sharing with her mother, the single quality in their relationship that Paige had longed for since childhood. When this occurred, Paige said that she began to trust others for the first time in her life. Paige stated that another change in the family's emotional culture was her decision to go "overboard" to be connected and show emotions. She consciously decided to be close with her own children, giving them the physical closeness she did not have as a child. She said she breast-fed her children "until they were bored with it."

Paige was judged preoccupied on the AAP. In general, we see how a reliance on cognitive disconnection eventuates in fragmentation of context, ideas, and verbalizations. As a result, reinterpretations of her responses are common along with response sequences that are diffuse, confusing, and entangling. Disconnected preoccupation with the self interfered with Paige's ability to maintain self–other boundaries during the AAP task, as evidenced by her overarching need to shift the focus to her own life in the majority of her responses. Agency of self, connectedness to others, and integrated synchrony were strikingly absent from Paige's transcript. In adult relationships, friendships are substituted for attachment relationships. She tries to coat her story deficiencies with a thin veneer of positive affects and outcomes. In this way, she skips over the integrated work that needs to be done; the goal is positive outcome, not resolution and integration. In the face of potential dysregulation, she falls back on a shallow confidence that things will work out in life, a stance of preoccupied individuals that gives them a false sense of their ability to make change. Only traces of clear self-protective agency in response to dysregulating anger are evident in her stories, although this protection is often undermined and ineffective.

Alone Stories

Paige's responses to the alone pictures typify disconnected passivity. Her attention is so dominated by affect that other story elements are blurred. She has trouble identifying the self characters, which are at best described as a person and sometimes only as "he" or "she." This confusion is partly due to Paige's inability to stay on task. In two responses, her preoccupation with self when attachment is activated distracts her to such an extent that she describes the personal experiences aroused by the picture stimulus. These personal intrusions create even more confusion about the elements of the hypothetical story. Story events are prototypically disconnected, as evidenced by themes of uncertainty and relationship entanglement, anger, and fear (i.e., disconnected segregated systems).

Paige's stories lack agency of self, with the exception of an act of self-protection described in the *Corner* story. Her stories also lack connectedness to others, attachment figures or otherwise. This is striking, given how sad her characters are when alone. Paige never clearly manages the characters' distress. Her story endings consistently refer to going "back," a state of mind that indicates in the AAP the absence of representational or behavioral change. Rather, the endings trick the self and the listener into believing that her life is going forward. It is obvious from these stories, however, that Paige has no clear idea about how or why this might occur.

> ***Window:*** That reminds me of a scene that [one of Paige's children] told me happened that I don't remember but she said this day that, that, um, she was at the neighbor's with me was a very rainy, um, gray day, that, I don't know I just think we might have been looking out the window. She didn't want to be there, I probably didn't want to be there, so we might have been looking out the window. Wishing we were somewhere else. (So what do you think is happening in this scene?) I think she's, she would rather, she's turned her back on whatever's in her house, she's looking outside and she's alone too. There's nobody with her so she's probably feeling quite alone. (What might happen next?) She's probably going to wait for the first opportunity to change her situation—and go back out, go run away from home, whichever, whichever the situation is she's going to try to create something else at the first opportunity.

The first attachment stimulus activates such intense personal distress that Paige cannot focus on telling a hypothetical story. It is also noteworthy here how Paige had not actually been aware of her daughter's distress at the time, which was marked enough for her daughter to remember it and later tell her mother, a common pattern when representation is defined by cognitive disconnection. The interviewer's prompt refocused Paige's attention to the picture stimulus. The character has turned away from ("turned her back on") something and needs to escape from traumatic feelings of being afraid that are somehow associated with being in this house ("run away from home"). The emotional intensity associated with these events interferes with her ability to define the self (described only as "she") or the context of the story. Without agency and having turned away from connectedness to others, Paige seems to know that real change is not possible, as demonstrated by her use of the term "back" at the end of her story. Paige does manage to pull the story together by using a defensive trick: the conviction of being able to make changes ("create something else at the first opportunity") contains and organizes Paige's distress, even though it is clear that she does not understand how the process of change is accomplished.

> ***Bench:*** It reminds me of my youngest daughter, she's very very very introspective—you know, it's too um . . . you see, I would think that person is sad but, when I'm sad . . . being an extrovert, I would probably put myself in the middle of people, instead of covering my eyes and—and being sadness. Um . . . (What do you think led up to that scene?) Something happened unacceptable, and, uh, and of course I always think about the relationship, issue, there was some relationship that that's going . . . either someone's died or left or . . . got angry or something went wrong in the relationship, 'cause those are the things that matter to me . . . (So what might happen next?) So he'll feel sadness and then figure out, um, sadness, desperation, aloneness, and then make some choices . . . But, not too soon because it's important to, ah, to be like that, sad for a time, you know so that's important—choices.

Again, distracted by her personal sadness of being alone, Paige only returns to the hypothetical story when prompted by the interviewer although she continues to have difficulty staying on task. Her response again centers on emotions, including traumatic levels of segregated helplessness ("desperation," "died"), about which there was no confusion. Uncertain about the precise precipitating event ("Something happened unacceptable"). Paige's anxiety is potentially dysregulating, and her descriptive statements become muddled before she continues with her story. Disconnected (cut off in midsentence: "relationship that's going . . . ") and confused, Paige lists a range of event possibilities ("died," "left," "angry," "something went wrong"), the feelings about which ("sad," "desperate," "alone") first have to be figured out before coming to a resolution of the story line, one of which is frightening separation ("died"). Similar to her *Window* story, the absence of agency and the failed connectedness to others (someone left the relationship), force Paige into another sleight-of-hand ending in which the character will somehow make choices.

> ***Cemetery:*** I guess somebody's lost someone, if it was a parent there, they might have a wife with them. That's old-fashioned graveyard. It's probably the parent, but that really is technical. This person's probably thinking about life and death and if there are any regrets that, they're thinking they are grateful. (What do you think might happen next?) Hopefully that person has a family to go back to, and hopefully they'll share some of what they've learned about life and death.

Interestingly, personal distress does not sidetrack Paige's response to the *Cemetery* picture. The self character is obscure, only identified indirectly by referencing another relationship ("they might have a wife"). The deceased is, however, identified as a parent, which is an unusual and meaningful specification for Paige. Although disconnecting processes interfere with real thinking (i.e., internalized secure-base agency) Paige's response does suggest some understanding of the importance of unspecified internal processes in working through the entangling feelings (regret) of this situation. However, similar to her *Window* and *Bench* stories, nothing about the self and attachment changes. This is indicated by the description of going "back"; the learning about life and death has the quality of a self-help book missive instead of genuine integrated understanding.

> ***Corner:*** The person is crying, oh, are they going to be hit? Why would they put their hands up they're backed into a corner. I guess they're trying to protect themselves from something, so somebody's angry at them, that kind of thing, but it's kind of like they're defending themselves instead of fighting back, they're not kicking and scratching and screaming. (What do you think might happen next?) I don't know, be a victim of something most likely because I don't see them fighting to get away. (What are they thinking or feeling?) For Heaven's sakes, fight back. (What do you think the child is thinking or feeling?) I think he's feeling defenseless and, um, powerless and he's given up. He won't even try to scratch his way out.

Again, feelings dominate Paige's response in this story. Dysregulated by traumatic helplessness ("backed into a corner" and "powerless") in response to an angry, physical threat ("hit"), Paige's first response is self-protective agency (capacity to act). This action reorganizes Paige's representation of attachment by containing her fear and preventing total dysregulation. But Paige also is aware that there is no recourse in this situation because of the character's helplessness. The character was forced to disconnect (give in). Finally, frustrated and dysregulated by the character's passivity, Paige jumps into the picture to demand that the person (her terrified self) fight back.

Dyadic Stories

Paige's responses to potential attachment dyads create situations that describe functional friendship and togetherness without integrated synchrony. Similar to the alone stories, her responses are all emotionally toned. While characters and events are somewhat better specified, key elements of the stories are often neglected or relatively diffuse in quality. Unlike the false reliance on self observed in her alone responses, Paige's representations of dyadic relationships are somewhat more satisfying.

> ***Departure:*** Um, he's leaving. What's he got . . . another suitcase? (It's up to you.) Um . . . well, a man and a woman, um, I don't know who's saying goodbye to who. I think they might both be, getting on the train, but each with separate luggage—so they might just be people who met on the platform and are waiting for the same train. (What are the characters thinking or feeling?) Well, when I first looked at it I thought that maybe it was a sad parting, but now I don't believe it is, there might not be, there might not be very much going on between them. (So what would happen next?) They would just both get on the train and travel together, maybe develop a friendship. Maybe just share the journey and talk to people. When I travel, lots of people . . ., it does look separate, I know (laughs). Well, that does look like a suitcase on the side or something.

Uncomfortable and confused by separation ("he's leaving," "who's saying goodbye to who"), Paige disconnected from the negative emotions associated with this theme and shifted to a theme with a more positive valence; strangers who happen to be waiting for the same train (disconnected uncertainty) develop a friendship. This relationship, in which attachment is redefined as a potential friend, is marked by physical proximity in the absence of mutuality ("talk to people"). Anxious about separation, seen in the abrupt but incomplete shift back to her own personal experience and stating "it does look separate," Paige maintains a false sense of mutual enjoyment and relatedness.

> ***Bed:*** Oh, that just reminds me of grandchildren always so delighted to see you. My friend has twins, they're adorable, but she also has the two girls. But it looks like people, uh, it looks like mother is just eager to greeting the day, eager to get out of bed, and get on with things. (So what might happen next?) Um, they get into the bed and have breakfast together, and go play in the backyard. Or maybe just have a hug first. Um, and then get to something.

The immediate self-focus observed in the alone responses is evident in her response to the *Bed* picture, but now she moves into telling the hypothetical story without a prompt. Paige again attempts to portray the synchrony of mutual enjoyment. On first reading, the story may appear to be very nice. It is not until one tries to figure out the details that the goal of creating positive affect is splintered by the disconnected and vague elements in this story. We know there are two people in this story (referred to as "they"), but why is the specification of the child character missing? Why is the mother described as eager to greet the day, but not the child? If the characters "have a hug," why doesn't Paige describe the hug in response to the obvious signal portrayed in the drawing? Why was the idea of a hug thrown in at the end of the story as an element of uncertainty? And why is the hug described so passively ("have a hug") rather than as an active form of mutual interaction (e.g., they hug each other, the mother hugs him)? Paige's efforts are fractured, and she is clearly confused about what elements in relationships contribute to positive synchrony.

> ***Ambulance:*** So is that a grandma and a child and something happens to the parent, because that would be significant that would be the stereotype for an older person. So, you know I don't know which person it is, um, but what would concern me about the picture, I would want those people to be right there in the ambulance with the person, whoever that may be. Um, more directly. (What do you think led up to this scene?) I think someone, oh I suppose it could be carrying someone out of the house, so there could have been someone ill in the house like grandfather, and they called the ambulance and they watched. Yeah, I guess that could be it, could be a grandfather or uncle, anyway a family member. The ambulance has come

to the house. (What are the characters thinking or feeling?) Um, puzzled, surprised, afraid of what's going to happen, and the fact that I want to be there, inside the ambulance. I'm trying to think of . . . (What do you think might happen next?) Um, well, there could be an arrival at the hospital when there could be, the anxiety level. And the person could come through this one, it could be death or a long illness, or a short illness. But I would want to know the strongest feelings, I would want to be there and be the first to hear. I don't want to be sitting at home waiting for the phone to ring.

Paige again shows in this story how confusing ("puzzled"), entangling ("anxiety"), and frightening ("surprised," "afraid") separation is for her as well as the centrality of emotions in defining attachment events ("I would want to know the strongest feelings, I would want to be there . . . I don't want to be sitting at home waiting for the phone to ring"). Although she is able to identify the woman and child in the picture stimulus ("grandmother," "child"), she is not able to identify the character who is going away (parent, grandfather, uncle, generic family member). By the end of the story, Paige is still confused about the nature of the precipitating event ("death," "long illness," "short illness"). Her anxiety is evidenced as well by disconnecting from storytelling and abruptly stopping midsentence while describing the characters' inner world ("I'm trying to think of . . ." [breaks off thought]). Paige seems to understand that functional behavior can help manage distress ("they called the ambulance") and keep her from becoming dysregulated by anxiety and fear. Functional care, however, only involves getting care for the patient; the caregiver never responds to the child's need. Once again, passive togetherness ("they watched)" replaced caregiving comfort.

Paige's AAI was judged as passive-preoccupied (E_1). The main qualities of her AAI classification were endless passive discussions that lacked specificity and detail. She was confused about some events, and memories were vague and incomplete. For example, she became confused about the nature of her parents' involvement in punishment and expressed puzzlement as to why she had difficulty remembering. "I was about to get my first spanking . . . and I can't remember which one it was, but the other one intervened. I remember someone was about to spank and I don't know what for, and the other parent said no. Isn't that funny I don't remember which one it was." She also sometimes cut off or shifted her attention away from the question's topic, thereby disconnecting from potential discomfort and anxiety.

Paige was grumpy and critical of her parents without becoming overtly angry. She vacillated between not being able to describe and not being able to understand major events in her life, such as her hospitalization and the effects of her parents' fighting. Longing for emotional honesty, Paige was in fact dishonest about her experience and seemed not to realize the wealth of the contradictions in her interview. One major contradiction was sloughing off her father's slap in the face, yet labeling it later as assault. Still another was circling around descriptions of her parents' fighting as just confusing and unpredictable, yet labeling their fights later as traumatic.

Paige's AAP was consistent with her AAI in that it also demonstrated the importance she placed on emotion in attachment relationships. Emotions were the only clear elements identified in her AAP stories. The AAP also evidenced Paige's desire for a peer relationship with her mother, which culminated in her adulthood as friendship. Friendship was the theme of the *Departure* story, the stimulus that portrays the attachment–caregiving dyad in adult partners. It should be noted that attachment–caregiving relationships defined as friendship is an important characteristic of the ambivalent-resistant/preoccupied state of mind (George & Solomon, 2008).

The AAP also permits us to understand more clearly some events in her AAI that were ill defined or circumvented during the interview. Paige diverted her discussion of trauma during the AAI to expressing her disappointment with her own childbirth experiences. The AAP provided clear evidence that Paige believed she did experience trauma during her childhood, and that it was associated with anger and being hit. Furthermore, in contrast to Paige's feisty proposal that she demanded and executed relationship changes in her life, the AAP demonstrated that Paige has no personal agency and little confidence in self and attachment figures in her inner world. The AAP showed that the changes Paige attributed to herself are in fact a disconnected defensive smoke screen that projects images of false agency and positivity. This cognitive disconnection seems to protect her from becoming overwhelmed by the intensity of her feelings and becoming dysregulated, which would otherwise have led to an unresolved classification (see Chapter 9).

Adam

Adam is a 27-year-old Chinese American male. He is a college student and engaged to be married. Adam has one older brother. The family lived in several locations during his childhood, and his father frequently traveled and stayed away from home for long periods of time. His parents separated at one point during his childhood and finally divorced when he was a young teenager. Adam and his brother lived with their mother. His father lived in the family home off and on for several years even though his parents were legally divorced.

Adam was puzzled when asked to describe his relationships with his parents. His childhood memories were contradictory and confusing. The first description of his childhood was of not having a relationship with his parents because the family was always fighting; yet he remembered feeling loved. He described himself as a self-absorbed child. He used to hang out with his brother despite the fact that his brother wanted nothing to do with him and Adam felt rejected. Adam often ended up playing by himself. He was confused about the origins of his parents' behavior, which he at times ascribed to their cultural background. Being the second-born son, he knew that he was not being scrutinized or molded, like his older brother was, to be the perfect son. He felt that his family loved him because he was cute and loveable. "I was the good little son." The cultural conflict was sometimes frustrating for Adam, as he explained, "I am not a Chinese son; I'm an American Chinese son."

He described his relationship with his mother as loving, clarifying that he used a Chinese cultural lens as his interpretive guide. He explained that Chinese mothers demonstrate their love by preparing food. Adam recalled family meals as happy times that often led to other activities, such as going to the movies together. Adam's primary descriptions of his mother were not as loving, however. He was cranky about the fact that his mother was not interested in him as a person, a personal hurt that he tried to circumvent by ascribing her behavior as typical for her culture. He recalled a time when he asked his mother if she wanted to come to his karate tournament. She replied, "No, you're not going to win anyway." "And I got two first places, and I'm thinking, 'There you go.' My mom has never been overly concerned with or interested in the things I was doing and what interested me." He also stated that there was a lot of "*reverse caring*" in their relationship. He remembered taking his mother's side when his parents fought because his mother was intimidated and frightened of his father's anger. He said that she would try not to show when she was feeling bad, but would quietly cry as she went about her day. Adam said that he would go out of his way then to help his mother out and tell jokes to make her happy and laugh.

Adam's father was a powerful figure. His father's male role as head of household was cemented by his Confucian orientation. His father directed how family members should live their lives, determined things that needed to be done, and guided intellectual and spiritual matters.

"Everything was a lesson. It's a philosophy and he makes it into a religion." Adam said he adored his father as a young child because of his father's involvement in the martial arts. Adam also became involved in martial arts, and this feature of his childhood had a prominent influence on their relationship because it epitomized his father as powerful.

Despite claims of adoring his father, Adam's personal memories of his father were conflicted, contradictory, and confusing. His father was usually nice to Adam, but yelled and verbally attacked the rest of the family. "It made me unhappy. Why was he being nice to me and why was he being so mean to everybody else? I wanted him to just be nicer to everyone else and he could be a little meaner to me. I wouldn't care. He had this switch he would just turn and it was creepy." Adam was also bothered by what he called their "parallel dialogue. We were always talking at each other or by each other but never to each other." Adam thought that his father, too, was disinterested in him as a person. "My dad would be around and always doing work. I remember he didn't come to my graduation when I was in the sixth grade. I was like, 'You're homem' and he said he had a home-based business. I didn't see why he couldn't just come." Adoration turned to resentment when his mother leaked information that his father had a wife and family in another country. Adam, then a young teenager, said that he was devastated by this news and became even more confused about his parents' relationship. He viewed his father as a hypocrite traveling back and forth between two families. Adam was angry as he stated, "I wanted him to stop yelling at people, but I also still loved him because he was so nice to me but then when I realized that he was hurting my mom like this, and the deception of leading this other life and just made me resent all of his morality preaching."

Adam evaluated these situations as mentally abusive and traumatizing for him. The intensity of his emotional reaction eclipsed his ability to describe the details of most of his childhood memories. He described himself as generally recalling being uncomfortable, sad, unhappy, and angry. He made no attempt in his discussion to circumvent the distress he felt growing up feeling alone in the shadow of his parents' marital conflict. He said that he discovered as a young child that they would stop fighting if he had a temper tantrum, so he developed quite a temper. Sometimes, however, he said he just cried in the corner of the room. As he got older, he would go outdoors and find something to do, such as climb a tree, go canoeing, or go to his neighbor's house and play with her pets.

When hurt or ill, Adam received functional care. He remembered one time falling out of a tree and going to the hospital to get stitches. His parents had to hold him down on the stretcher while he was "bawling and crying." His mother's response when he was sick was either "don't get me sick" or "get better quick."

Adam's most difficult separation experiences were related to his parents' initial separation following a big fight. He remembered that his mother quietly took Adam and his brother away to live with a relative. Overall, Adam did not seem to be upset about the separation. His father had typically been absent for months at a time before the separation. His father used to call during these separations and they would talk on the phone when Adam was a child. As he got older, Adam said he was not interested in these phone conversations anymore. The only other separations Adam described were elementary-school-age sleepovers with friends. He liked going to other people's houses and see that they were not always yelling at each other.

Adam's only experience with loss was his grandmother, who had died when he was 18. He had not known her very well. He stated that attending her funeral was fine, except the open casket made him uncomfortable.

Adam stated that he has "more or less blocked out much of his childhood. It was just not a happy time, so why revisit it?" He now saw his mother weekly. He continued to be ambivalent about and annoyed with his father. His father lived abroad and sent e-mails that Adam had not bothered to read. Adam said he has had tried to talk with his father about his childhood dissatisfaction. He said, "We talked about why he did what he did to my mom and the family and what did he think about how badly it hurt us. I have dissatisfaction with his answer because his answer was so what, big deal, you know I had another wife and kid, you know I could have just abandoned you guys and been with this other family and I didn't abandon you so I was thinking 'Yeah, you're not winning any father of the year awards at the same time.' I just didn't like his answer to my questions so I'm just never you know . . . the older he gets the more Confucian he gets, and I'm just like please . . . I feel bad for my father because he's really put himself in this lonely situation by his inability to talk to people: 'I'm the father and I'm Chinese and I can't talk, tell anyone to, it's like my father never talked to me.' So I find that to just be bullshit, you can go beyond your programming, you know. It would force him to look at himself and hear criticism from someone that he's not willing to accept."

Alone Stories

All through Adam's alone stories, we will see reliance on defense by disconnection manifest in diffuse, affective responses. As a result, the contextualizing story elements are often fragmented and poorly articulated, or more typically, not explained at all. While he is able to identify the character in each alone story, he has difficulty specifying precipitating events and outcomes. The first two alone stories are masterpieces of confusion. The last two alone stories express Adam's conflict between the desire for connection and his need to deactivate and create distance in relationships, including pushing others away for self-protection. Agency of self is limited to the capacity to act, which is minimally functional and emotion focused rather than problem focused. The capacity to act helps him make connections in relationships, although he is confused as to what actions or relationships would accomplish this end result. In *Cemetery* and *Corner*, he uses the capacity to act to deactivate potential entanglement or threat. Most of all, Adam's representation of the self in these stories is one of utter aloneness.

> ***Window:*** Okay . . . little girl looking out a window . . . I don't know, to me seems like the girl's sad, she's just kind of looking out, there's no one around her, no one to play with. She's just thinking she, wish she had a friend, somebody to play with. (What led up to the scene?) She's stuck at home, so . . . she's kind of bored, as little kids get, and she wants somewhere to go, someone to play with. (What might happen next?) She's going to wander around the house, or go to her parents and see if they can take her out somewhere, or maybe she'll try calling a friend or something but seems like she wants to go outside, so maybe she'll talk to a parent or go outside and play.

This response provides a classical statement of uncertainty and lack of clarity observed when cognitive disconnection is the main organizing defense. The girl is confused ("wish," "bored," "wander") and even a bit frightened (segregated systems—stuck) by being at home and must figure out how to remedy her sadness. Although the potential to take action to remedy attachment distress is suggested, Adam can neither decide on which action to take (confused agency of self) nor which relationships, if any, are desirable (attachment figures or friends).

> ***Bench:*** Uh, seems like a very, very unhappy girl sitting on a bench, uh, crying. She seems like she's kind of doing it in a pretty open place, so maybe she just got hurt by somebody out in an open place and she's just kind of . . . uh . . . expressing her grief in this place or maybe, uh, you know she found out some tragic news about someone and she just doesn't know how to deal with it . . . um, the thing that happens next? She'll just, uh, continue crying for a while until

she feels like she's done and she needs to move, then she'll probably go somewhere else and be unhappy, but . . . yeah.

The main theme of this story is emotional catharsis and confusion ("she . . . doesn't know how to deal with it"). The girl is unhappy because of some dreadful experience, the nature of which is only implied in dramatic descriptors ("tragic news," "expressing her grief"). The depth of her unhappiness renders her incapable of agency and connectedness. She does not think, repair, or consider constructive action; she shows no desire to be connected to another human being. Suspended in unhappiness, Adam is left with no solution other than to abruptly disconnect from the stimulus ("and be unhappy, but . . . yeah").

Cemetery: Person is visiting, looks like a man, is, uh . . . visiting a tombstone of a relative, possibly a father or mother, and doesn't look like it's being very well taken care of, tombstone seems to be kind of slanted so maybe the person hasn't visited in a while, hasn't taken care of the gravesite. Seems kind of cold, the person's got both hands in their pockets, and they're just kind of standing on the gravesite, kind of weird, uh . . . just maybe having a talk and saying why they haven't visited or is having some trouble in their life. (What led up to the scene?) Something . . . not so good happened, or just made this person, made this guy feel guilty that he hasn't visited the gravesite in so long and left it in neglect, just wants to come back and, uh, make amends to it or, uh, say, uh, talk to the person. (And what might happen next?) Person will talk for a little while, they'll, uh, try to clean up around the area, probably go back to not paying very good attention.

The conflict between closeness and distance shows itself in this story. Bowlby (1973) posited that this type of conflict originated in contradictory caregiving experiences, which subsequent research demonstrated as characteristic of ambivalent attachment (Ainsworth et al., 1978), the child attachment group analogous to preoccupied adult attachment. Adam is conflicted between his negative evaluation of self for wanting distance (deactivation, "hasn't taken care of the gravesite") and not wanting to be entangled ("guilty"). The response demonstrates, too, that Adam seems to understand how unnerving this dilemma is for him, calling the situation "weird," and describing a dysregulated spectral state ("having a talk") as he tries to make sense of it. Similar to his description of the girl's unhappiness in the *Bench* story, his response falls just short of acknowledging how frightening separation in attachment relationships is for him. Personal agency invested in taking care of the relationship ("clean up around the area") relieves his guilt for being inattentive. As discussed previously, agency of self bespeaks the ability to make changes in attachment relationships; it also keeps attachment organized in the face of potential dysregulation. Adam is only able to accomplish one of these tasks. His actions prevent dysregulation; they do not result in moving forward. In the end, nothing has changed; the man goes "back to not paying very good attention".

> ***Corner:*** This looks like a kid being afraid of somebody. They're standing in a corner, they're kind of, their head's turned off to the side and they've got their hands up and they're saying like no, stay away. Looks like the child's possibly, uh, got into a, uh, something with somebody, um . . . they don't show another person, so it could be an adult or a child, I don't know, but looks like the child's not fighting back, and they're just trying to like you know, uh, please stay away from me, don't hurt me kind of attitude. (What might happen next?) Um . . . kid's probably going to get hit, and is probably going to huddle up into a ball if he does get hit, and just kind of let it happen.

Adam is immediately dysregulated by this stimulus. The child is frightened ("afraid") and helpless ("huddle up into a ball"). Although Adam describes protective action in an attempt to deactivate the intensity of the threat ("no, stay away"; "stay away from me, don't hurt me"), his efforts are disconnected and the kid gives in ("let it happen"). While he clearly specifies the self and emotional content of the story, the specifics about the circumstances and other person are disconnected and blurred out. His action prevents dysregulation, although once again we see that nothing has changed. Adam is entangled in a relationship in which he has no recourse for change ("the child's not fighting back").

Dyadic Stories

Adam's responses to stimuli portraying potential attachment relationships accentuate his confusion about the elements of relationships that contribute to synchrony and mutuality. Similar to the alone stories, his responses return to the much-emphasized negative emotions. Dyadic togetherness engenders themes of separation, and story characters are unhappy, needy, confused, and frightened. Such solutions to attachment distress as suggested seem relatively minimal attempts to reestablish calm, and certainly are a far cry from characters engaged in sensitive and mutual synchrony.

> ***Departure:*** These are, uh, two people that are not comfortable with each other, uh, they're leaving, going off somewhere, each both of them going their separate ways . . . uh, there's a piece of luggage in front of the girl and kind of separates her and the guy, and both their hands are in each other's pockets . . . are in their pockets, so they don't feel too comfortable with the whole situation that they're about to leave. (What led up to the scene?) Um, seems like it's a breakup, it's a relationship that kind of went its course and the people don't feel comfortable with each other but they still kind of care for each other but, uh, nothing's the same anymore. (And what might happen next?) They'll go their separate ways and be pretty unhappy for a while, then probably get better.

Emotions once again take center stage in this story. We know that there are two people in this relationship. Disconnected for contextual detail, Adam provides no information about the nature of the situation itself. This story epitomizes the inability of preoccupied individuals to withstand relationship problems. The solution is failed synchrony. There is no goal-corrected synchrony in this relationship; the couple's problems are not a topic for thoughtful discussion. Instead, dissolution of the relationship (i.e., separation) is the ultimate path to happiness, even if the people in the relationship still care for each other.

> ***Bed:*** This is a child wanting a hug from his or her mother before they go to bed. Mom was just, uh, having a talk with the kid, maybe the kid was feeling down or something and the mom looks like she's kind of comforting and sitting and having a good talk with the kid and the kid just wants some physical contact. Because they're kind of far away from each other so it makes me think maybe the kid, they got into an argument or something. Now the kid just wants a hug and wants some attention. (What will happen next?) The mom will give the kid a hug.

Bowlby (1973) described anger in relationships as potentially destructive, which, if not repaired, ultimately engenders ambivalence and mistrust. George and Solomon (2008) described how the accumulating experiences of attachment and caregiving mismatches, evident in

Adam's responses, are the foundation of ambivalent attachment. The child–parent dyad in this story is disconnected by anger ("argument"), which Adam describes as undermining spontaneous synchrony. Adam's first response to the stimulus clearly describes the child's attachment signal ("wanting a hug"). Yet the mother's response to this signal is the last element in the story, which is specified only when Adam is prompted by the interviewer to provide an ending to the story ("The mom will give the kid a hug"). The sequence of verbalizations in this story describes the contradictory miscues and responses that characterize the relationship. The boy wants a hug because he is sad ("feeling down"); his mother talks to him. The mother is "comforting" and "having a good talk with the kid," yet they had an argument. Is this the reason, then, that the child is sad and needs a hug in the first place? The anger generates a sense of separation ("they're kind of far away from each other"), and the child's signals are amplified as their uncomfortable separateness increases.

> ***Ambulance:*** Uh, looks like somebody is going off to the, uh, hospital and . . . a family . . . and oh, looks like someone actually rather just died so the family, the people seem to be staying here instead of getting into the ambulance, um, looks like a younger person's sitting down, looks like a much older, maybe a grandma or something standing up. Uh . . . the thing that'll happen next is they'll call up people they know and tell them that this or that person just died, or is in the hospital or maybe the other family members like the parents, this looks like the grandparent, the parents are going to go off to the hospital with the person, I don't know if they're living or dead, but perhaps seems like they're possibly dead. (What are the characters thinking or feeling?) Uh . . . the child has no clue as to why all of this is happening and the adult has seen it before and is trying to comfort the child and tell them things like it'll be okay, or . . . or what . . . just listening, or just being there with the child as that child cries.

Confusion and dysregulation run through Adam's response to this picture. A momentary strengthening of defense against the frightening theme of separation (death) is followed by confusion as to whether the separation is temporary or final ("person just died, or is in the hospital"; "child has no clue as to why all of this is happening"). Although he identifies the self and attachment figures in the story ("child, grandma, parents"), he is unable to maintain their clarity as he tells his story. In contrast to his responses to the other two dyadic stimuli, Adam cannot maintain the character's identities ("other family members, family, person, adult"). Consistent with his responses to *Window*, *Cemetery*, and *Corner*, the events leading up to the story are especially entangled and fuzzy, almost incomprehensible ("call up people they know," "the parents go off to the hospital"), although the emotional tone of sadness is clear ("the child cries"). Adam tries to describe sensitive synchrony (adult comforts the child), but as he goes on the caregiver's response to the child becomes increasingly passive ("listening, or just being there").

A pseudo-analytic overlay utterly fails to conceal his anger about his parents' disinterest in his childhood self and the continuing anger with his father. Such nonobjective, preoccupying anger is consistent with an AAI E_2 subcategory classification.

Consistent with individuals manifesting prominent, pervasive cognitive disconnecting emphases, Adam's AAI was an unintegrated puzzle of contradictions, some of which he was not cognizant of during the interview. As expressed in the AAP content, Adam could describe emotion-laden memories generically, but when asked to provide specific examples he typically replied, "I just remember times like these, this was a time like that and it is not a one-incident thing." The presence or absence of attachment figures and the contextualizing details of particular incidents are often blurred together to form a vague, but highly distressing, pervasive memory. Blurring and disconnection increased as Adam became more anxious. For example, in describing his parents' first separation, when his mother took the children to live somewhere else, Adam recalled, "That was very very gray. Everything was just I remember as being very gray. I think I just, I don't know, kind of shut down. We just didn't say anything about it. What was there to say, it was just ah . . . " He became so distressed that he cut off his sentence. Although such passages are evaluated as incoherent or sometimes as passivity of thought in the AAI coding system (Main & Goldwyn, 1985/1988/1994; Main et al., 2003), these kinds of discourse errors are prototypic examples of cognitive disconnection in the AAP.

From Adam's AAI, we expected to observe an accumulating emphasis on emotional elements in his AAP responses. It is also noteworthy that Adam's AAP stories brought out the most explicit evidence of his unhappy aloneness and whose diffuseness of self interferes with the ability to maintain a coherent representation of attachment. The passivity of self is particularly striking, such that his thinking seems to have remained vague, fragmented, and confused: "I know growing up I didn't know what I wanted to be, ah, as a job I didn't know what kind of person I didn't want, what kind of person I wanted. I knew what I didn't want to be, you know, and what I didn't want and so that was good because . . . " In the end, Adam's AAP stories certainly confirmed the view of his parents' rage as traumatic and mentally abusive.

CONCLUSION

We have considered the AAI and AAP records of Adam and Paige, both of whom manifested prominent, pervasive cognitive disconnection emphases. Confusing, unpredictable, and contradictory attachment conditions in which the attachment figure was sometimes responsive, sometimes rejecting or threatening, eventuated in an uncertain and ambivalent state of mind with regard to attachment. Whereas dismissing individuals set aside attachment difficulties and deactivate attachment-related feelings, we have seen that Paige and Adam were unable to separate themselves from their attachment experiences, and the topic of attachment (including all of the details and the emotions associated with it) was open for them. Both of them were beset by a preoccupying enmeshment with their past attachment experiences. In his AAI, Adam's enmeshment was accompanied by intensely angry affect. Conversely, Paige's enmeshment was expressed as a passive, somewhat distracted continuing involvement with attachment events or attachment figures. Both Adam's angry preoccupation and Paige's passive preoccupation meant that neither of them had been able to integrate their attachment experiences into their representation of attachment. This lack of perspective-taking was borne out in their AAP stories in which the ability of characters to explore their internal world (internalized secure base) was strikingly absent.

When we speak of cognitive disconnection, we are ultimately referring to the underlying uncertainty in thought and the aforementioned absence of thoughtful integration in the preoccupied individual's AAP responses. As seen through all their stories, unfinished thoughts, empty phrases, wandering off topic, and floundering about the identity of characters and precipitating events prevail. In these vague and affect-laden responses, there is minimal evidence of agency of self in their stories' actions. Thus characters do not enter and actively explore their internal worlds of attachment and they are rarely depicted as capable or confident in making things happen. Despite this general ineffectiveness, both Adam and Paige's defensive operations succeed in mastering the breakthrough of threatening themes, and they are not overwhelmed by attachment distress.

9

Dysregulated Segregated Systems

Unresolved Attachment, Failed Mourning, and Preoccupation with Suffering

In 1995, when we began development of the AAP, this chapter would have been mainly concerned with the assessment of the unresolved attachment group. Today, more than 25 years after the identification of the unresolved classification group, the field's understanding and our own thinking of what it means to be unresolved has expanded and, in some ways, changed direction. No doubt these developments should be seen in the light of the history of the unresolved attachment concept.

Unresolved adult attachment was first identified from the AAI (Main et al., 1985); it is not isomorphic with unresolved or complicated grief as defined in the grief literature (e.g., Hamilton-Oravetz, 1992; Parkes, 2006). As is well known, the AAI classification groups were empirically derived to mirror infant Strange Situation classifications (Hesse, 2008; Main et al., 1985). Thus each AAI transcript in Main's original Berkeley sample was painstakingly examined to develop analogous adult categories that matched a mother's state of mind regarding her own attachment experience with her infant's classification in the Strange Situation (Main et al., 1985). One group of mothers seemed to be derailed by discussions of parental loss, and their infants' attachment strategies were similarly derailed in the Strange Situation. These infants were designated as "disorganized" (Main et al., 1985; Main & Solomon, 1986, 1990). The unresolved classification was designated as the adult analog of this high-risk infant attachment group, thus establishing the conceptual postulate that unresolved and disorganized attachment (originally abbreviated U_d) are essentially child and adult forms of the same phenomenon.

In this chapter, we first of all examine the AAI criteria for identifying unresolved attachment and other risk-related AAI classification groups. We are next concerned with the definition of attachment trauma. This concept is used to identify high-risk experience but is loosely employed in the field of attachment and has not been clearly defined. Finally, we present examples of the four attachment trauma groups identified with the AAP—unresolved loss, unresolved trauma, preoccupation with personal suffering, and failed mourning. We focus only on the core issues related to assessment. Readers interested in the details of the etiology of unresolved and disorganized attachment are referred to comprehensive discussions in other volumes (George & Solomon, 2008; Hesse, 2008; Lyons-Ruth & Jacobvitz, 2008; Solomon & George, 2008, 2011a, 2011b).

UNRESOLVED/DISORGANIZED ATTACHMENT: JUDGING AAI LACK OF RESOLUTION

Individuals are judged unresolved in the AAI if they receive a rating of midpoint or above on one of two lack of resolution rating scales—loss (the mourning of a death) or abuse (Main & Goldwyn, 1985/1988/1994; Main et al., 2003). Lack of resolution of mourning is evaluated from descriptions of loss at any time during the lifespan with the exception of the loss of a child for parents. Unresolved loss is designated when discourse features during the interview indicate notable "lapses" in reasoning (e.g., speaking as if the deceased is still alive; confusion between the deceased and the self; unwarranted belief of causing the death), absorbed or dissociated shifts of attention (e.g., unusual attention to details related to the loss; prolonged silences; invasions of discussion of death without logical introduction), or descriptions of extreme responses to the death (e.g., attempted suicide; behavioral collapse in response to a subsequent death). Lack of resolution of abuse is evaluated for reported experiences of physical, sexual, or emotional abuse, defined as hitting that leaves a physical mark, bizarre or extreme punishment, parental suicide attempts, parental rage directed at the child, and seduction or sexual interaction. Unresolved abuse is designated by discourse features during the interview that indicate attempts to deny abusive events or their intensity, viewing the self as causal or deserving of abuse, descriptions of dissociated behavior during abuse (e.g., mind going somewhere else), and strong or disoriented visual imagery of abusive situations.

Subsequent research that demonstrated a significant correlation between disorganized childhood attachment and unresolved loss and abuse on the AAI provided the first empirical evidence for the attachment premise that childhood attachment experiences have an intergenerational effect on parenting (see Hesse & Main, 2006, for details). Although the evidence does not support a simple parent-to-child transmission model (see George & Solomon, 2008; Solomon & George, 2011b, for detailed discussion), this research helped establish the AAI as a valid and reliable developmental adult attachment assessment tool and opened up new avenues for research (van IJzendoorn & Bakermans-Kranenburg, 1996). One such important avenue was the ability to examine empirically the attachment correlates of adult risk and psychiatric symptoms, one of Bowlby's (1980) original goals for attachment theory (Allen, 2008; Dozier, Stovall-McClough, & Albus, 2008; Hesse, 2008).

As a result of this body of research, many expert and novice researchers and clinicians alike who use the attachment construct in their daily work equate adjustment and psychiatric problems with the unresolved attachment group (e.g., Moran, Bailey, Gleason, DeOliveira, & Pederson, 2008; Riggs, 2010). However, the unresolved classification is best viewed only as a risk factor; it does not follow, in other words, that every individual designated as unresolved is beset by psychiatric symptoms or problems (Bakermans-Kranenburg & van IJzendoorn, 2009). In this regard, we found no statistical differences in our studies among attachment groups on any of the main symptom indices of the SCL-90-R (see Chapter 5).[1] From a developmental standpoint, attachment theory is a context-sensitive model; that is, specific attachment experiences are moderated by other factors, including the caregiving environment and other attachment relationships (Solomon & George, 1999). From a psychometric standpoint, the assessment of unresolved attachment using a biographical interview requires that the interview actually contains discussion of traumatic material for evaluation. Spieker and colleagues (Spieker, Nelson, DeKlyen, Jolley, & Mennet, 2011) described interview problems in their discussion with regard to AAI stability in their sample

[1] Other researchers similarly report no differences in symptom reports between U and non-U adult attachment groups in community samples (Dr. K. Petrowski, personal communications, August 10, 2011).

of high-risk young mothers. They noted that these mothers were especially inconsistent in bringing up risk experiences during the interview. They suggested that the mothers' decisions regarding discussion topics changed depending on what they deemed relevant to their current life events, including the transition to parenthood (see also George & Solomon, 2008; Waters et al., 2000). Lyons-Ruth, Yellin, Melnick, and Atwood (2003) added a trauma interview to the AAI to obtain more information about traumatic experiences. Following their lead, we too always include a trauma interview when we use the AAI to obtain biographical information about an individual's attachment past so as to maximize our ability to get a more complete chronicle and detail about events a person considers traumatic.

It seems unlikely that the unresolved attachment group is the only group associated with risk. Another psychometric issue, therefore, is how to identify other risk classification groups. Main identified the first non-unresolved risk group in her Berkeley sample (Main et al., 1985). Specifically, a group of mothers appeared mentally overwhelmed and preoccupied with regard to topics of abuse rather than unresolved. Termed "fearfully preoccupied by traumatic events," this group is designated as a preoccupied subgroup (E_3) (Main & Goldwyn, 1985/1988/1994). The E_3 classification is relatively rare in community samples and more prevalent in psychiatric and abuse samples (Fonagy et al., 1996; Patrick, Hobson, Castle, & Howard, 1994; West & George, 2002). The correlates associated with this subgroup are not, however, well understood in part because researchers typically combine E_3s with the other two preoccupied subgroups or combine E_3s with other insecure classifications when reporting results (see Chapter 8). These analysis techniques obscure the meaning of the E_3 group, including evaluating whether or how individuals who are judged E_3 differ from individuals who are judged unresolved. Indeed, individuals judged E3 are often also judged unresolved (i.e., E_3/U or U/E_3).

Other AAI risk classifications have emerged in response to reported problems in applying the AAI classification scheme to high-stress/risk samples (e.g., incarcerated criminals, adolescent psychiatric inpatients, severe maltreatment, Holocaust survivors (Schuengel & van IJzendoorn, 2001; Turton, Gauley, Marvin-Avellan, & Hughes, 2001; Wallis & Steele, 2001). Main created a fifth AAI classification group, designated "unorganized/cannot classify" (CC) (Hesse, 1996; Main & Goldwyn, 1985/1988/1994; Main et al., 2003). The CC group is defined by a different quality of discourse anomalies than those used to designate the unresolved and E_3 classifications, such as evidence of simultaneous discordant states of mind during the interview (e.g., secure and insecure), apparent attempts to frighten the interviewer, or periods in which the individual seems unable to speak. This latter "freezing" quality appears to us to be analogous to the representational constriction indicator we define as evidence of segregated systems in our AAP coding based on validating research that has established the link between constriction and attachment and caregiving disorganization (George & Solomon, 1999; George & West, 2001; George et al., 1999; Solomon et al., 1995) (see Chapter 4). The increased use of the AAI in risk samples has led researchers to develop additional supplementary rating scales or new AAI classification schemes (Crittenden, 1997; De Haene, Grietens, & Verschueren, 2010; Lyons-Ruth & Spielman, 2004).

The above review of the literature suggests that the refinements of the AAI classification categories are increasingly driven by an overly empirical approach and lack a theoretical rationale. This approach raises some practical and conceptual problems that have been virtually ignored in the field to date. One such problem is determining the place of unresolved trauma in understanding the attachment contributions to developmental and psychiatric risk. This determination is difficult because researchers normally combine the anomalous classification groups and refer to the resultant collection as "attachment trauma." Another difficulty results from variations among researchers as to what constitutes attachment trauma. Some limit attachment trauma only to the unresolved abuse classification group. Still others combine unresolved loss and unresolved abuse, placing a case in the trauma group using the highest lack of resolution score. In addition, some studies include CC classifications in the trauma group while other studies set the CC cases aside on the basis that this group is poorly understood and has not been evaluated psychometrically (Hesse, 2008). Moreover, recent research has demonstrated that the criteria used to delineate the AAI lack of resolution of abuse scale are too narrow. This scale especially falls short by not evaluating emotional abuse or other frightening and disorganizing experiences (e.g., parental rage not directed at the child, failed protection, and out-of-control family members; Solomon & George, 2006, 2011b; Zajac & Kobak, 2009).

All of the questions and problems generated above are a problem only for those who are interested in the nuances of attachment trauma. Broberg (2001) reminded the field that the approaches directed at solving attachment classification problems were developed primarily for research purposes. From a practical standpoint, researchers typically report findings in terms of differences between secure and insecure participants or, especially in studies of parenting, differences among the four standard adult attachment groups (secure, dismissing, preoccupied, unresolved). They usually only report the results of non-unresolved risk classifications when the study was specifically designed to investigate the correlates of the attachment state of mind of participants in high-risk samples. From a clinical standpoint, however, psychotherapists have expressed the concern that attachment assessment runs the "risk [of] reducing complex human experience to typologies" and have limited utility (O'Shaughneessy & Dallos, 2009, p. 559). We propose that one source of the problems of these clinical complaints is the lack of specificity and adequate theory building around what constitutes attachment trauma.

The assessment approach detailed above has produced a wealth of information about the correlates between frightening attachment experiences and unresolved attachment. Yet the conceptual distinction between unresolved attachment and the collection of classifications that are considered reflective of attachment trauma are obscure. It may be argued that these distinctions are unnecessary because all of these subgroups and variations address attachment trauma. Turning specifically to the AAP, the issues associated with assessing risk have played a central role in developing the AAP coding and classification system. Our challenge was to develop a representational coding scheme that retained the integrity of the AAI unresolved classification group but at the same time identified non-unresolved traumatic risk.

ATTACHMENT TRAUMA: DYSREGULATED ATTACHMENT AND PATHOLOGICAL MOURNING

What is attachment trauma? Webster's dictionary defines trauma as a violently produced physical or psychological wound that is accompanied by shock. In psychiatry, trauma is defined in part by the enduring emotional effects of shock and alarm, including chronic debilitating anxiety, fear, and anger. The conceptual foundation for defining attachment trauma is disorganization, an explanatory model that draws on Bowlby's seminal discussion of the place of separation fear in attachment theory (Bowlby, 1973; Main & Solomon, 1990). The ultimate separation in Bowlby's view is loss, which he viewed as a form of attachment trauma (Bowlby, 1980). Although trauma is clearly related to separation and fear, we find that the current approach to attachment trauma as analogous to disorganized attachment falls short of Bowlby's goals. It is insufficient for theory building, assessment, and clinical application. In this section, we attempt to advance the attachment model of trauma in light of Bowlby's thinking about mourning and defense.

Current thinking about the concept of attachment disorganization provides a solid beginning. Disorganization expands on Bowlby's position that separation is instinctively frightening; separation events signal dangerous threats to survival and activate the attachment system (Bowlby, 1973). From an evolutionary perspective, for children and adults alike, reunion and regained proximity to attachment figures, the set goal of the attachment behavioral system, is the only solution to assuage fear.[2] Attachment is such a powerful motivator that attachment goals instinctively override other forms of mammalian fear survival mechanisms, such as escape, freezing, or avoiding the frightening stimulus. Attachment disorganization is conceived as the "collapse" of organized behavioral attachment strategies when children are extremely frightened and without attachment figure accessibility (Main & Solomon, 1990). For infants, attachment behavior can literally collapse, such as is observed when an infant freezes or "melts" instead of seeking closeness to the parent. The physical or psychological inaccessibility is in itself a separation, and attachment behavior and organized strategies to regain proximity break down when attachment figures are consistently unavailable or impervious to attachment needs (Main & Solomon, 1990). Researchers have shown that frightening, threatening, and extremely anomalous interactive communication disorganize the attachment system (Lyons-Ruth, Bronfman, & Parsons, 1999; Main & Hesse, 1990; Solomon & George, 2006, 2011b). What is important to our thinking here is that these experiences are traumatic; they instinctively signal extreme danger. Following Bowlby's model, attachment is disorganized by the separation fears generated when attachment figures fail to provide protection and abdicate the caregiving role (George & Solomon, 2008; Solomon & George, 2000).

The behavioral collapse that defines disorganized attachment in infancy has a representational counterpart in older children; in the doll play assessment procedure disorganized children exhibit the inability to contain their feelings of being out of control, frightened, and abandoned (Solomon et al., 1995). At the behavioral level, these same children develop rigid forms of controlling behavior (Cassidy, Marvin, et

[2] We showed in Chapter 4 that the AAP concept of internalized secure base is essentially an integrated reunion with attachment figures at the representational level.

al. 1987–1992; Main & Cassidy, 1988), and caregiving and punitive controlling strategies that are futile behavioral attempts to guarantee attachment figure proximity (George & Solomon, 2008).

In adults, AAI discourse anomalies associated with unresolved loss and abuse provide evidence of representational disorganization, a collapse of adult meta-cognitive thinking and memory processes; these anomalies are analogous to behavioral collapse. These collapses indicate dissociated or absorbed mental processing states and short-term memory interferences associated with trauma (Hesse & Main, 2006). They are likely related to imbalances in limbic system–cortical functioning and limbic–hypothalamic–pituitary–adrenal stress regulation dysfunction (Buchheim et al., 2008b; Buchheim, Erk et al., 2006; Gunnar, Brodersen, Nachmias, Buss, & Rigatuso, 1996; Pierrehumbert et al., 2009; Schore, 2001).

In considering the developmental and clinical approaches to attachment and trauma, Solomon and George (2011a; George & Solomon, 2008, 2011) proposed that disorganization represents a fundamental *dysregulation* of adaptive behavioral, representational, and biological processes. In turn, they demonstrated that the failure of attachment figures to buffer children from "toxic levels of stress" brings about traumatic homeostatic dysregulation at all response levels. From an evolutionary perspective, therefore, we emphasize that the core element missing in current views of attachment trauma is the individual's experience. These authors emphasized that experience, and later representation, is characterized by dysregulating fear that is associated with *attachment figure abdication and caregiving helplessness*. The perception of being abandoned and alone consequent to failed protection by attachment figures, whether abusive or not, compromises psychological safety, self-integrity, and ultimately survival. This conceptual framework defines attachment trauma.

We are now at a point where Bowlby's concept of segregated systems in relation to loss may provide the key to understanding and defining the AAP indices of dysregulation and attachment trauma. According to Bowlby, loss "is one of the most intensely painful experiences any human being can suffer. And not only is it painful to experience but it is also painful to witness, if only because we are so impotent to help" (Bowlby, 1980, p. 7). The impotence to which Bowlby (1980) refers is what Solomon and George described as blocked access to attachment figures and the helplessness of others to assuage attachment pain and despair (Solomon & George, 2011b). As a result, attachment trauma leads to "the persistent and insatiable nature of the yearning for the lost attachment figure" (Bowlby, 1980, p. 26) and the quality of persistent dysregulated fear that we posit as the foundation of all attachment trauma (i.e., loss, abuse, rage, abandonment). Bowlby proposed that homeostasis is reestablished through mourning, the process of updating representational attachment models. Representations of self must be reorganized and reintegrated to match the reality of their attachment figure's inaccessibility. Using AAP terminology, mourning involves transforming perceptions of the abandoned, unprotected, and helpless self into a representation of self as organized by constructive agency (i.e., perceptions that actions and future plans are the consequences of one's intentions and the internalized reunion with attachment figures) and connected to available attachment figures.

When mourning is incomplete, representational models of the self and attachment figures remained unchanged and failures of the past continue to "haunt" the present. The failure to accomplish reintegration, in which the individual's internal world is experienced as incoherent and chaotic, begets helplessness, futility, and isolation. Bowlby referred to this state as pathological mourning and described two main forms that he believed were powerful explanatory tools for understanding debilitating psychiatric and physical symptoms.

One form is failed mourning, or a state of "prolonged absence of conscious grieving" (Bowlby, 1980, p. 152). Failed mourning reflects defense by segregated systems buttressed by strong deactivation that is expressed as a detached psychological state likened by Bowlby to a "protective shell" (Bowlby, 1980, p. 154). Individuals who exhibit failed mourning outwardly appear unaffected by the loss and deny any feelings related to it; they continue with their normal lives and are proud of working hard to move beyond the past. They appear strong and in control, and actively avoid situations or reminders associated with the loss. Observable evidence of emotional distress is unusual, but deactivating defensive exclusion may occasionally be ineffective and distress is not altogether staved off. Individuals in failed mourning are susceptible to anniversary reactions (i.e., strong distress on the anniversary of the loss). Signs of sadness and depression sometimes seemingly appear out of nowhere and that then seem to disappear (e.g., crying and bouts of depression). Bowlby suggested that failed mourning is the source of problematic personality characteristics such as compulsive self-reliance, compulsive caring for others in distress (deflecting personal need to care for others), or depersonalization. He also suggested that failed mourning contributes to problematic physical stress reactions and some eating problems, which has been supported in studies that assessed failed mourning

(DiRiso et al., in press; Hamilton-Oravetz, 1992; Sagi-Schwartz, Koren-Karie, & Joels, 2003).

Bowlby (1980) described the other main form of pathological mourning as "chronic mourning," a state that is characterized by more readily observable signs of disorganization and despair. In contrast to failed mourning, chronic mourning is outwardly intense. It often begins abruptly and is evident in a prolonged immersion into the memories and emotional details of the loss, accompanied by a confused yearning and search for the lost attachment figure. One manifestation of chronic mourning is marked by emotional breakdown, together with lapses and interruptions in the ability of the individual to function and relate to others. Another manifestation is marked not by lapses and flooding, but by "preoccupation with personal reactions and sufferings" (Bowlby, 1980), a representational state that we conceive of as "living in the war zone." Both manifestations of chronic mourning are characterized by disorganized behavior and endless searching for attachment figures, pining, and anger.

Chronic mourning reflects defense by segregated systems reinforced by cognitive disconnection. Cognitive disconnection interferes with the reintegration required to complete mourning by disconnecting incompatible and contradictory representations of the self and the deceased and blocks the recognition of entangling resentment and anger. For individuals seemingly stuck in mourning, "the mental situation remains unstable" (Bowlby, 1980, p. 236).

We have covered a good deal of theoretical ground in the above discussion of attachment trauma. The section that follows presents the case studies of the four main forms of attachment dysregulation. Before proceeding, it will be useful to summarize briefly the dynamics of the segregated system concept that were outlined in detail in Chapter 5. This summary should facilitate the transition to the case studies.

The essential purpose of defense by segregated systems is to "package" and "lock away" trauma-related memories and emotions in a separate representational model that is kept inaccessible to consciousness. Importantly, a central feature of this defense is that it is an extremely brittle form of exclusion. When the attachment system is activated, and defense begins to fail, we may anticipate the breakthrough of frightening or traumatic imagery. Finally, and very important, there are varying degrees of success among individuals in containing the breakthrough. The success of containment usually spreads out over a continuum from effective containment to ineffective efforts to contain the threatening material. In the instance of failure of defense by segregated system, that is, in the instance of ineffective efforts to contain attachment fear, the individual is designated as unresolved.

The following cases present examples of four representational forms of attachment trauma assessed using the AAP. The first three cases are variations of chronic mourning: unresolved loss, unresolved abuse, and preoccupation with suffering. These examples demonstrate representations of attachment in which individuals are caught in an unending or continual state of attempting to manage segregated attachment affect and experience. The two unresolved cases demonstrate the representational inability to contain segregated systems material. The case that demonstrates preoccupation with suffering shows how maladaptive cognitive disconnection processes splinter and filter segregated systems material to such a degree that disconnected transformations are dysregulating because the individual lives in the memories of trauma (see Chapter 8 for examples of normative forms of cognitive disconnection). Defensive attempts to disconnect distressing experiences from attachment figures backfire, creating a state of mind in which the individual is immersed in and confused by traumatic experience. The fourth case is an example of failed mourning. This case demonstrates representational attempts to "clamp down" and normalize traumatic segregated systems material. These attempts also backfire, and the individual is flooded by segregated rage and yearning that requires extreme defensive management to prevent becoming overwhelmed by distress.

CHRONIC MOURNING CASE EXAMPLES

Unice: Unresolved Loss

Unice is a 55-year-old married Caucasian woman with two adult daughters. She is the eldest of five sisters. Her father's job required the family to move several times across the country throughout her childhood. Her mother did not work outside the home. Relatives and her parents' friends were an important part of Unice's life, although none were supplementary caregivers.

Unice's mother and father were her haven of safety and secure base. She frequently described events with both parents together, suggesting that parents were equally present in her mind. She remembered her childhood as happy and peaceful, a quality of family life she said she only fully appreciated and understood as an adult. "I was just, um, a happy kid, I mean I don't remember anything unhappy, really, about Mom and Dad. My mom and dad were wonderful. I don't want it to sound like my parents were perfect but hey, well, they were pretty good." Because her mother was home full-time, she turned more to her mother when she was upset but said she also never hesitated to go to her father. "They'd make things better, help make you feel better." She said she had difficulty understanding people who didn't cry when they were sad. "Where I grew up, you were sad, you cried, simple," and she felt she was lucky to have her parents because they had showed her how to comfort others.

Christmas was an especially happy family time for Unice. She remembered helping her mother bake the Christmas cake. She was so excited on Christmas Eve that she could not fall asleep and bounced in and out of bed. Her mother would tell her to go back to bed, which her mother explained to her later was to allow her father to lay out the presents for Christmas morning. "I remember one Christmas, oh, I was so excited and woke up at one o'clock in the morning and my dad, he didn't say no, back to bed. He said, oh well, we may as well get up, so we got up we opened everything and went back to bed." Her father used to nail the children's stockings to their bedpost. She had one bittersweet memory of being awakened by her father's stifled yelp as he hammered his finger instead of the stocking.

Unice described her parents as encouraging and trusting. "I was always encouraged, she always encouraged me. I was never stopped from doing, anything. I never grew up thinking that oh gee, I should be a nurse as opposed to a doctor, we were never told that the world, you know, when you get out into the real world females get a rude awakening, we never knew that, we had no idea." Her parents' overall message about their family, and people in general, revolved around trust. She said that it was a "shock" to her when she got her first job to realize that there were people who could not be trusted.

She remembered her household as peaceful. She never saw her parents argue. Her mother has since told her that the parents worked out disagreements when the children were not at home. She said it was a "shock" to her when she first saw other parents arguing.

Unice described her relationship with her mother as understanding and praising. She remembered an incident as a young girl when she was not able to open the heavy entrance door to her elementary school. She ran home worried about being late. "My mom said, 'Don't worry, I'll take you to school,' and she took me to school and opened the door for me." She said her mother was always pleased with her report cards and never scolded Unice for less than outstanding grades. She recalled that her mother resolved tussles with neighborhood kids by telling Unice to invite them to play at her house. Her mother allowed them to be messy and play on the grass, which the neighbor kids' parents did not allow. "We put our toe on the grass because we were so scared we wanted to see what would happen, because we really believed you know if you step on this grass, boy, something's going to happen and we didn't know what, so we did it and nothing happened. Anyway, not in our yard."

Unice remembered her relationship with her father as comforting, encouraging, and filled with humor. She loved the feeling of her father's hands on her stomach when she had a stomach ache. "My dad would come home and he'd come in there in the bedroom and I'd say would you please put your hand on my stomach, oh, he always would do that. It used to feel so good." Her father was very involved in report card day. "I used to be happy when it was report card day because I would read it to my dad and he would always be so happy." She described her father's sense of humor as doing fun things. He liked to dress up and put on funny skits or kid around with his children. She fondly recalled one time when he crawled around on the floor at the dinner table looking for a mouse under the table. "I remember we laughed, oh, we thought that was wonderful."

Discipline was her mother's job. Her mother has since told Unice that her father could never bring himself to reprimand his children. Unice could not recall any spankings. Her mother used to "flick" their noses to get their attention and, if they were really naughty, they had to weed the garden. When asked to give an example of discipline, she recalled a situation where she was sure she would be spanked or scolded but was not. A neighbor's mother caught Unice and her son in the middle of a childhood prank. "I waited all day long, you know, for the boom to fall and I waited and waited and nothing happened 'cause this kid's mother, there's no way that she wouldn't have told my mom about what happened, and I waited and I waited and finally my mother was tucking me into bed and still nothing was happening, and all she said was something about that I wasn't, um, that wasn't to play with Person 1 under the blanket anymore, so I got off easy on that one. You know, my mom doesn't even remember the incident now. No, she doesn't remember, so I was waiting for, you know, all hell to break loose but it never happened."

Unice said she was never separated from her parents as a child. "My mom and dad were homebodies; they didn't go very far." Her first separation was at age 18 when she met the man she married. Defying her father for the first time in her life, Unice decided to return to her then boyfriend after her father's transfer moved the family to a new town. Her mother finally accepted that she was serious about moving back and helped her pack. They spent a long day worrying about her father's response to seeing the packed trunk and what he did when he arrived home that day surprised both of them. She said he was stern but kind, and he lent her some money with the directive that she had a month to get a job, or she had to move home. Unice knew that she would not return home, but did not argue. She said she cried every day after she moved "because I missed them, no I was, into the next phase of my life, and I mean it would have been nicer if they had been there, but ah, I would not have changed what I did, I had to do what I did. They missed me a great deal. I'm sorry that it hurt them, I know why they opposed it, I know very well why they did, they were afraid for me, but I would not have done it differently, and, um, I do not regret doing it—um, even though there were a lot of difficulties, and so when my mother and father, you know, became accepting I was just happy."

Unice did not experience loss until her grandparents died when she was in her late teens. Her paternal grandparents visited the family often during her childhood, and she had fond memories of the games her grandfather played with her and her sisters. She remembered this loss in particular because her grandfather died overnight on one of his visits. She laughed as she recalled a gopher-catching technique he invented just for them. Her grandfather gave them a string with a noose that they put into the gopher hole. He cautioned the girls to be very quiet so they could snag the gopher as soon as his head popped up out of the hole. She understood now that catching gophers with a noose on a string was impossible, but her grandfather had been so convincing. Her mother told her the news of her grandfather's death and how her family's comfort had helped. Although she claimed that she had moved forward in a few months, she recalled, "I still remember him just like the last day I saw him. He's just as clear and real to me even though that's, um, 35 years ago."

Unice's father died 15 years ago. She said she felt the same way about his death as she had about her grandfather's death. "I don't mind talking about my father. He's with me every day. If I have a problem I always think to myself, what would my father have said what would he have told me to do? No, he still is as real to me as he ever was." Her father died following major surgery for a congenital medical condition that worsened quickly as he aged. Unice said she felt helpless; there was nothing she could do to help him. He had had multiple small surgeries throughout his life, but had to have major surgery because he was getting increasingly sick. He died suddenly in hospital while recovering from the surgery. "We were called to the hospital and, um, and before we got there he died. I didn't get to say goodbye to him, but you know, he knows he sees me in the, I know where he is and he sees me, and he knows that, um, we tried to get there but we could not have gotten there because those things they're instant."

Unice still very much misses her father. In this regard, she said that she thought for a long time that she would cry forever. She said too that caring for her mother following her father's death was traumatic. "We were afraid she was going to die after my dad passed away. My mother was lost, totally completely lost." Unice and her sisters put her mother into a care facility because they were worried about her health. "I would never presume to tell my mother what to do," but they hoped that the shock of moving would "bring her around." Her mother adjusted and moved into her own apartment. "And we would never have done it if we hadn't honestly thought that she was going to die."

Unice was judged unresolved on the AAP based on the overwhelming sadness unleashed by the *Cemetery* picture and her ineffectiveness to contain and reorganize her dysregulation in that response. All of Unice's responses demonstrate the importance in her mind of attachment figures and caregiving experiences in her representational model of attachment. Her responses also show a range of adaptive and defensive resiliency. Her *Window* and *Bed* responses are characterized by integrated agency and synchrony, which gradually give way to stories in which characters neither have the capacity to act nor the capacity to find comfort as the attachment stimuli portray increasingly distressing scenes. The reliance on cognitive disconnection, reinforced at times by deactivation, succeeds in helping her to mute and integrate attachment feelings in many responses. But the *Ambulance* and *Cemetery* pictures overwhelm her capacity for organized defense, and she describes how alone she feels with her grief. Her organizing defenses are unstable, as evident in her inability to maintain the personal–hypothetical boundary in some of her stories. This gives way to the instance of the failure of organizing defense to contain her distress noted above in her *Cemetery* response. Also consistent with her attachment tension and anxiety, Unice blurs identification of the "projected" self seamlessly from personal experience statements (e.g., *Bed*), or does not identify the projected self at all (e.g., *Ambulance, Corner*).

Alone Stories

Attachment–caregiving relationships are depicted in all of her alone responses. Unice's responses evidence the complete range of AAP agency and connectedness coding elements. Characters demonstrate agency in the forms of internalized secure base and the capacity to act. These stories exhibit connectedness to internalized attachment figures and the use of affiliation relationships (i.e., affiliative system) to cope with moderate levels of attachment distress. As attachment distress mounts, integrated personal agency and connectedness begin to disintegrate. Unice's primary defensive approach is cognitive disconnection. There is some evidence of deactivation attempts to "cool down" attachment distress, as seen in her *Bench* story. The instability of cognitive disconnection blurs representational self–other boundaries in two responses. In *Cemetery*, disconnection fails, leading to dysregulation and the representational inability to contain the segregated feelings associated with the loss that she is trying so hard to manage. The spectral segregated systems evidenced in Unice's personal story represent the intensity of the wish for reunion with her dead father.

> ***Window:*** Um, a little girl, she's looking outside, she wants to go out and play, and she's, she's already dressed, I think she's got a dress on, she's, she's thinking probably she wants to go out and play and thinking about what she might, um, like to do, go and play with her friends. I don't know what else (laughs). She's sitting there by herself, I don't know if that's significant. Or her sisters are probably in the other room. Or her mom's probably off, I know her mom's off baking some cookies or something, and she's just, ah, she's just deciding like, oh I know she's deciding whether she'll play in the house or whether she'll go outside, but it looks like a nice day, the tree must be summer, yeah, she's going to go out and play she's going to call on her friends. That's it.

The first attachment stimulus is not overtly distressing. Unice's story captures the girl at the moment when she is trying to decide what to do. The first elements of the story clearly depict agency of self; the girl's thinking indicates representations of attachment figures as an internalized secure base. The girl's dilemma is to play in house or go outside. The tension of this uncertainty, defined in the AAP as an element of cognitive disconnection, supports Unice's thinking processes by delineating the problem. The moment of uncertainty gives her time to pause. Thinking leads to more agency and connectedness in relationships—she goes outside to play with friends (i.e., affiliative system). Unice's representation of self demonstrated that she has the capacity to be involved in other important relationships drawing from the secure base provided by internalized attachment figures, even when real attachment figures are busy elsewhere ("her mom's off baking some cookies"). Unice completes her story quickly, but there is some indication of tension due to her understanding that AAP task asks her to elaborate on the story details. She disconnects this tension ("I don't know what else"), which again gives her pause to think, and she tells the same basic story with added detail. This suggests to us that the most important feature of Unice's story is her representational capacity for personal agency and connectedness.

> ***Bench:*** She's tired, she's resting. She has been working really hard and so she's just taking a moment to put her head down and rest a little bit. Getting her second wind, that's it, maybe she's a young mother and she's been chasing kids all day. Like my daughter (laughing), so she's just taking a minute, you know, for herself maybe to recharge her batteries. (What might happen next?) She'll get up and go on doing what she was doing.

This is a story of a mother resting from the stress of taking care of children. This alone stimulus activates more obvious tension than the *Window* stimulus. The mother has "been chasing kids all day," is "tired," and "resting" (cognitive disconnection). We see in this story how Unice ascribes the tension to the effort associated with trying to deactivate attachment—the mother has been "working really hard" and needs a "second wind." Cognitive disconnection processes momentarily undermine Unice's capacity for self–other differentiation, blurring the boundary between the hypothetical mother and descriptions of her own daughter. Efforts to balance attachment and defensive exclusion support representations of agency of self. The mother gets up (agency–capacity to act). We note, however, that the attachment distress activated by pictures of the alone self is increasing. In contrast to the integration of internal and external agency and connectedness demonstrated in *Window*, Unice's representational resources portray what we consider in the AAP to be only a minimal form of agency. The act of "getting up" represents the ability to keep moving, but it neither depicts progress away from the source of distress (i.e., the bench) nor results in connectedness with others. Nothing has changed; the mother is alone and goes "on doing what she was doing."

> ***Cemetery:*** Oh, that's sad—I, um, I've never been to my father's grave, I really don't feel the need because I feel he's with me. I don't have to go to the grave to be with him, to be close to him. And one

> of my sisters does like to go. But I've never felt, like I said he's close to me all the time, so I don't feel like I have to go there. But it's possible this man, because he looks unhappy to me, I'm not sure what about exactly. Maybe just sad because somebody he's cared about has passed away. (What might happen next?) He might get some comfort from, going there, hopefully he'll go back to his family and tell them he's sad and they'll make him feel better.

The *Cemetery* stimulus was too close to Unice's own experience. Her defenses fail and she is flooded with memories of her own loss. She describes her spectral relationship with her father (*dysregulated segregated systems*) without contextualizing her feelings in space and time before telling a hypothetical story. The man in her story depicts her own sadness—"somebody he's cared about has passed away"—and the importance of family in helping the man "feel better." Her story is disconnected, however, from her reality ("I'm not sure what about exactly"), and she is only able to label the deceased as *somebody*, rather than identifying the deceased as the man's father. The two response lines (personal vs. hypothetical) are in evidence in the AAP of Unice's nonintegrated selves. The hypothetical projected self has agency; the man tells his family that he is sad and is comforted by them (capacity to act and haven of safety). But the personal experience self lacks agency in this ethereal relationship with her dead father.

> ***Corner:*** Ooh. He's probably been bad, standing in the corner. He's got his hands up like he's . . . I don't know. He's got his hands up like he's defending himself but I don't know against what . . . oh maybe there was something he had for dinner that he didn't like, maybe someone's trying to get him to eat his veggies, that's it, he's not necessarily, I think it's a corner but not necessarily, he needs to, you know, eat his veggies. (What might happen next?) His mother will say just some of them. No dessert until you've eaten some of them.

The reason the character in the *Corner* response is standing in the corner is that he has been bad. Unice describes the boy's action as a response to being threatened ("defending himself"). She immediately disconnects from this tension to create a pause to figure out how to continue with the story when she abruptly stops speaking and says "I don't know." Unice's response again shows how cognitive disconnection defenses are used to support representational organization and the ability to keep on task. We note also that the identity of the projected self is blurred to a "he." The failure to specify the character as a hypothetical person is an indicator of the underlying tension in Unice's response. Unice's story portrays the firm kindness of attachment–caregiving compromise. Faced with the boy's refusal, the mother suggests that eating some of the vegetables will suffice for the child to get dessert.

Dyadic Stories

Unice's dyadic responses again all depict attachment–caregiving situations. The responses to *Departure* and *Bed* indicate mutual enjoyment, although the clear elements required by the AAP coding system to code integrated synchrony are absent. In *Ambulance*, presumably a more intense stimulus for Unice, functional care for the person on the stretcher undermines the capacity for comfort. Cognitive disconnection defenses seamlessly blur Unice's real personal experience with characters and events in the hypothetical story. The dyadic stories demonstrate the capacity to maintain some representational distance from feelings and experience through deactivation, a defensive process element that was not evident her responses to the alone stories.

> ***Departure:*** Oh look at that, I'm, they're at the airport, they're leaving for Hawaii, she's got a coat on but that's 'cause it's cold, and you got to wear your coat to the airport. That's what we did and then my sister took our coats (laughing), you know, after we got on the plane. Oh no, they're packed they're going off, I bet you it could even be they look kind of young, maybe it's probably a second honeymoon, we used to go on like a honeymoon every year, at first, all we could afford was a weekend in a tent, you know, my mom used to take the kids, my mom and dad, but of course as we got, the kids left home, you know, we'd go to Hawaii or . . . Yeah, they're going on a second honeymoon. (What might they be thinking or feeling?) They can hardly wait to get out of those winter coats because they're going where it's warm and they're going to have a wonderful time. We had such a good time in Hawaii (laughing). Yeah, they're happy.

Unice is quite distressed in response to what is typically viewed as a very mild attachment scene. Unice launches into two parallel stories of couples going on a second honeymoon, failing to identify either couple. Their relationships evidence functional synchrony, although their excitement hints at mutual enjoyment in the hypothetical story without describing real togetherness. The response theme deactivates attachment by turning attention to the romantic implications of a second honeymoon. References to the sexual system in the AAP demonstrate representational attempts to neutralize attachment tension by refocusing on the sexual system. The desire to go someplace warm is also another sign of deactivation.

> ***Bed:*** Oh there's me. There's me and my dad, he's just got home from work a little bit the cold hands. Okay, and I'm happy to see him because he's going to put those cold hands on my stomach. (What might they be thinking and feeling?) They're obviously to see each other, oh, I know what might have happened, maybe the father had to work late, that's it, and the kids already had to go to bed so he's just come in, like, to say goodnight and they're happy to see him and they're going to tell him a bit about their day or whatever and then they'll go to sleep.

Attachment is activated by Unice's memories of her and her father in a mutually enjoyable, goal-corrected partnership. The description of father–child reunion is spontaneous, and the child is happy to see the father in both the hypothetical and personal experience story lines. The response also demonstrates the centrality of deactivating defenses in her representation of her relationship with her father (achievement–work; sleep). There is no evidence of cognitive disconnection or segregated systems in this response.

> ***Ambulance:*** Oh, somebody somebody's sick and they had to go in the ambulance . . . but that's okay, um, the ambulance will take them to the hospital and their family will go and visit them and they'll be fine. (What might they be thinking or feeling?) Oh, oh, they're probably worried or they're scared that something might be wrong, you know, they'll be much happier when they find out what's wrong but, um, once they do then they'll be fine.

The distressing story theme is this response is defined as illness. Distressed, Unice fails to identify the person on the stretcher, and the description of the two characters at the window is vague. They are presumably the sick person's "family." The stimulus dysregulates Unice's organized defenses; Unice's representation of illness generates fear. The family engages in functional care (they go visit). Unice's shift of attention to the sick person from the self is striking. Disconnected (worry) and deactivated (wrong), Unice circumvents the need for anyone to care for or comfort the child.

Unice was judged unresolved for loss on the AAI. Her interview demonstrated that she continued to be unsettled and somewhat disoriented regarding her father's death. Although there was some disorientation also evident in her discussion of her grandfather's death, her unresolved state of mind is clearly linked to her father.

The AAI coding rules require that all unresolved or anomalous AAIs are assigned an underlying (called "alternate") organized classification. Unice's underlying organized classification is secure. Her interview demonstrated many of the key features of security described in Chapter 6, including valuing attachment relationships and integrative thinking about her adult self in relation to her past. She stated that she was satisfied with her relationship with her mother now, saying that it was basically the same kind of relationship that she had with her mother when she was a child. "And even now if I if I have troubles I go to my mom, she always listens. She never tells me what to do." Unice genuinely values how her childhood upbringing has influenced her own parenting. She said that she gave her children the same things that her parents gave her.

The parallels between Unice's AAP and AAI are striking. Her stories depicted several satisfying attachment–caregiving interactions, and her response themes presented both a child's and a parent's perspective. The parent's behavior in *Corner* is not unlike her father's firm but kind response when she chose to leave home to go to her boyfriend and future husband. Her open distress and indices of representational dysregulation were evident only in those stories most closely associated with her personal history—her father's illness in the *Ambulance* story and her response to his death in *Cemetery*. Her response to the *Ambulance* scene is understandably more difficult for her, knowing the history of how her father died.

There was more evident distress in the AAP than in the AAI. Unice was not able to fully describe the qualities associated with integrated attachment agency and synchrony in any of the responses that followed the first stimulus. The AAP demonstrates a prominent underlying "layer" of tension and anxiety that is not evaluated in the AAI and would, therefore, be missed. Unice's struggle with her father's absence is noted as she corrects herself in *Departure* to include "dad," which she omitted in her parental statement. She consistently fails to identify characters, especially the projected self character. Her representational aloneness and inability to maintain self–other boundaries would not be evident in the

AAI. The AAP also revealed a defensive shift that seemed to be related to Unice's representation of self when alone versus when attachment–caregiving relationships are present. When others are present, Unice demonstrates a capacity for deactivation and distance (perhaps in support of perspective taking). When alone, Unice's main defensive strategy is to disconnect, often to pause to think, but also leaving her susceptible to segregated systems flooding.

Abby: Unresolved Abuse

Abby is a 49-year-old Caucasian woman, the eldest of three children. Her father's work took him away from home for long periods of time. Her mother had problems with alcohol and illness, and did not work outside the home. Her father had problems with alcohol, gambling, and womanizing. Her paternal grandmother took Abby and her siblings to live with her when she was 4. The children lived with their grandmother for 4 years, during which time her parents divorced. The children subsequently lived with their father and stepmother. Abby never married, although she had several long-term relationships with men. She did not have children.

Abby's description of her life as a child is a chronicle of terror and parental caregiving abdication. The first 4 years of her life were austere. Her mother was an alcoholic and always pregnant or sick; she could not work outside the home. Her father made good money, but Abby said his financial support was either "feast or famine," mostly famine. Abby's parents lived in many different communities during her early childhood. Their homes were big, beautiful houses that she called "a shell with nothing in it." The family owned very little furniture and they rarely had heat, food, or warm clothing. Abby's main memory of these years was "always being hungry, cold, and scared of my father."

Abby was unable to settle on how to describe her relationship with her mother. Her discussion portrayed her mother as both succeeding and failing to protect her. Her first memories of her mother were of her as a haven of safety—as Abby's only source of protection from her father's abuse. She described her father's presence when he was home as "a cyclone . . . he was so mean, he was scary, scary, frightful, I was frightened of him, my mother was frightened of him." Abby thought her mother had taken the brunt of his violence in order to protect her. Abby said her mother's protective stance began at the very beginning of her life when her mother refused her father's directive to have an abortion. Born in the flurry of her parents' move to a new community, Abby said she almost died at birth. She still remembered her mother holding her tightly and feeling protected. She described several incidents growing up in which her mother would shove her into small physical spaces in the house to block her father's attack. She thought their combined survival of her father's violence defined their strong mother–daughter bond. Yet she was also confused by the fact that she was not sure whom her mother was protecting. She said her mother was a "fragile," slight woman who did not have the strength to stand up to Abby's father. "So I don't know if she really was protecting me or protecting her so it's hard to know. I mean, if you're going to hide a kid in the basement, it's going to stop anybody in their tracks, don't you think? Him from hitting her and coming after me, I just don't know." Abby also stated that she knew that her mother couldn't protect her from her father forever. She hoped that the birth of her siblings would mean she would not be alone and would not get hurt anymore.

Her parents' marriage deteriorated and, at the risk of being placed in foster care, Abby's paternal grandmother raised the children in her home for 4 years. Abby and her siblings returned to her father's home when she was 8 years old. Her father's cruel physical abuse continued until she was a teenager. She described her stepmother as her father's jealous and spiteful collaborator. "He's a very violent man, and sometimes he would walk by and he would just hit me he would just catch me by the chin and my head would just go back and hit the wall . . . I can remember screaming at the top of my lungs while my stepmother is standing there with a smile across her face. My dad would be beating my brother to the point that he was bleeding, I swear to God they wanted to kill us. I, I do, I believe that to this day they really just didn't want us around, you know."

In spite of his brutality, Abby described how very much she wanted her father's love. She adored him as a young child and was heartbroken by his cool distance. She remembered sitting at his feet and gazing up at him or crawling up on his lap telling him that she loved him. She said he would usually swish her away. She remembered that even if she managed to get into his lap, she was confused by the fact that, while he was supposed to feel like her father, he felt like an "alien." She recalled feeling like she was being seduced when he came to give her a hug and then all she wanted to do was to get away from him.

Abby was closest to her paternal grandmother. "She said I wasn't going to let any one of my grandchildren go and be orphans, so she took us. We were fed, clothed, warm, and Grandma loved us." Abby remembered that her grandmother cared for her when she was sick; she bought

Abby books to read in bed when she had the measles. Her grandmother also intervened on the children's behalf when her grandfather threatened them with harsh spankings. Abby's grandmother, however, was not always a safe haven. Abby remembered her grandmother's punishment as painful. She said her grandmother would punch her or make her kneel on rice: "I remember picking rice out of my knees when I was a kid." Her grandmother was unsympathetic to anger and distress. Abby said she was once seriously hurt when she angrily punched her fist through a door. Her grandmother blamed the injury on Abby's anger and was not sympathetic. Abby said her only respite when she was distressed or angry was to hide under the bedcovers.

Separation punctuated Abby's childhood. Her mother was frequently hospitalized because of illness or childbirth; Abby stayed with her grandmother during these separations. Abby was frequently hospitalized as the result of her father's physical abuse. She said that being in the hospital was frightening and isolating. She had no memory of either parent visiting her in the hospital. She only remembered nurses "sewing her up." The nurses told her to close her eyes when she was frightened, but Abby said she could not close her eyes because not knowing what was going on was worse than seeing them treat her wounds.

Despite all of her hospitalizations, nobody ever said anything about Abby being abused. As a child, her best escape was to run to the park. "My escape was to a park, it wasn't too far from where we lived, and I used to get on the swing and I used to swing so high that I was hoping somehow by some grace that I would just fall off the swing and go to the sky and be gone." Her father's physical abuse became so bad when she was a teenager that she threatened to kill him. "My dad had just beat the living hell out of me and I said to him, next time you do that, I will kill you." Her father never hit her again.

Abby was sexually abused beginning in toddlerhood by her father and maternal grandfather. She said of her father, "Mmmm. I remember. I just wanted to be loved by him, I just wanted to be loved." The sexual abuse was not a central element in her interview; Abby noted as if listing a series of life events and provided little other information.

When asked about loss, Abby described her mother's and later her brother's sudden disappearances from the family. Her mother disappeared after one of her hospitalizations. She said this was confusing because she was a young child and her mother had always come home. She remembered the morning she discovered that her mother was missing. Her mother had gone into the hospital the day before and Abby found a new woman in her father's bedroom. Suddenly, without explanation, her mother was no longer there. Abby's brother disappeared when she was in high school. She said that she went to school to find him when he did not come home from school one day. The school counselor called home when Abby inquired about his whereabouts at school. "All hell broke loose for me doing that, I just, you know, what it is very hard, I just accepted that my brother was gone. It was devastating. I went to school and then he wasn't there."

Abby did not experience death when she was a child. Her grandfather died when she was a young teenager. She said she was "shaken up" when he died because she had dreamed about him the night before. An aunt died when she was in early 20s. She said she was not affected by her death.

Abby's adult life continued to be traumatic. She suffered from depression, and an eating disorder that began in middle childhood continued into her 40s. She has been in several abusive adult relationships and miscarried several times. She proposed that the miscarriages were ultimately a good thing because she was terrified of being an abusive mother. Her father, temporarily estranged from his wife, tried to seduce her during this time.

Abby's descriptions of her current relationships with her parents were haunted by the past. She said she had tried on several occasions to build an adult relationship with her mother. She said each time she would become frustrated and break off their interaction because her mother only wanted to dwell on her own victimization. Abby had not seen or talked with her mother for more than a decade before her interview. In a state Abby described as new "awareness" and "forgiveness," she had recently written to her mother asking for renewed contact. She was not hopeful that her mother would reply.

Abby had an adult relationship with her father. They talked on the phone or she visited him only when her stepmother was out of the house. Her father was unhappy that Abby was not married, telling her that he didn't want her to be alone. She said she told him to stop pestering her and reminded him that she had survived on her own her whole life. Abby sees her grandmother as her only real connection to the family. She said that she sends the family greeting cards and letters; although nobody replies, she said she had not given up hope.

Abby was judged unresolved on the AAP. Attachment figures who are frightening and abdicate their caregiving roles dominate her stories. Ominous elements of segregated terror, from helpless isolation to numbness, are conspicuous in every response. Her AAP responses demonstrate a representational cycle of dysregulation and containment. Although the characters in her stories are unable to signal their attachment distress to caregivers, there is some suggestion of protective maternal care and connectedness to alternate caregiving figures. In spite of these relationships, Abby's responses predominantly reflect her struggle with feelings of horrific isolation.

Alone Stories

Abby's representational self is beset with feelings of fear and isolation. The opening theme in each of her alone stories is the self in danger. The segregated systems material expressed in these stories are unusually extreme as compared with typical AAP responses. Abby struggles with multiple and contradictory representations of self and attachment figures. Although she shows some capacity to handle distress, her stories suggest that she can only hope that attachment figures will detect her distress because she is unable to communicate it to them. She is not able to recover from the feelings of intense isolation and numbness associated with *Bench* and *Cemetery*. In the end, Abby demonstrates that her survival depends solely on her ability to protect herself. She relies on defensive cognitive disconnection. Not a sturdy defense in the face of fear, disconnection at least defuses and blurs Abby's state of fear into confusion.

> ***Window:*** Oh man . . . this is a little girl looking out for someone, to come and be with her—she looks very forlorn there, alone . . . she doesn't have any shoes on, that's familiar, and it even looks like her hands might be in her pockets, although I'm not able to see her face I think she's a sad little girl. (What might have led up to the scene?) Something could have happened, she could have been disciplined rightly or wrongly . . . she could be missing her mom or her dad, or she could just simply be taking a quiet moment out, I mean there's a lot of ways of looking at this. More so I say this is a sad thing, that something has happened that she's been disciplined in some way and probably wants to get away, maybe wants to be on the outside instead of on the inside. (What might happen next?) Well, maybe Mom will come up to her and put her arms around her and ask her if she's okay or maybe Dad will come up and say get to your room, you're wasting time. Yeah.

Abby immediately becomes dysregulated. The girl is "forlorn" (segregated system), a frightening emotional state that goes beyond sadness. We observe that the intensity of the girl's hopeless and desperate situation is indicative in the AAP of intense dysregulation that we have found to be associated with physical and psychological trauma. An attempt to organize distress by creating emotional distance backfires; the girl's discipline (deactivation) is identified as the source of her forlorn state. Only disconnecting defenses help Abby stay organized. Portrayed as disconnected representational opposites, the girl's hope for the mother's care (haven of safety) directly conflict with her father's cruel rejection. Representations of mother and father are not integrated and agency of self is undermined—the girl does not have the agency to remove herself from the source of her distress (i.e., no capacity to act).

> *Bench:* This is [sister], oh my, it's [my sister] allright, this is how [sister] spent her years as a teenager learning how to hide (crying), she just didn't feel she had anything to offer, to give, that she was a bad person, sad and lonely, asked too many questions couldn't do anything right . . . had no friends, had very few friends, she's very dejected, rejected. (What might happen next?) She might just get up from that bench and walk away, without really acknowledging where she was, how she was really feeling.

This scene of the alone self essentially renders Abby defenseless. Overwhelmed by the stimulus, Abby's is flooded by segregated affective memory. She is quite distressed as she exclaims, "This is [sister] oh my, it's [sister] allright." She portrays her sister as hiding because she felt so "very dejected" and "rejected" (segregated systems), thus isolated without connection to other people. Abby seamlessly shifts to describing the hypothetical character after the prompt, presumably with feelings about her sister's desperation serving as the background for the remainder of her response. There is no evidence of organizing defenses in either the personal or the hypothetical threads. Abby can envision the projected self as having the capacity to act and move away from the source of her distress. She gets up (agency). Agency is defined as the representational state of taking action to create change. Abby describes the character's action as if she was numb, "without really acknowledging where she was, how she was really feeling" (segregated system), which undermines agency. Neither the personal or hypothetical threads of this response are contained. Segregated feeling continues to flood Abby and her response is unresolved.

> *Cemetery:* So it looks like that maybe Mom might have died, if we're to take it from this picture. This is obviously a man, he's at a

> graveyard and someone close to him has passed on, and ah, he looks like the, he's sad he's lonely—empty, what do I do now . . . maybe even confused, at a loss. And he might just walk away without feeling all those feelings and he'll move on with his life or he'll stay with the parents, or he may not even be feeling anything, maybe he has no concept of what he's really feeling, it's so he's a little better although he's got his hands in his pockets, it could be a sign of holding something back.

Abby is immediately dysregulated as indicted by the personal intrusion statement "Mom might have died." She tries to recover with the phrase "If we're to take it from this picture"; however, the absence of a specifying pronoun (i.e., the mom) is evidence in the AAP of an intrusive shift in attention to personal experience. The process of telling this man's story (i.e., her projected self) unleashes feelings of intense isolation associated with his loss (segregated systems). The remainder of the response illustrates Abby's struggle to disconnect from and contain the emptiness. Abby contextualizes his confusion (cognitive disconnection) in numbing fear—he is "confused" (segregated systems). Representational fear is contained and reorganized by the man's potential to stay with his parents (capacity to act). As in *Window*, Abby fractures representational agency (cognitive disconnection by introducing another story ending) and the numbness of being "without feeling" leaks back into her story (segregated systems). Abby seems to know that she is on the edge of disintegration at the end of the story as evidenced by her description of the man as "holding something back" (cognitive disconnection). The story is judged unresolved because the intrusion of her mother's possible death at the beginning of the story is never contained.

> ***Corner:*** Oh, this is in a different light . . . he keeps putting his hands up to protect himself from being hurt some way, and ah . . . (What might they be thinking or feeling?) I think he's feeling very frightened and, ah, so frightened that he can't even look at the one who might be coming at him, ah, he's got his hands up and it could be to protect him but it's not going to help, and he's thinking, ah, I'm toast, I'm going to get it so I may as well just not look at and just take it, just take it. (What might happen next?) He'll get very hurt, physically . . . he'll just get crushed and will turn back. Well, that was real positive (laughing), no, I'm just thinking of myself, that's really interesting.

Abby is very distressed by this stimulus and immediately launches into a story of the potential annihilation of self. The boy character is desperately frightened by the threat of being hurt and crushed—"I'm toast" (segregated systems). The character and perpetrator are never identified clearly. Abby's representation of protective agency of self is the only action that keeps him alive—"he keeps putting his hands up to protect himself." This active protective attempt does describe agency in the form of the capacity to act in the AAP, even if it does not stop the abuse. It is this act of self-protection that keeps Abby going forward. As with her other alone responses, Abby is not able to stay completely attuned to the hypothetical story without being distracted her own memories. The self-reference is oblique and she is not flooded, but the intensity with which these stimuli flood her consciousness is clear.

Dyadic Stories

Abby's responses to the dyadic stimuli depict parental figures as cruel and isolating. Segregated systems material is visible in each story and is unusually intense. The level of overwhelming fear activated by representations of dyad relationships is almost impossible for Abby to contain. The *Ambulance* story demonstrates her representational capacity to view care as functional, but there is no evidence in these dyadic responses of representations of self as involved in integrated dyadic synchrony (i.e., comfort or mutual enjoyment). As in the alone stories, Abby's main defensive posture is cognitive disconnection. The deactivation evident in the *Ambulance* story shifts attention away from potential self distress and, given the intensity of the story, is likely an indicator of Abby's failed mourning of her mother.

> **Departure:** Hmm, this looks like my father who's just leaving his date (laughing) for the day or whatever that might be, I've seen this so many times. Um, hands in their pockets so they're keeping their distant, there's sadness there, there's, um, emptiness, loneliness, seems as though they might have had an argument or don't want to part but have to, um . . . (What might happen next?) Oh, they'll go their separate ways, the woman may be crying or just on the verge of crying and the man could be sad too, or maybe walk away knowing he's had a great success that he's got another woman to cry over him.

Abby's is overwhelmed by her father's cruelty (segregated system) and anger (cognitive disconnection). She again seamlessly shifts from the personal story to the hypothetical thread, continuing to be dysregulated by the representational presence of her father's malice and power to make a woman cry (segregated system). Abby unsuccessfully attempts to disconnect segregated fears by introducing a story line in which the characters are so unhappy that they are forced to part. The segregated story line overwhelms her and she cannot shift away from it. Neither the personal nor the hypothetical threads contain or reorganize Abby's traumatic dysregulation. The response is judged unresolved.

> *Bed:* Hmm . . . this is me wanting [stepmother] to kiss me good night, to tuck me in, to tell me sweet dreams to tell me that she loved me (crying), to just say throughout the night I didn't have to beg my dad, and that's her she's just sitting there and I'm reaching out reaching out, taunting me with her presence, oh . . . she'll just leave the room, I'll lay down and cry, bang my head, rock myself to sleep.

This stimulus is so overwhelming that Abby can only describe her personal desperation. Her pitiful craving for her stepmother's kindness to save her from her father is answered with taunting cruel silence (segregated system). Abby describes her only resource as self-harm.

> *Ambulance:* Well, it looks like a grandmother. Looks like somebody is, ah, going to a hospital, this could be my mother. Having gone to the hospital and I didn't get to see her. I don't know, in this one it looks like the person might have died . . . just by the posture of the paramedic, and the posture of the grandma and the posture of the body there, looks like more of a final thing than just someone going to the hospital, I'm thinking, I don't know. Well, she might get to go live with Grandma, or not, or they might be stuck with whoever's there whether it's Mom or Dad on that stretcher.

As Abby begins her response, she is flooded by the memory of not being able to see her mother when she went to the hospital. She shifts back to the hypothetical ambulance scene as she discusses the potential theme of death, disconnecting from the stimulus intensity and creating a moment of emotional distance by describing paramedics, a typical element of ambulance-based care (deactivation). Identifying the child character as "she" (the projected self), Abby is confused by the representational opposites (cognitive disconnection). The potential for the grandmother's functional care (functional synchrony) is threatened by the possibility of being stuck (segregated system) living with the parent.

Abby was judged unresolved for physical abuse on the AAI. Her continuing disorientation with regard to her father's abuse, despite claims that she was reorganizing her life, was evident in the interview. Furthermore, although she professed to understand that her abuse was not her fault, her discussion was unconvincing. She continued to believe that her father's attacks were caused by something she did wrong as a child, but she was unable to figure out exactly what this was because his rage was so unpredictable. Her father never acknowledged his abuse at any point in Abby's lifetime, and she had never been able to confront him or even talk to him about it. Abby's mother was absorbed in her own victimization, which Abby claimed blinded her to Abby's victimization by her father. She said that her mother only wanted a relationship based on past violence and Abby wanted to get beyond this and build what she thought might be a real mother–daughter relationship. Another indication of Abby's unresolved state of mind was her fear of becoming an abuser in her own relationships and her confusion as to why she chose adult partners who terrorized her.

Abby was not judged unresolved with regard to sexual abuse. She was not demonstrably overwhelmed when asked to describe these experiences. She has since learned of generations of male sexual abuse in her mother's family. Her brief discussion of molestation by her father in toddlerhood was confused with her desire for love. She declared that she had "turned the tables" on her father when she knowingly permitted him to seduce her as an adult. She said that her decision placed her in the position of taking revenge on her evil stepmother, even though neither she nor her father ever spoke to anyone about their affair.

Abby was not unresolved for loss. Abby's only real losses were her grandfather and her aunt. These deaths really did not affect her, even though she was somewhat disoriented by the memory of her grandfather before his death. Rather, her representation of loss was the disappearance of her mother and brother from her life as a child, which she likened to actual losses. Abby later accidentally found them while trying to correct some family legal documents. Her brother rejoined the family, and she has since learned the details of his disappearance. This was not the case for her mother.

Abby was judged "failure to mourn" regarding her mother.[3] Her descriptions suggest that she continues to be numb regarding her moth-

[3] Hamilton-Oravetz and George (1991, published in Hamilton-Oravetz, 1992).

er's "loss." She either has not been told anything about the context of her mother's disappearance and/or she has no memories of it. Until Abby was asked about her current relationship with her parents, there was scant mention of her mother during the interview after describing her mother's disappearance. Clearly, her parents had divorced and her father remarried, and she had visited her maternal grandparents. But her mother seemed to have become invisible to her until her discovery in adulthood.

Abby's inability to maintain boundaries between her own story and the AAP stories confirm the degree to which the AAP responses portray her experiences with attachment figures. She was judged unresolved in the stories in which she depicted cruelty in the absence of caring adults. Her view of her mother as protective and comforting in the AAI is confirmed by the image of the mother in *Window*. Her stories echo, both in the personal experience and hypothetical threads, her father's and stepmother's cruelty, confusion about discipline, her grandmother's functional care, and her view of herself as her only protector. The feelings associated with loss in response to her mother's disappearance are evident in two responses. In *Cemetery*, Abby's intrusion confirms her feelings that her mother was dead. Abby's failure to mourn this loss is evidenced in *Ambulance*. The death theme and the terror of living with the surviving parent are distanced by deactivation, which is the prototype of failed mourning in the AAP. The failed mourning is evidenced also in that Abby seems to know that the projected self in this response is holding something back.

The AAP shows a somewhat different representational self than that portrayed in her AAI. Abby claimed with great pride during the AAI that she could now stand her ground with her father and not succumb to being driven "crazy" by his cruelty and rejection. She also claimed that she still adored her father, but that she drew the line with him finally when he refused to respect her privacy. "He'd say, well, we're family, you don't need privacy, yeah I do, he would just not take no, finally I looked at him what part of no don't you get, and he said you know, I got to teach you, and I said there is nothing that you have to teach me."

By contrast, Abby's AAP responses demonstrate that she neither has agency nor personal strength with regard to her father. There is no evidence of fatherly adoration in the AAP. Instead, Abby was overwhelmed by terror and threatened annihilation in response to scenes she associationed with her father. The AAP responses show concretely just how little progress Abby has made in reconstructing her disintegrated self and mourning her mother's loss.

Paul: Preoccupation with Personal Suffering

Paul is a Caucasian 30-year-old college student and the youngest of three siblings. His father, a minister, and his mother, a teacher, divorced when he was 7. His father soon remarried. Paul and his siblings all lived with their mother until Paul was 11 years old, at which time his brother left to live with their father.

Paul has few distinct memories of his parents before their divorce other than unpleasantness because he said his parents "did not get along." It was clear from his AAI that his parents were neither a haven of safety nor a secure base. After the divorce, his mother tried to prevent the father from seeing Paul and his siblings. He recalled that his father once broke into the house in order to see them. Paul said that he "shut down" after the divorce and became quiet and introverted. His grandparents were not present in his life. Elderly friends of his mother acted as "surrogate" grandparents, but they were not involved in a caregiving role.

After the divorce, Paul described his relationship with his mother as one of "incomplete trust" and himself as his mother's "surrogate husband." He took care of her. Their discussions centered on practical family matters, such as finances. He made meals and played the piano to soothe her to sleep at the end of a tiring workday. He said that he did not mind going along with this new role because he tends to be a "pleaser" and shied away from angry confrontations. He wanted family life to "flow along smoothly."

Paul lamented that his mother was a shallow communicator, which he interpreted as the result of her personal life stress. She also frequently yelled at him. He said that she would later explain that she wasn't really yelling at him but was frustrated and tired by work. This was a logical explanation, but not an apology. Paul said that she yelled so often that he learned to "tune her out to shut her off."

Paul believed that one of the biggest issues in their relationship was his mother's inability to discuss sexuality and sex when he was a young teenager. She was unwilling to answer his many questions. He was angry, disappointed, and frustrated by his mother's unwillingness to talk frankly about sex. Instead, she would give Paul directives about healthy male behavior, which she would not explain. "I had a lot of questions, especially sexually related, and, I mean I threw her an easy tester question, and she wouldn't even answer that one, so, it was like how could I trust her with any other questions, that were impacting me a lot more. So I essentially just gave up on her from that perspective."

Paul was unsettled during the interview, noticing that his descriptions of his mother were primarily negative. He stated that he needed to think of some "wonderful" descriptors for her as well. This produced descriptions of his mother as encouraging him and being proud of his accomplishments in school and the arts. Yet as he described her in this more positive light, he remembered that she primarily expressed her pride only in public settings where other people could hear her talk about her son. He wished she would have told him directly and lamented that he did not understand why that was so hard for her. Compliments directed toward him, such as "I still love you" or "I'm still really proud of you" were embedded in her chronic complaints about her life.

His mother provided functional care when Paul was sick. He remembered that she stayed home from work. He said that he had to go to bed, but had a bell that he could ring if he needed her. She would bring Paul ginger ale or chicken soup to help him feel better.

Paul thought he grew up in his brother's shadow. His brother was sickly as a young child, and Paul remembered playing alone on the sidelines while his mother cared for his brother. When Paul went to school, his brother was popular and he said even his own friends preferred to play with his brother. Paul said he did not have "the space to define who he was until his brother left" to live with their father. In short, Paul's memories suggested that he rarely had satisfying interactive experiences with his mother or his peers.

Paul's relationship with his father was even less satisfying. He described their relationship as distant, and Paul had no memories of his father prior to his parents' divorce. He said that he missed his father when he left and hoped he would divorce his new wife and return home. He said their physical and emotional distance made it difficult for him to tell his father about his life. He only visited his father a few times a year, and when he did, Paul was hurt that his father did not make a special time for them to be together. "It wasn't that he took time out of his schedule to spend time with us, but rather he just kind of brought us along with whatever he was doing. That was kind of frustrating because, it's like, he seemed to make very little time."

This distance fostered what Paul called a "shallow" relationship. According to Paul, they talked very little and were always interrupted. "Even then, that didn't always happen because—I mean, we were sort of, doing what, you know, whatever we were doing at home and he was packing getting ready to and do, you know, go to church, to run some errands, or go into town to buy the groceries or go to the garbage dump, whatever, and then bang, okay, so—we were all busy getting ready to go and do that, and then bang we'd be in the car, and he'd sort of, almost, switch gears and assume that I was ready to just be open and talk about whatever, and—obviously you know, most people aren't just able to switch gears off the cuff like that, and so—I mean, sure, there were the times when we were able to talk during car rides, but there were times where I wasn't able to."

Paul said he longed for a real father figure in his life. He sadly recalled that a family friend took him to father–son camp. Although impressed that the friend thought he was important enough to spend time with, he also had to face the fact that his father did not feel the same way. Paul believed that his father tried to buy his children's affection to make up for his unavailability. But he complained that the presents his father sent never arrived on time, or he would just send money.

Paul didn't recall going to either parent when he was hurt. He did not remember getting physically hurt much as a child, so there would have been no reason to seek their care for injuries. He said that he did not see much point in telling his parents about emotional upsets because, for example, his "mother wouldn't know what to do anyway." His remedy was to go to his room. He managed his upsets by punching a pillow or playing games. "I would play one person as my left hand, and one person as my right hand . . . emotionally just to deal with stuff, I would—I mean essentially shut down, from either parent, and just go pull out a board game and go to my room, and play by myself, and avoid the . . . it was probably a safe haven, so to speak, it was a place where I felt I could go, and be unheard, unseen, unspoken, whatever, and probably at times, hopefully unnoticed."

Paul's only memory of separation involved his parents' divorce, which he said seriously affected him. When asked about loss, Paul's immediate response was to describe the divorce. "I really didn't understand what was going on, all I knew was . . . I was . . . not comfortable and I couldn't understand what was going on, and it was confusing and it was frustrating, and I'd just wish he was there . . . I almost wonder sometimes if that was so impacting that anything before that got blotted out of my memory."

Paul's only experience with death was the loss of older relatives and friends. His grandmother died when he was 5. His family had visited her regularly but Paul said he was not close to her. His other grandmother died when he was 19. Paul's surrogate grandparents also died around this time. He described feeling hurt by the fact that he was not able to visit his surrogate grandfather much when his health started to decline. Paul cried at the funeral and his death "allowed me to realize that it was okay to have feelings. And, and that was probably one of the first times, I got an inkling, or a grasp of, what love actually means. What it meant to love someone. And how it really hurt, to, to feel that loss when they, when they died." What impressed Paul most about his surrogate grandmother's funeral was that listening to what people were saying about her made him realize he really did not know her.

Paul vaguely alluded to physical mistreatment as a young child, but his memories were obscure. He could not describe the experience, and he could not figure out whether it was abuse. He remembered in his mind's eye having bruises on his legs and arms around the time his parents first separated when he was a young child. He thought that his mother was the mostly likely source, which at one point during the interview he associated with his what he called his mother's "physical assault." He was adamant, though, that he did not have the "slightest clue" how often this occurred or if his siblings similarly had bruises. He remembered being uncomfortable, but did not know what he did about these injuries. "I think part of it too is that, I wouldn't have known what to do, or how to react". He thinks his response to these experiences was to "shut down" and he had no idea if he was outwardly emotional or not.

Paul was sexually molested at age 12 by his cousin when he was visiting his father's home. He addressed the experience directly during the interview, but did not provide much detail. He explained that he did not feel threatened or frightened. He said he just went along with it because he trusted his cousin and he got used to it. He said their trysts made him feel like a man. His cousin abruptly curtailed their activities, which left Paul terribly confused. He then pursued several other teen boys but could not understand their shocked reactions and the imperative to keep their sexual activity a secret. Paul's confusion about sex and sexuality only increased. He said that he had a lot of questions and was distressed by being alone without anyone to talk to. "So like, for my, the sexual abuse, it only ever happened three times, but it was, very, very significant, so it made a huge impact. These events were very sexually repressing because I wasn't allowed to talk about it, I was supposed to just grow up and deal with it myself, without anybody telling me."

Paul recalled that he had not thought his cousin's sexual behavior was abuse until he read about the definition and signs of sexual abuse in an educational pamphlet. He said he was stunned by the revelation that his cousin's acts were considered sexually abusive. His self-view had suddenly been redefined as an abuse victim and subsequently as a perpetrator. Paul sought spiritual guidance and had attended sexual abuse and sexual dysfunction groups for the past 5 years. He was resolute that these therapeutic experiences provided him with a more solid understanding of these experiences and also the capacity for forgiveness. He said he had since forgiven his cousin, and his therapy had given him more perspective on his emotional life. "I got a better grasp of my emotions . . . I was so distant from my parents, did that sort of, somehow shove down my sense of, feeling emotions. And therefore my emotions either—weren't there, or didn't react, or came in kind of later (laughs) after the fact. And were delayed somehow."

Paul firmly stated that he was not emotionally close with either parent as an adult. He wanted to forgive them but had not yet achieved this goal. He thought he had made more progress in this direction with his father. He had talked to his father about his therapeutic transformation, which led his father to express his regret that about his absence in Paul's childhood. Paul was disparaging when he described his father's ignorance of the meaning of relating. He said that he had let go of his desire for his real father. As the result of therapy, he turned to his spiritual "father" to answer his questions. Paul had made little progress in forgiving his mother. He said he continued to be affected by how much she yelled at him as a child and he did not want to spend time with her. "It's going a lot slower, in terms of being able to love her or appreciate her. I still have a lot of low-lying or residual, um, anger I guess, frustration toward her, that, that I, not fully letting go of yet."

Paul's AAP indicated traumatic preoccupation. We see in Paul's responses how his reliance on cognitive disconnection is ineffective in staving off intense feelings of helplessness and pain. Indeed, disconnection fractures themes of attachment failure to such an extent that he has no representational capacity to "see" it, even though these elements are plainly visible in his responses. It may be said of individuals with dysregulated disconnecting defenses that they are "living in the war zone" of their trauma, often without realizing the extent to which their trauma defines attachment relationships and the self. As we noted in Chapter 5, one defining feature of cognitive disconnection is the unintegrated representation of opposing feeling states. In this regard, Paul's transcript is striking in the juxtaposition of terror and hope. Although elements of dyadic interactions are similarly disconnected, his stories nonetheless suggest that attachment figures and surrogate attachment figures provide the functional care he needs to keep his terror at bay.

Alone Stories

The most striking feature of Paul's alone responses is disconnection from fear and helplessness in an effort to create an illusion of safety through hope. The alone responses neither demonstrate clear agency of self nor connectedness to others in meaningful relationships. Attachment figures, when identified, are dangerous, and neither the capacity for action nor the ability to signal for help is evident in his stories. In the face of trauma, dysregulated disconnecting processes mask the vulnerability and terror of finding himself alone. Paul is unable to confront his fears with agency of self. With no ability to reorganize and integrate his own distress, he is threatened with feelings of fragile aloneness. His primary strategy is hope, hoping that he can decrease the visibility of fear and pain until someone notices and saves him. He is not confident, though, but he believes that chronic hope will keep him from becoming totally helpless and out of control.

> ***Window:*** A girl staring out the window, that kind of brings back the whole concept of my dad leaving, you know, kind of like, a child, a child standing at the window, it looks like it's, it's probably a child standing there being reflective, thinking about something, that happened, or looking out the window noticing something that's going on and, and, not being involved. Possibly, um, one of those, daylight hour things, where it's 11 o'clock at night and the sun is still shinning, and the kid doesn't understand why they have to go to bed (laughs), when other kids get to stay out and play (laughs). (What might happen next?) In that specific situation? They probably have to go to bed because it's late.

Paul's mention of his own father at the beginning of the response suggests that this element figures prominently in the telling of his hypothetical story. Without knowing Paul's personal story, we would not know that his father's leaving was viewed as akin to his father having died. He leaves it to the interviewer to interpret the meaning of this event rather than describing it explicitly. The story epitomizes AAP representations of a passive, incapable self. The girl in this story ends up doing something that she does not want to do. References to potential actions and outcomes are almost meaningless because cognitive disconnecting defenses severely fracture and confuse the situation. Paul seems to know that "thinking" is important, but his empty and convoluted description of internal work belies evidence of an internalized secure base. In other words, Paul does not have the capacity in this situation to explore and potentially transform the self. His response shows layer upon layer of cognitive disconnection that can only increase the confusion about what is going on. Her stares (cognitive disconnection) lead to two plot lines (cognitive disconnection). The description of the girl's internal work is diluted by pseudo-thinking language (reflective); she is reflecting/thinking about some unspecified topic. We note how the second plot line suggests that she has only noticed something going on, an activity that has the quality of distraction because of her lack of involvement. There is no evidence of Paul's capacity to represent the self as engaged in active agency. The girl's final activity does not originate from within the self—they have to go to bed. The origin of her behavior is unknown. Did someone else tell her to go to bed? Or perhaps she went to bed because this was the general expectation. What we do know is that she is disconnected from this action because she goes to bed somewhat unwillingly and does not understand why (cognitive disconnection).

> ***Bench:*** That looks like a woman who's been abused (laughs) in some way or another, either, uh, not necessarily, but could be. Could also be some woman who's just simply upset or disappointed, needs some time (laughs) alone. (Now, can you tell me a story about it?) Well, let's go with the abused one (laughs). Um . . . (What lead up to this?) She's probably been, um, through a situation of abuse, whether it be a husband, or a boyfriend, or, some other, I'm, I'm just sort of, assuming, and, a male abuser. Um, and uh, so she's finally gotten to a point where that abuser is no longer around and she can cower (small laugh), hide, and cry, and . . . attempt to deal with the emotional stress of what has just happened. (What will happen next?) In the majority of situations (laughs), the abuser will come back and it will go on again. Um, my hope for her would be that she might finally be at a place where she can realize that she doesn't have to put up with this anymore. And that there are people out there that she can call and talk to, and, hopefully get the, you know, dealt with, and sorted with, sorted through whatever. And at least begin the long painful process of recovery.

Paul is immediately dysregulated. He begins with the story describing the projected self as abused and helpless. He shifts away from this frightening theme by introducing a different, less distressing story line (cognitive disconnection). He had the opportunity to change the story, but returned to the abuse theme following the prompt. Fears associated with attachment figure abuse (husband or boyfriend) elicit images of the woman cowering and hiding, rendered helpless by her fear (segregated systems). Paul then mutes the tension by shifting away from the story to describing what he understands to be a well-known rule regarding abusers. The woman's future hinges on the hope that she will get help and find people she can talk to in order to understand her situation. There is a hint of potential agency as he hopes the woman "can realize" that she can get help by connectedness to helpful strangers (i.e., not people in the committed relationship). Paul's hope that the woman can take action (agency) contains his attachment distress and prevents him from having to face vulnerability and fear. In the story ending, he parenthetically acknowledges that "recovery" involves more pain.

> ***Cemetery:*** First thing that jumps into my mind is a man whose wife has died. And, is, uh, is feeling a deep sense of loss, uh, from no longer having someone who he has deeply loved, to be with him. Um, it's, I mean, I, there's no kids in the picture, so whether he has kids or not, is hard to say, but, um, obviously if he did, then, you know, the thought of having to be a single parent, and all the plethora of stress (laughs) that could bring on. If there were no kids involved then, and um, possibly just, wondering what's going to happen next being alone, and to have to face being alone, to not have someone to be with anymore.

Paul's response focuses on the emotional intensity of loss. Although Paul introduces possibilities for what might come next in the man's life, his disconnected defensive transformations essentially render the man conflicted and caught between two life or story endings (cognitive disconnection). Paul's description of each possible ending introduces another layer of cognitive disconnection as he becomes increasingly confused and distressed. The possibility of being a single parent is stressful (cognitive disconnection). The possibility of being alone without children is confusing (cognitive disconnection). In the end, the character lacks the agency required to handle his distress. We are left with the image of a confused and distressed man not knowing what to do as he confronts his loss.

> ***Corner:*** Uh, um (laughs), that looks like, another abused kid, standing in the corner, possibly, um, even still current, probably still in some kind of a, a situation that is currently happening, that is some kind of abuse. Um, whether it be verbal, or possibly emotional, or physical, um, perhaps sexual, but it, but because he's standing up with clothes on I would (small laugh) probably say not. Um, but, you know, could be. Anyway, um, just having the sense that whatever is

> going on, is not right. But having no idea what to do, nowhere to go, no one to go to, no ability to keep that person from doing whatever to this little boy, person, girl, child, helpless confusion, whatever. So essentially completely defenseless. (What happens next?) In this particular situation, probably the abuser comes in, and, once again, does whatever kind of abuse that they do, to this child . . . You kind of hope for this child that there's going to be someone else, somehow intervene and, and find out what's going on, so as to stop it from happening. Um, kind of hope there's going to be someone there that's going to be able to somehow counsel this child into gaining some kind of an understanding of what's been happening, and what's happened and how to get over it . . . I mean it, it looks like in the near future, for this child, that, you know, the abuse will probably continue, but again, you hope that that's (laugh) not going to go on forever.

Paul immediately identifies this stimulus with ongoing abuse, describing the situation as "still current" and "currently happening." He stumbles through a long description of segregated systems indices of terror, fixated on the child's feelings of confusion, helplessness, and vulnerability in this cycle of abuse. The kid has "no idea what to do, nowhere to go, no ability to keep that person from doing." He is "completely defenseless." The "abuser comes in and . . . does whatever kind of abuse that they do." This quality of repeated and intense description in the AAP is often associated with extremely frightening experiences, even though the details of the abuse are not described (Buchheim et al., 2008a; Buchheim & George, 2011). The child in this story has no agency and is essentially at the perpetrator's mercy. Paul's solution is to try to disconnect from the trauma and save the child with the hope that the situation will not go on forever (cognitive disconnection—uncertain). Once again, we see how cognitive disconnection transforms terror into hope to create a situation in which someone will notice Paul's distress and intervene on his behalf when he is incapable of even the slightest agency to signal his need for care.

Dyadic Stories

In contrast to the threats associated with being alone, Paul's representations of dyadic relationships suggest feelings of safety through proximity to others. The interactions in these relationships demonstrate functional synchrony without evidence of integration. That is, the projected self receives basic care without mutual enjoyment or comfort. Again, Paul's main organizing defense is cognitive disconnection. His confusion blurs his ability to see what is really happening. Fractured and unsettled, the tension and nervousness described in the dyadic responses belie underlying trauma.

> ***Departure:*** That looks like either, parents going on a trip, or it could be, it almost looks like two university-age people, possibly going to university, or something. Um, I'd say it looks more like the latter, because they look more younger than older, so it's almost like, um, two college-age people, heading off to university, or getting home from university or whatever. Um, one of those, sitting at the bus stop scenarios, waiting for the bus to come. (What are they thinking and feeling?) If I were to relate that, to times when, um, like okay, um . . . if, if we say that it's, um, going off to college, or whatever, with suitcases, then he's probably thinking of, what's gone on in the last few days, or the last week, whatever, however long he's been, for example, he's been at home, I mean that's just, what I would think from my, situation. But uh, um . . . kind of a little bit of anxiousness about what's going to happen, uncertainty about what's going to happen, um, knowing that it's time to move on. And that whatever has happened is, you know it's essentially got to be over so, for the sake of, moving on and . . . (What will happen next?) Well, either the bus comes along and takes them away or they carry the luggage up to their new university room (laughs) and go their separate ways, and uh, go on with whatever life, new phase of life they're going to experience, whatever.

Paul's response represents the hope associated with beginning a new life using functional synchrony in the peer group (i.e., affiliative system) as an instrument of change. These peers are beginning their life as university students. The potential for change is simultaneously anxiety provoking and exciting. Settling on this plot line is evidence of Paul's ability to create distance from parents by focusing his attention on achievement goals, which are associated in the story with references to going to university (deactivation). Paul's attempt to deactivate parental distress, however, is incomplete as it leaks through into the situation and the new peer relationship. He develops two opposite story ideas—the characters are either heading off to or arriving at university (cognitive disconnection). The characters are waiting, which introduces an element of pause that is evidence of uncertainty in the AAP (cognitive disconnection). The situation is associated with anxiety, which is evidence of entangling relationship tension (cognitive disconnection). The story is now quite fractured, and we see that Paul is not able to maintain the idea of the projected self in a functional dyadic peer relationship. The students either stay together on the bus or they go their separate ways and start their new lives alone (cognitive disconnection).

> ***Bed:*** That looks like, uh, the parent has just finished reading a story to the child, and the child is now wanting his final goodnight hug and kiss before she tucks him in, or he tucks her, or him in. I don't know, so, before she tucks him in, tonight, to, or for bed, for the night, she shuts off the light. Then she tucks him in and he goes to sleep. (What are they thinking or feeling?) (Laughs) The mother's thinking, oh, I'm so exhausted, will you please just go to sleep, so I can have, uh, a few minutes, to, to get, to catch my breath from the day. And (laughs) the kid is thinking, um, um, I love you Mummy and I'm scared of the dark, and I don't want you to leave, but . . . I know it's time to go to sleep, so I'll go to sleep (laughs).

Paul describes a common AAP nighttime scene. A child is going to bed and signals his need to complete the separation from his attachment figure with affectionate caregiving. The boy wants a "final goodnight hug and kiss." Paul immediately interrupts his description of child–parent interaction (cognitive disconnection) and shifts his attention to the details of the mother's lengthy preparatory activities. The mother finally "tucks him in, which" demonstrates that she has capacity to accurately interpret his bid for closeness. He portrays the mother as entangled (cognitive disconnection) in the relationship to the extent of exhaustion and craving relief. The projected self risks dysregulation during the moments of separation by his mother's tension and insensitivity, and his incapacity to tell his mother that is afraid. Typically, fear in response to this AAP stimulus is implied (e.g., bad dream) or described as a nightmare. This boy is afraid of the dark. Bowlby (1973) described being alone in the dark as one of the most frightening of human experiences. The mother's functional care before leaving is sufficient evidence in the AAP to demonstrate that the boy's fear was contained. Functional care can keep fear at bay in the absence of sensitive comfort. We also see from the description of the boy's "thinking" that he knows what is expected of him—he is expected to go to sleep (deactivation). Paul's view of functional dyadic care is that he ultimately must distance himself from his fear in order to manage his fears with little help from attachment figures.

> ***Ambulance:*** That looks like, probably a grandmother and a grandson, looking out the window, and probably, or assumingly it could

> be, one of his parents. And possibly the grandmother's son or daughter, who for some reason is going into the ambulance, and being taken off to the hospital, um, for some reason or another. Obviously, some physical ailment, that's (laughs) . . . (What are the characters in this story thinking or feeling?) They're probably, the grandmother and grandson are probably both scared and nervous, um, the . . . the boy's probably wondering if his mom or dad is going to die. And the grandmother, um, has probably been around enough to realize that they're probably not going to die, but it's uncertain as to what the outcome may be. And uh, she's probably been around long enough to know that things like this happen, and would somehow be able to give some kind of words of encouragement to the grandson. (What will happen next?) Depends on how skilled they are at the hospital. Um, obviously there's going to be some time of nervousness and uncertainty, until they actually hear back from the hospital- to know, what happened, what's going on, or how, if there's any kind of surgery that has to go on, you know, what's going to happen there. So obviously there's going to be some, emotional roller coaster that perhaps both the grandmother and the grandson will be feeling, until they actually get some kind of word back. Uh, obviously if it's good word back from the hospital then, um, they'll both be relieved, and happy. And if it's not, good words, like if it's something bad that's happened, then uh they may be just really stressed out, (laugh) and want to cry, and have to phone someone else to talk about it.

The grandmother and grandson in this story are frightened and confused by death (segregated systems, cognitive disconnection). Once again, the AAP stimulus unleashes "roller coaster" levels of fear, suggesting that these feelings are potentially uncontrollable. Paul reorganizes and contains these feelings by drawing on the functional synchrony depicted in the grandmother's encouragement. Her ministrations are not sufficient, however, to reduce the tension created by wondering about the outcome of the situation (cognitive disconnection). Paul's reliance on disconnecting defenses again leaves the characters immersed in their tension as he describes two incomplete and opposing story endings. One ending describes the characters as potentially relieved (cognitive disconnection). The other describes the flip side of relief; the characters remain stressed out (cognitive disconnection). Cognitive disconnection essentially leaves the characters confused and standing at the window immersed in their distress at the brink of becoming overwhelmed.

Paul was judged as "fearfully preoccupied by traumatic events" (E_3) on the AAI. Paul's experiences of attachment trauma for the purpose of rating included loss through death, potential physical maltreatment, and sexual abuse. His discussions of these experiences did not qualify him to be judged unresolved for loss or abuse. To Paul, loss was identified as his father leaving home. He was unable to elaborate on the possibility that he was physically maltreated by his mother. Although he openly acknowledged his cousin's sexual abuse, he did not describe these sexual acts. The defensive disconnection from his cousin's trysts leaves these sexual activities as somewhat of a mystery. Yet he did not hesitate to describe the details of his sexual encounters with his peers, which involved what is commonly viewed as male sex-play behavior. Furthermore, Paul could not decide whether this sexual activity or his parents' unwillingness to discuss sex and sexuality was more distressing. Paul was definitely confused and preoccupied with suffering.

Paul's underlying or alternate classification on the AAI was "passive preoccupation" (E_1), as indicated by his vague memories, contradictions, and the unsuccessful struggle against portraying his parental attachment figures in a negative way. He frequently attempted to demonstrate during the interview that he had engaged in the self-transformation needed to understand the past and construct a new connected integrated self. For example, he figured out that his inability to "stay tuned in when people are talking to him" resulted from his response to his mother's yelling, but then told the interviewer that he was not having trouble concentrating on their conversation. He was proud of becoming a "forgiving person" through his spiritual therapy and not clinging to what he called "false expectations" of how people should have treated him. Yet he had not completed this developmental task. His childhood remained a collection of representational pieces.

There are clear parallels between Paul's AAI and the AAP responses. Paul willingness to cooperate, even if he did not want to, was demonstrated in the *Window* response. His description of being alone to manage his own stress is evident in the *Bed* response. The *Window* and *Cemetery* responses confirmed the intensity of his experience of "loss" when separated from his father by his parents' divorce. The *Bed* and *Ambulance* responses confirmed that Paul was not able to receive the care he needed from his mother but could count on some minimal care from surrogate caregivers. The *Departure* response demonstrated his hope for a new life when he left for university. His *Corner* response demonstrated his intellectual knowledge regarding patterns of sexual abuse, likely gained from his initial exposure to this information through an educational pamphlet and his years of recovery therapy.

The AAP responses demonstrate how hard Paul must work to tell the story of his life to quell attachment distress without becoming overwhelmed and flooded by attachment trauma in order to maintain the illusion of self-transformation. Unless trauma is directly described in the AAI, the judge must infer trauma from evidence of "unconscious preoccupation" or "traumatic memory loss" (Main et al., 2003). No inference is required to interpret Paul's AAP responses. The haunting image of helplessness and vulnerability that dominate his *Bench* response and his *Corner* response demonstrate the extent to which abuse dominates his self-view. Contrary to his claims in the AAI, there is also no evidence of parental forgiveness in the AAP. Often overwhelmed (or on the brink of being overwhelmed by intense emotions), the AAP shows the breakdown of organizing cognitive disconnection defenses in the face of trauma. We witness a quality of conflicted confusion such that characters were rendered immobile. More generally, the AAP responses demonstrate Paul's hypersensitivity to attachment distress to a large range of hypothetical attachment situations. Frightening separation, attachment figure abdication, and the absence of personal agency and connectedness are evident in his stories. Paul is "living in the war zone," caught in a chronic cycle of fear and helplessness for which he can neither clearly identify the source nor "see" how it affects him.

FAILED MOURNING CASE EXAMPLE

Magna

Magna is a 36-year-old Latina woman who never married and has no children. She has a younger sister. Magna's father was a shoe salesman. Her mother worked outside the home, but Magna was unsure of what her mother did for a living. Her family moved frequently during her early childhood and lived with her paternal grandparents for several years when Magna was 7 years old because of financial difficulties. These problems and her father's affairs led her parents to divorce when Magna was 8. She and her sister continued to live with their grandparents for 2 years. She lived with her mother until she was a teenager and then moved in with her father. When asked who raised her, Magna replied, "I would say I pretty much raised myself."

Magna described the years before her parents' divorce as good. "I don't have any terrible memories of my parents doing evil things to me or behaving badly." She claims to have been unaware of her parents' problems until she heard them fighting while she waited for them to take her on an outing planned for her eighth birthday. She described life after her parents' divorce as less stable.

Magna's described her relationship with her mother as a young child as creative and fun. Magna loved the attention she received in the years prior to her sister's birth. She cheerily recalled a Halloween costume that her mother made for her when she was 3 and that she and her mother went trick-or-treating together. Her mother played board games with her. Magna recalled her mother watching from their picture window as she splashed in puddles outside. During the period Magna and her sister lived with their grandmother, Magna's mother picked them up on weekends, when they would splurge on special dinners and stay up late watching TV. Magna also remembered feeling bad for her mother because of her unremitting financial woes.

Magna's mother could also be threatening, although Magna said that she did not feel abused or endangered. She described what she called "an ugly story." Before going out for the evening, her mother had instructed Magna, age 6, not to eat the chocolates she was saving for Magna's father. When her mother came home, she did not know that the teenage babysitter had eaten the chocolates while her parents were out. Her mother accused Magna of eating the candy and lying. "They come back and she's like, 'Where's the chocolates, you ate the chocolates, I told you not to eat the chocolates.' 'I didn't eat the chocolates.' 'You're lying to me. I don't care if you ate the chocolates. I just want you to tell me you ate the chocolates.' 'I didn't eat the chocolates.' And this went on for quite some time and she became progressively angrier and more bizarre and ended up saying, 'I'm going to paddle your behind because you're basically lying, you're lying to me, and that's what's bothering me is that you're lying to me.' And she went and got the paddle and she did, she paddled me and I was screaming and crying and she said, 'Okay now you, now can you tell me that you ate the chocolates.' And I said, 'I didn't eat the chocolates.' And then she was just livid and ended up calling the babysitter asking the babysitter if she ate the chocolates. She said yes. So she was pretty threatening there standing there with the paddle. (Laughs)"

Magna's father traveled away from home quite a bit when she was a young child and, in addition to living in their home, had a place of his own for several years before their divorce. They would all visit him there, and her father came home on weekends. She described their relationship as distant and recalled that he was frequently absent when she needed him. "He's not here to take care of this for me and that's weird he's always gone, he's never here . . . When we lived at my grandmother's house, he was supposed to pick us up at a specific time to spend the weekend. This happened ninety-seven thousand times. 'Yes, I'll pick you girls up at 7 o'clock after I get off work and we'll spend the weekend together.' So we're dressed up cute and waiting to be picked up, and then at 3 o'clock on Sunday afternoon we get a call that he's not coming because something happened, so that's where we were, it wasn't just one specific time, it was just all the time."

Her father wanted Magna to do well in school and expected nothing less than perfection. Her father had no use for any grades less than an A on her report card. "It wasn't, 'You're awesome, you got an A, you got six A's.' It was, 'Let's talk about the B's.'" She thought his expectations exceeded what she could deliver and sometimes his emphasis on her achievements put her in embarrassing situations. She described a time when her father introduced her to his coworker when she was 10 years old. "He told him I spoke German completely out of the blue, it had nothing to do with anything and then the guy started talking German to me and I totally didn't want to embarrass my father and I responded like immediately in Spanish because my brain, I don't know just it, I didn't do it on purpose, and then I was totally embarrassed. But I was also kind of pissed off that he would do that. He tended to do things like that to me, but I don't think he was evil, he was just so proud of me and sometimes he just forgot she really doesn't do that or she doesn't speak that language or she doesn't really have black hair or whatever."

Magna's other memories of her father were more descriptions of his personality than their relationship. She thought he was funny and he could make everybody laugh. "He was hilarious and I was just in awe of how he totally charmed [this lady], and he was like that with everybody. He could charm the pants off anybody and thinking that was cool and that I really liked that about him."

There is no indication in Magna's description of her childhood that her parents were a safe haven or secure base. Yet Magna said she felt safe with her mother, likely because her mother provided some instrumental care. When she cut her foot on a piece of sharp metal, her mother "rushed me to the hospital." She remembered having the flu and lying on the couch thinking it was cool that she didn't have to go to school. She never described her father as taking care of her when hurt or sick, and even her mother was not always available. She recalled a time when she was frightened terribly of a centipede and neither her mother nor her father was available to help her. "It was the hugest centipede I've ever seen in my life. It was in my toybox and I saw it and it was crawling at me and I thought, 'Oh my God, it's going to kill me.' I went running out of my room and realized, 'Who's going to save me. Who's going to save me from this centipede?' My dad's not here and my mom's sick, she had the flu and she'd been in her room for 2 days."

Magna identified two protecting childhood "caregiving figures." The most important was her paternal grandmother. Magna and her sister lived with her father's parents for a few years after her parents' divorce, at which time her grandmother stepped into the primary caregiving role. She says her grandmother was crazy, though, "not diagnosed but lots of delusional bizarre and comical things that aren't dangerous." Despite these problems, Magna remembered her grandmother as being "solid as a rock" in the midst of her parents' chaos. "She cooked dinner every night, bathed us, put us to bed at night, and combed our hair in the morning . . . even though she pulled my hair really hard and I didn't like it. I remember her being totally solid and there for us, which I appreciated." Looking back, Magna says she really appreciated her grandmother for buffering her and her sister from their parents' problems. Her mother had a nervous breakdown and, although Magna had no memory of her mother's condition or how long it lasted, she said that her mother was unavailable during that time. Her father starting taking drugs and became a serious drug addict. She said the reason she did not feel rejected as a child was due to her grandmother's sturdy care.

Magna's other childhood caregiving figure was her father's girlfriend. "She was independent, gorgeous, had a great job, a great car, and was funny and smart. She was just great." Magna said she owed her self-esteem to this woman because she took the time to remind Magna that she was a great kid and treated her like an adult. She introduced Magna to makeup and treated her like a friend; they shopped and lunched together. Magna said this was an important influence because she had assumed a parent/adult role with her own mother after her parents' divorce.

Magna lived with her father during her teen years, although she did not explain why. She said that she liked living there because he was never home and she was free to do as she pleased. Her father let her be totally independent, and she said she got into a lot of trouble. No further explanation was provided.

Magna had several inappropriate sexualized experiences as a child. There is some suggestion in her interview that Magna's relationship with her father as a child was sexualized, although not in sexually explicit ways. She recalled him being very proud of her beauty, and she was an early maturer with noticeable breast buds at a young age. Magna's grandmother dressed her up and her father took her with him to a sleazy bar. "I had frilly little ruffles at the bottom and the top was completely inappropriate for an 8-year-old girl, thinking back on it. It was like the dress the waitresses wore in the restaurant and it was like off my shoulder, very bizarre. I felt cute and it was fun, but weird in the context of the restaurant where the waitresses are like falling out of their thing and they got these dresses off the shoulder and they're, you know, seducing the customer for their tips, just bizarre. I had my hair all fixed and I probably looked like I was, you know, 27 and I was 8. He bought me a Shirley Temple and we were chit-chatting and hanging out. God only knows, I don't know if he knew, but I think that was inappropriate."

Her relationship with her stepfather was also inappropriately sexualized. She and her mother moved in with him when Magna was 9 and her mother married him a year later. She described interactions with him as having sexual overtones. "I don't feel that he was evil, but he definitely had his issues. I didn't feel like he was going to come into my bedroom and rape me in the middle of the night, but when he put his hands on my breasts and said, 'His tits,' that was physically threatening, inappropriate, how can I extract myself out of this situation, this is a weird thing. And I think it was his way of showing his affection toward me. It was also my number one interest from age 8 to 14 to be beautiful. I would just do anything. I was really into makeup and how I liked fixing my hair, attention from boys, men, this was my number-one objective. So I think that was also difficult for him to deal with."

Magna also recalled being touched sexually at daycare when she was little. It was difficult for Magna to pinpoint how old she was at the time, suggesting that the experience may have caused her grandmother to take her to the doctor when she was masturbating as a young child.

Magna says she did not tell her mother about any of these incidents until she was 20. She says it is hard to know how this and her stepfather's behavior affected her. "I don't think it was that big a deal."

Magna witnessed a lot of domestic violence after her mother remarried, and she did not mention any abuse directed toward her. Magna developed an "attitude" in her tone as she recalled these experiences during the interview. "He was a huge guy. And he would be sitting on my mom's back and beating her. I felt physically threatened and threatened on her behalf, and felt helpless and stressed, and what do you do? I just wanted to kill him and all that and she's a, she's fucking crazy too, to stay with him and she's just, she must be just a big loser."

Magna experienced two deaths in her life. One was the death of her maternal grandmother when she was 10. Magna said the loss was not hard for her because she had not seen her grandmother when she was sick. The other was her father's death. He died of AIDS when she was 20, probably contracted from years of drug addiction and unprotected sex. She and her father had a "falling out" many years before he died and she had not seen him for quite a long time. They oddly came together in her late teens to resolve a problem she was having with her car insurance, during which time her father apologized at the time for his inconsistency during her childhood. "I told him it was okay and it didn't matter to me. And then I left him and everything was groovy." She learned about her father's disease from her grandmother. Magna had seen him about 3 months before he died, but did not go to the hospital to see him as his health deteriorated. "I figured he was out of his misery. I think everybody has their time to move on and if you walk out in the street and you get hit by a truck that's really shitty and the people that are left behind are going to be really shocked and dismayed to find out that you were just killed by a truck. But on the other hand, it's part of the cycle of things, and so especially because he had been so sick, I thought it was that it was like kind of for the best."

Magna had a poor adult relationship with her mother. She said they did not get along and that their relationship waxed and waned. They recently had a disagreement and their relationship was nonexistent.

Magna was judged dismissing with failed mourning on the AAP. Unlike other individuals in the dismissing group, Magna's deactivating defenses are dysregulating in the attempt to maintain a wall around pain. Magna's deactivating armor is not impenetrable. Bowlby (1980) described the explosive potential associated with failed mourning. Magna explodes with fear and fury during the AAP that threatens self-integrity and would, if Bowlby is correct, plunge her into mourning if attachment is sufficiently activated by another loss. Overall, Magna views relationships as tense and threatening. Drawing on her capacity to create representational distance through deactivation, she either manages her distress with agency through action, including rejecting others for self-preservation, or the help of a caregivers' functional care.

Alone Stories

Magna's alone responses indicate her capacity to handle stress alone, even when she becomes dysregulated and is out of control. With the exception of her *Window* response, all of the other scenes elicit extreme segregated systems material. Each self character is portrayed as having the capacity to reorganize by defensively deactivating the emotional sting in the situation and having the capacity to act. There is no evidence that Magna's defensive posture permits her to think about these situations; there is also no evidence that she is connected to others in supportive relationships that might help her. Relationships with attachment figures are infuriating and, therefore, kept at a distance.

> ***Window:*** That's a little girl looking outside her bedroom window, and she's looking at a house and a tree. And it's a very clear day, and it's nice, and she has the whole day ahead of her. (What led up to the scene?) She got out of bed in the morning. (What is she thinking or feeling?) What an awesome day. It's really clear outside. (And what's going to happen next?) She's going to get dressed and prepare for her day, she's anxious to go outside. (Anything else?) She has a backyard view, nothing other than that.

Magna tells a straightforward story about a girl who is looking forward to beginning a new day. The girl seizes the opportunity and gets dressed to prepare for her day (agency—capacity to act). We note a bit of anxiety associated with this action, which is evidence in the AAP of disconnected entangled tension.

> ***Bench:*** This is a woman sitting on a bench with her head down on her knees, relaxing or thinking, and she appears to be outside and maybe she's in a really nice nature area that you can't see in this picture, and she's tired or might need some time alone to think and that's why she's taking this kind of . . . looks to be uncomfortable position but kind of shutting out the rest of the world. (What do you think led up to the scene?) Stress in her, her normal life and she came upon this bench and thought wow that looks really comfortable . . . I can go there and kind of shut the world out. (What do you think the character is thinking or feeling?) Just relief, she's just in her own little world, relieved. (What do you think might happen next?) That she's come back to reality after her meditation and go back to her hectic life.

On the surface, this is a story about a woman sitting on a comfortable bench enjoying nature to refresh the self. However, the underlying elements in this response tell a different story. This story describes a cycle of dysregulation. The cycle begins with two nonintegrated plot lines (cognitive disconnection), one of which suggests that the woman's tension might be managed internally by thinking (agency—internalized secure base). As the tension increases and becomes "uncomfortable" (cognitive disconnection), feelings of dysregulating isolation emerge. Magna describes the woman as "shutting out the rest of the world," "in her own little world" and "her hectic life" (segregated systems). The representational self is now at risk of losing control, from which Magna quickly recovers and contains the emotional intensity of the situation by returning to reality (deactivation). We note that in the second iteration of this cycle Magna states that the woman comes "back" to reality, a word that indicates that nothing has changed. In short, the story is resolved, but nothing has changed.

> *Cemetery:* This is a guy standing, looking at a gravestone in a cemetery, and he has a big jacket on so it's probably cold outside. And . . . he probably knows the person that he's standing in front of the gravestone, and maybe he's talking to the person in his mind, "Well it's pretty cold outside and I came by to tell you that I love you, and that I miss you," or maybe he's telling the person, "You were a bastard and I hate you but I'm coming to pay my respects because that's what I'm supposed to do. I wish you were here so I could smack you around or tell you what a bastard you were." I don't know what he's thinking. (What led up to the scene?) He felt obligated or he felt like he should go to the cemetery. (What do you think he's thinking or feeling?) Um, again I think he's either thinking, he's probably thinking "I wish you were here." Either "I wish you were here because I love you and you were groovy to me and I miss you," or or maybe, actually, "You're in a better place now. I love you and I'm glad you're in a better place now, but for selfish reasons I miss you." Or he's thinking, "I wish you were here so I could smack you around because you were a bastard. I didn't get a chance to tell you what a jerk you were when you were here." (What will happen next?) He'll turn around and leave and go home.

The loss stimulus unleashes a quality of fury that is rare in the AAP. We note how Magna carefully keeps her rage under metacognitive control. The man at the grave talks "to the person in his mind." Again, we see the cycle of cognitive disconnection, dysregulated segregated systems, and deactivation. The tone of the man's thoughts vacillates between tender yearning and rage (cognitive disconnection). Magna becomes confused after describing the man's tirade and disconnects from the stimulus—"I don't know what he is thinking." This pause gives her the opportunity to create emotional distance, ultimately deactivating distress by contextualizing his visit to the graveyard as an obligation. When prompted to delve further into the man's thoughts or feelings, Magna cannot manage her rage and she becomes increasingly dysregulated. Attempts to express her love for the deceased dissolve into fury. Dysregulated attachment rage is contained by the capacity to go home (agency of self—capacity to act), but the rage seethes beneath the surface and follows him home.

> *Corner:* This is a little boy standing in the corner and it reminds me of my sister standing in the corner, she would never stand in the corner, and my mother would have to say, "If you don't stand in the corner I'm going to *stand* you in the corner." And he's saying, "I will not stand in the corner, you can't make me stand in the corner," and he's just really stubborn. (What do you think led up to the scene?) He did something bad. He . . . he refused to go to bed or something, he watched TV and wouldn't go to bed. (What is he thinking or feeling?) "I will not stand in the corner, it's boring and you can't make me." (What do you think will happen next?) His mom or dad or whoever is over here will come and take his shoulders and make him stand in the corner and he'll be furious and fuming, but he will stand in the corner.

Magna begins her story with a reference to her own experience of authoritarian parental power. She then smoothly shifts to the hypothetical story and describes the prototypic elements of the attachment deactivation–rejection cycle that maintains physical and emotional distance in attachment relationships. The boy's distance is defined by multiple images of rejection (deactivation), which also serves as the motivating force of his personal agency. He is defiant and rejects his parent's wishes. He refuses to go to bed and uses his agency (capacity to act) to refuse to stand in the corner. His parent, however, has the power to "make him stand in the corner." Magna's story also describes in this response the classic disconnected emotional undercurrent in rejecting relationships (George & Solomon, 1996; Solomon et al., 1995). Magna describes the boy as "stubborn" (cognitive disconnection). Unique to Magna's attachment representation, the boy's anger is out of control; he is "furious and fuming" (segregated systems).

Dyadic Stories

Magna demonstrates in these stories that physical closeness in relationships generates tension and representations of being too close cause feelings of entanglement to surface. This tension is handled by deactivation defenses that create the distance needed when relationships are too close. The stories portray functional synchrony; attachment figures are never portrayed as comforting or enjoyable.

> ***Departure:*** Two people going on a trip, it's a couple going on a trip, and they're standing on a train platform with their luggage, packed with luggage, and they both have their hands in their pockets, so it seems like they've been waiting for a while for the train to come . . . and the man is looking down to see if the train is coming and woman is looking somewhere else ahead, the opposite way, and it looks like it's cold outside because she has a jacket that has, looks like it has a little fur thing. (What led up to the scene?) Uh, they decided that they wanted to go on a train trip. (What are they thinking or feeling?) When is the train coming? It's cold out here. That's probably why, too, they have their hands in their pockets, because it's cold and they're anxious for the train to come. (What will happen next?) Hopefully the train will come soon and they'll get on and they're excited about their trip.

Magna's story is a straightforward description of a functional relationship. The couple is going on a trip and they get on the train when it arrives. There is no evidence of mutual enjoyment generated by being together. Embedded in this simple story line is Magna's attempt to deactivate the tension in the relationship. Contextualizing their physical posture as cold (deactivation), Magna successfully distances herself from relationship tension and describes the couple as moving forward in time. The deactivation attempt is not totally successful, however. Relationship tension is transformed into a positive; the couple is excited (cognitive disconnection).

> ***Bed:*** This is a woman and her son, her son is in bed and he's sick, and he has a cold, and his mom is making chicken soup, and although she has her slippers on, so . . . yeah, they're both ready for bed, he's going to bed and she's going to bed but she's made him dinner first, which is chicken soup, chicken with soup, and she's bringing it to him and he's excited to have it. (What led up to the scene?) She was in the kitchen, he has Campbell's chicken soup and he was lying in bed. (What are they thinking or feeling?) He's excited to have soup, and she's happy that he's eating. (What will happen next?) He'll spill the soup on his blanket, a little bit, and she'll have to clean it up and he'll eat most of the soup and she'll be

relieved that he's finally eating, and then she'll go to bed and he'll go to sleep too.

Magna tells the story of a woman caring for her sick son. This response again illustrates deactivated tension. Although implied, the woman is never identified directly as his mother. The synchrony in this relationship takes the form of functional care and does contain the boy's attachment distress. Once again in Magna's representation of attachment figures, there is no evidence of mutuality, enjoyment, or maternal sensitivity. The mother's behavior is defined by social stereotypes (deactivation); she brings her son a tried and true cold remedy and the most well-known brand of chicken soup in the United States. There is a tense undercurrent in this robotic caring relationship, as she suggests that the mother and child are too close. The boy's excitement (cognitive disconnection) causes him to spill his soup. The mother experiences relief (cognitive disconnection) when the boy cooperates and eats her remedy. Momentarily caught in close proximity, Magna introduces the physical distance needed to manage potentially entangling distress. The mother leaves and he goes to sleep (deactivation).

> ***Ambulance:*** This is a grandmother and her grandson and . . . someone is dead, it appears that they're dead because it looks like they're covered, and they're being taken away in an ambulance, and the little boy is thinking hmm, someone's dead and they're being taken away in an ambulance. And the grandmother's saying yes, just trying to talk to him about it, yes this person's dead, and I don't think the person was related to them, and I think this because if they were, they wouldn't be sitting inside the house looking at this happening out the window, they would actually be outside involved in the process. So I think it's like a neighbor or someone across the street or something, or maybe if there was a car accident or something, but the person in front of their house, and the person got killed and is being taken away. (What are they thinking or feeling?) Well, I think they're like rubbernecker kind of people, they're like sticking their nose in, very curious about this thing that's taken place outside their window. And the little boy's a little bit confused, maybe about death, and he's saying, "But why is their head covered?" And the grandma's saying, "Well, because the person's dead, and they don't need to breathe anymore, so . . ." (What will happen next?) The paramedic, ambulance people will put the dead body in the back of the ambulance and drive away. The grandma and the kid will go on

with the rest of their daily business. (Anything else?) The kid will tell his parents about it when the parents get home.

In this story, the grandmother and her grandson witness an ambulance taking an acquaintance away after he has died in a car accident. Although the story of a death is a common response to this AAP stimulus, the theme of being killed in a car accident while in close proximity—"in front of their house"—is an atypical and more extreme reaction. The stimulus requires Magna to examine the loss that is right in front of her nose, so to speak, and this is distressing. Magna tries to disconnect from the risk of becoming flooded by these feelings by splintering the elements of the story, thereby introducing uncertainty and confusion into the story. The deceased is identified as a "neighbor or someone across the street," the dyad is "curious", and the boy asks about a detail—"But why is their head covered?" Magna uses distance to shift attention away from their confusion to the action taking place. Magna again portrays characters acting according to their social role (deactivation), describing paramedics and what happens to dead people when the ambulance comes—"ambulance people will put the dead body in the back of the ambulance." The child does not express overt distress and, therefore, the grandmother's comfort is unnecessary. Magna's images of the next events are guided by deactivation. The grandmother creates emotional distance and normalizes the situation by explaining the meaning of death and they "go on with the rest of their daily business." The boy can now tell his parents about the episode without the risk of becoming upset.

Magna was judged dismissing on the AAI, "restricted in feeling" regarding attachment (Ds_3) and occasionally "derisive and derogatory" toward both parents (Ds_2). Magna did not fully dismiss her childhood relationships but, with the exception of the years when she lived with her paternal grandparents, she portrayed herself as a strong, independent person who took care of herself. Although she referred to some situations as weird, embarrassing, or inappropriate, in the main, attachment feelings were notably absent from her descriptions. She sometimes made "over-the-top" remarks about situations when being derogatory. Her discussions of her mother's harsh treatment and the sexual molestation did not evidence the quality of thinking required to be judged as unresolved for abuse on the AAI.

Magna received high rating for absent grief/failed mourning.[4] She described her response to loss as generally lacking feeling. She wondered

[4] Hamilton-Oravetz and George (1991, published in Hamilton-Oravetz, 1992).

in response to her grandmother's death, "why, since it was the first death that I experienced that I can remember, why I didn't cry and why it didn't bother me." Magna seemed even more anesthetized to her father's death. Her relationship with her father was complicated by sexual boundary confusion, an experience that has been described in other failed mourning cases (Buchheim, George, & KŠchele, 2008). Magna dismissed her father's attempt to apologize for his inconsistencies. She did not visit him in the hospital and she received the news of his death in a phone call from someone whom she failed to identify. Although she said she was upset by his death, she summed up her reaction by saying "he was pretty much gone as far as I was concerned."

Magna's descriptions of a sturdy self supported by her grandmother's functional care are evident in her AAP stories. When attachment distress is low, Magna likely responds to life like the girl in the *Window* scene. She has the capacity to act and gets ready to greet a new day. The AAI does not capture the degree to which Magna is potentially derailed by feelings of isolation in reaction to having to take care of herself and her failure to mourn her father's death. Deactivating defenses have created a superficial shell that Magna uses to protect herself from becoming overwhelmed by segregated fear and rage. Nothing has changed in Magna's representation of attachment to allow her to acknowledge the pain of death. The *Bench* stimulus activates feelings of isolation. The need to deactivate feelings in order to maintain relationship distance is evident in response to the death theme she develops to the *Ambulance* stimulus. Like the boy in the *Ambulance* story who could tell his parents about the death, Magna demonstrates the importance of maintaining distance from her father's death so that she can acknowledge it. Her feelings of yearning, love, and rage erupt and are totally out of control in response to the *Cemetery* stimulus. The combination of out-of-control rage suppressed by a relationship defined by mutual rejection and distance is evidence of Magna's failed mourning in *Corner*. In summary, her AAP responses demonstrate Magna's fragility and susceptibility to breakdown from the failure to mourn her father's death.

CONCLUSION

Bowlby (1980) laid down the conceptual foundation for defining attachment trauma and pathological mourning. He described trauma as the outcome of an unstable and brittle defensive exclusion that interfered with the representational reorganization and reintegration required to complete mourning. Through the complex interaction of deactivation and cognitive disconnection, defensive exclusion supports an extreme form of repression that leads to a segregated representational system that contains and organizes attachment fear and painful experience, rendering them inaccessible to consciousness thought. These processes contribute to a state of mind he termed pathological mourning. We must remember, however, that Bowlby's ideas were formulated from his clinical experience with individuals who presented severe psychiatric symptoms. We must also remember that Bowlby's approach was context sensitive. The occurrence of trauma is but the first step toward evaluating pathological mourning. The next step requires understanding the place of trauma in an individual's attachment history, particularly "assaults" to attachment associated with caregiver "abdication" (George & Solomon, 2008; Solomon & George, 2000, 2011a).

The cases presented in this chapter raise important conceptual, assessment, and clinical questions about pathological mourning, especially the relation between unresolved attachment and other attachment trauma classifications. What have we learned about attachment trauma based on the AAPs of these four individuals? Is unresolved adult attachment the representational equivalent of attachment disorganization in children?

Unice's AAP record was quite different from the AAPs of the other three cases. We might ask now what the emergence of segregated systems material in her AAP record signifies in terms of defensive failure and attachment trauma. More simply, was Unice's state of mind an instance of traumatic failure of organizing defensive processes? In many respects, the answer to this question must be no; she succeeded in recovering from the breakthrough of traumatic material fairly well, even though she was not able to reorganize her own grief in the personal experience thread of the *Cemetery* response. Indeed, her loss was traumatic in the classic Bowlby sense. Unice is in a state of chronic mourning. But we must consider this state in relation to Unice's underlying secure attachment representation. Unice's underlying representation of attachment evidenced her capacity to think about and draw on attachment figures to provide comfort and care. Her stories depicted agency of self, including the internalized secure base, which in the AAP is the capacity to think about attachment distress by using internalized attachment figures as a representational secure base. Her stories depicted the importance and accessibility of real-life attachment figures. Even in *Cemetery*, in which connectedness is not coded in the AAP, Unice depicted the projected self as expecting comfort in that the character told his family about his sadness. Unice's childhood caregiving experiences are a far cry from those of the other individuals discussed in this chapter. In her case, the death of a loving father was experienced within the context of descriptions of an otherwise sensitive and protective parent–child relationship. The source of Unice's unresolved attachment representation is her inability to say goodbye to her father. Her mourning was not complicated by experiences of either attachment assaults or failed protection. Using Bowlby's (1980) language, Unice continued to yearn and search for reunion with her father so that she could acknowledge their separation and finally say goodbye. What we learn from Unice's case is that her AAP record indicates underlying defensive instability rather than far-reaching failure of defense that is more likely to be associated with more severe and complicated attachment trauma.

On the continuum of attachment trauma, we suggest that the other three cases demonstrate more severe and potentially more debilitating forms of attachment trauma than "simple" loss. Magna was in a state of failed mourning. She outwardly appeared to manage the intense pressure of attachment distress reasonably well. Magna's kind of "lonely courage" adaptation, with the setting aside of attachment difficulties and detachment from attachment-related feelings, together made it possible for her to recover and contain attachment distress at the representational level. Her defensive posture is a kind of "hyperactive" deactivation, that is, dysregulated attempts to create representational distance in order to clamp down and dismiss conscious consideration of the effects of childhood trauma on the self and other attachment relationships. These defensive operations foster pathological mourning because defense by deactivation, although successful in containing segregated fear, blocks integration of traumatic experience and affect. Furthermore, Magna's AAP record showed the imbalance of deactivation and cognitive disconnection defensive processes, the effect of which was the unleashing of segregated affect in vehement bits and pieces.

Based on her AAI, Magna was judged dismissing and would be considered for all intents and purposes in the attachment literature as an instance of a normative dismissing attachment pattern (see Chapter 7). Magna's trauma experience was formally evaluated for death and abuse. Her interview did not qualify for placement in a trauma classification category using traditional AAI coding (i.e., unresolved loss, abuse, CC, E_3). Yet her AAP literally cries out with trauma. What is Magna's trauma? Unlike Unice, it is not simply loss. Magna has not only failed to mourn her father's death, but that relationship was complicated by inappropriate sexualizing and parental abdication. We also cannot ignore sexualized experiences in other adult caregiver relationships, combined with unwarranted maternal rage, abdication, and parental divorce. The breakthrough of intense anger and fury in her *Cemetery* and *Corner* stories suggest defensive failure in that she is vulnerable to literal disintegration, just as Bowlby (1980) described the risk associated with failed mourning. Magna's deactivation strategies seem to prevent her from being "bothered" by attachment (e.g., *Ambulance*), unless attachment cues more directly activate feelings of isolation, threat, and loss.

Abby and Paul seem the most loosely integrated of all the individuals described in this chapter. Their attachment representations indicate forms of chronic mourning associated with "hyperactive" cognitive disconnection. Their AAP records demonstrate patterns of dysregulated segregated fear and pain that is splintered and embedded in layers of confusion. Unlike Unice, these individuals appear more like the examples Bowlby (1980) used to describe pathological chronic mourning. Abby and Paul are caught in their isolation and terror, which Paul transforms into hope. In Abby's case, where traumas were repeated and persisted throughout her childhood, traumatic experience became the fabric of her attachment self. Again and again, we saw the failure of regulating defense that led to the appearance of a sense of surrounding threat together with fear. Only traces of agency of self are present amid the desolation of her adjustment efforts that have left Abbey an empty shell.

The problem of overlap and differentiation between AAI classification categories of unresolved abuse and preoccupation (E_3) is brought to the fore in the case of Paul. Paul's AAP also showed how traumatic experiences defined the self. The important question to consider for assessment is whether this is a design flaw in the evidentiary system (i.e., the AAI) or a necessary consequence of the underlying problem. When we approach the overlap between unresolved and traumatic preoccupation attachment from an instrument-centered point of view, we ultimately run the risk of what may be called an "AAI theory of attachment patterns." Instead, we have argued here that the overlap is a necessary consequence of the underlying attachment phenomenon. In this respect, we went back to Bowlby and reviewed his thinking about the ways individuals respond, and sometimes adapt, to attachment trauma. As we discussed above, this review suggested to us that Bowlby's notion of segregated systems associated with chronic mourning is the most adequate conceptualization of these phenomena. And in Paul's AAP stories, there is a kind of "living within a segregated system" quality to his responses. Thematically, the stories he told reflected miserable feelings of isolation and of having been abandoned. The characters in his stories seem to be saying, "I am alone; the world is barren and empty." Although his stories were overrun with segregated system material, he did show some degree of defensive containment, which protected him from becoming completely disorganized and more overtly overwhelmed.

Finally, we must return to one of the essential developmental assumptions of unresolved adult attachment. Is unresolved adult attachment the representational equivalent of attachment disorganization in children? We suggest that this equivalency model is too simplistic and does not the address the complexity of traumatic adult attachment. In some basic sense, the four forms of trauma representation described in this chapter fit the basic notion of disorganization. Disorganization is defined by the inability to gain access to attachment figures when frightened by parental abdication and inaccessibility at the moments of greatest need. All of these cases fit this description, yet the context of childhood experience also defines the capacity or incapacity to develop a defensive structure to manage such intense fear. Therefore we conclude that, if we are to understand attachment disorganization in adults, we must move beyond the unresolved classification and other anomalous interview-based classification categories and reexamine the fundamentals of grief and mourning as described in Bowlby's original work.

Perhaps from a clinical standpoint, we may understand the variants of mourning seen throughout these cases by uniting two propositions: (1) Individuals who come for therapy do not believe that it is obligatory to say goodbye to lost attachment relationships; and (2) the phrase "out of sight, into mind" (i.e. negative working models of the self and others) captures the effects of this inability to say goodbye. Using Bowlby's attachment framework, these reactions are called pathological mourning. The task is to move pathological mourning toward grief and resolution; that is, to help the individual renounce the past, forgive, forget, and reintegrate the internal world and the sense of self, emerging sadder and wiser. This task is made all the more difficult when attachment relationships are complicated by unpredictable rage, unexplainable events, a climate of parental conflict, and other events that assault attachment and render attachments figures helpless and unable to provide the protection and comfort needed to assuage feelings of terror and isolation.

10

Using the AAP in Neurobiology Research

Anna Buchheim and Carol George

This chapter discusses the use of the Adult Attachment Projective Picture System AAP in neurobiology research. According to attachment theory, the attachment behavioral system evolved in ways that influence and organize motivational, cognitive, emotional, and memory processes from "the cradle to the grave" (Bowlby, 1969/1982, 1973). Bowlby (1973, 1980) conceived of attachment as one of the primary elements that contribute to biological homeostasis, including modulating physiological stress, emotional balance, and overall mental health. Homeostasis and stress are defined in attachment theory as threats to the self and the attachment relationship. The most distressing contexts are defined in human evolutionary history by fear, especially fear of being alone when separated from attachment figures (Ainsworth et al., 1978; Bowlby, 1973, 1980). According to Bowlby (1973), fear is the root source of feelings of anxiety, depression, and anger. Developmental attachment researchers have carefully crafted assessments following the original Ainsworth Strange Situation (Ainsworth et al., 1978) such

Anna Buchheim, PhD, is Professor of Clinical Psychology, Institute of Psychology, University of Innsbruck, Innsbruck, Austria.

that the assessment measures present individuals with a range of attachment events that activate low to high levels of threat and fear (George & West, 2001; Solomon & George, 2008). How individuals respond to these events is shaped by experience, underlying defensive structure, and attention modulation capacities (George & West, 2001; Hesse & Main, 2006; Solomon et al., 1995). In order to understand the complexity of the neurobiology of adult attachment, it is essential for research to describe responses when the attachment system is activated and also describe the response patterns associated with different attachment patterns in a range of attachment-activating contexts. Otherwise, neurobiological patterns cannot be differentiated from responses generally associated with intimacy and sociability in human relationships. Researchers in the adult attachment domain use a variety of methodologies, ranging from procedures that are carefully grounded in attachment theory concepts to innovative procedures that substitute creativity for validity. Moreover, even when valid methodologies are used, most studies examine overarching attachment correlates, and the field knows very little about the neurobiological patterns associated with individual differences in attachment security across a range of attachment situations.

The chapter begins with an overview of the methodology and findings in attachment-related neurobiological research. We then discuss how the AAP provides a unique opportunity to examine individual differences of the neurobiological correlates of attachment while the attachment system is activated by a range of theoretically defined stressful attachment events. A complete research review of attachment and neurobiology is beyond the scope of this chapter. Readers are referred to other reviews for more comprehensive discussions (Buchheim, Taubner, Fizke, & Nolte, 2010; Coan, 2008; Schore, 2001; Siegel, 1999).

BACKGROUND: ATTACHMENT AND NEUROBIOLOGY RESEARCH

Kraemer (1992) stated that the attachment system is not only an organizing feature of basic neurophysiological function but also the central organizing system in the brain of higher mammals. The mother–infant relationship regulates the infant's neural system, especially orbitofrontal cortex in emotional regulation; its loss or dysfunction implies poor modulation and coordination of physiological function, affect, and behavior, (Hofer, 1995; Schore, 2002). Although some deficits in attachment behavior (e.g., disorganized attachment, autism, reactive attachment disorder) may have regulatory genetic links, the quality of interaction with the attachment figures plays an important role in expressed behavior (Gervai et al., 2005; Moles Kieffer, & D'Amato, 2004; van IJzendoorn & Bakermans-Kranenburg, 2006).

Basic animal studies and human imaging studies have contributed to our understanding of the psychobiology of intimate relationships and attachment. There are overlaps and distinctions in the neural circuitry of maternal love, romantic love, and long-term attachment relationships. In these circuits, important molecules that have been demonstrated to play a role in the psychobiology of social bonding include dopamine, serotonin, opioids, oxytocin, and vasopressin (Carter, Lederhendler, & Kirkpatrick 1997; Lim &Young, 2004; Panksepp, Siviy, & Normansel, 1985).

The main body of neurobiological adult attachment research with humans has used functional magnetic resonance to examine attachment-related brain activation patterns. This research is represented by three research threads, all of which make claim to attachment theory. The overarching goal of the first thread, conceived broadly as "attachment neuroscience," is to develop models to understand the neurobiological underpinnings of attachment-like characteristics in human conspecific bonds by integrating the findings of studies related to human social bonding, sexual pair bonding, and attachment bonding (Coan, 2008; Gillath & Schachner, 2006). These studies mainly focus on describing brain patterns associated with social affect regulation and emotion perception (e.g., detecting masked emotions emotion regulation). Most of the studies in this thread assess adult attachment using romantic attachment personality style measures (anxious or avoidant personality traits).[1] These studies typically report the brain correlates of anxious and avoidant traits in young adults' (average study age, 25 years) responses in the scanner to a range of social perception tasks (Suslow et al., 2009; Vrticka, Andersson, Grandjean, Sander, & Vuilleumier, 2008). Lemche et al. (2006), who did not use attachment style assessments, measured attachment security "by proxy." Attachment security was defined as the calculated reaction time difference between neutral and stressful condi-

[1] We discussed the differences between the Bowlby–Ainsworth derived model of attachment status and the personality trait attachment style model in Chapter 1. Developmental and social personality theorists now agree that attachment style and developmental attachment tap different aspects of relationships (Crowell et al., 2008). Developmental adult attachment measures were derived and validated based on behavior and mental representations of attachment based on childhood experience and secure base/haven of safety balances in reciprocal adult relationships. Attachment style measures were derived and validated based on sexual satisfaction in romantic relationships (Crowell et al., 2008).

tions in a conceptual priming task. The neutral prime condition typically paired nonsense statements with self- or other-directed statements, such as "Ym ymu jrecest em" paired with "My friends like me." The stress prime paired relationship oriented self- or other- directed statements, such as "My mum rejects me" and "Other people like me."

Three studies in this thread examined adult's responses to attachment events. Coan, Schaefer, and Davidson (2006) investigated 16 married women's (average age, 31 years) experience of their husband as a protective attachment figure. Attachment was activated by subjecting women to the threat of electric shock by attaching electrodes to their ankles. Shocks were administered at the end of an anticipation period that lasted between 4 to 10 seconds. Women's responses in the scanner were evaluated in three conditions. The first condition was while holding their husband's hand, defined by the researchers as the women's access to their adult attachment figure. In the other two conditions, the women held the hand of an anonymous male experimenter whom they could not see, or no hand at all. Women's responses when holding their husband's hand were influenced by marital quality such that higher marital quality was associated with neural activation patterns indicating reduced stress and threat (e.g., right anterior insula, superior frontal gyrus, hypothalamus).

Two attachment style studies examined brain patterns associated with imagined or real separation and loss of attachment figures. Benetti et al. (2010) described the gray matter volume patterns in a sample of 32 young adults (average age, 25 years; 17 women) as related to anxious and avoidant attachment style traits, and the interaction between attachment style and reported "affective loss" (e.g., separation or loss of loved one or friend within 5 years of the study). Avoidant attachment style (i.e., placed in the avoidant style group) was not related to brain gray matter volume; however, avoidance ratings and loss experience were related to gray matter volume in the left cerebellum. Gray matter volume was higher for individuals with low avoidance ratings and lower for individuals with high avoidance ratings. Anxious attachment style (i.e., placed in the anxious group) was associated with differences in gray matter volume in the right temporal pole and left lateral orbitofrontal cortex; however, there was no association between anxious attachment ratings and loss.

Gillath, Bunge, Shaver, Wendelken, and Mikulincer (2005) examined emotion regulation patterns associated with attachment style in 20 university undergraduate women recruited from a psychology department research participant pool. No information about participants' romantic attachment (e.g., married, level of commitment, length of relationship) was reported, so it is difficult to determine whether this study primarily tapped the sexual system in this age group (which would be developmentally appropriate) rather than committed attachment. Attachment was activated in the scanner by instructing the women to "think about" and then "stop thinking about" a range of positive and negative (e.g., conflict, breakup, death) relationship scenarios with their romantic partner. High avoidance ratings were associated with significantly less brain deactivation than expected (e.g., subcallosal cingulated cortex, lateral prefrontal cortex). High anxiety ratings were significantly associated with a strong reaction to imagined loss and an underrepresentation of responses in brain areas thought to be associated with negative emotion management (e.g., orbitofrontal cortex).

The combined results of this thread of research suggest the advantages of marital satisfaction and disadvantages of trait insecurity, and to some extent low attachment trait avoidance, on regulatory neural systems supporting the brain's stress response, including the affective component of pain, severe attachment distress (e.g., loss), and negative emotion. These researchers consistently use the developmental concepts of attachment to fortify their conclusions, including constructing confident statements that childhood attachment experiences significantly contributed to the observed patterns. These arguments nod to the importance of development, but the research designs and findings were couched in models of conspecific bonding and romantic sexual system bonding that fundamentally beg developmental attachment questions.

A second thread focuses on mothers' responses to their babies, mislabeled by many researchers as "maternal attachment." From an attachment theory perspective, these researchers are studying the maternal caregiving system (George & Solomon, 2008). The basic methodological design used in these studies is to present mothers with visual images (e.g., pictures, video clips) of their own children in the scanner. This design likely activates the mother's caregiving system, similar to other caregiving assessment paradigms (George & Solomon, 1996, 2008). The children were usually infants, ranging from 3 to 15 months; one study used images of children ages 5 to 12 years (Leibenluft, Gobbini, Harrison, & Haxby, 2004). Some studies compared mothers' responses to images of their own children with their responses to images of unfamiliar or acquaintance children, or unfamiliar adults (Bartels & Zeki, 2004; Leibenluft et al. 2004; Loberbaum et al., 1999; Nitschke et al., 2004; Strathearn, Fonagy, Amico, & Montague, 2009). The combined results of these caregiving system neuroimaging studies suggest that mothering is associated with specific hypothalamic–midbrain–limbic–paralimbic–cortical circuit activation patterns. Images of one's own child as compared with images of acquaintances or strangers activated stronger responses in emotional brain areas, including deactivation of negative emotion (e.g., orbital frontal cortex, amygdala, insula) episodic memory (e.g., cingulate and precuneus, anterior paracingulate, hippocampus, dorsolateral prefrontal cortex), cortical–limibic areas associated with motivation and reward, and mentalization (i.e., thinking about the mental states of others) (Bartels & Zeki, 2004; Leibenluft et al. 2004; Nitschke et al., 2004; Swain 2008). Swain, Lorberbaum, Kose, and Strathearn (2007) suggested that infant stimuli activate brain circuits and regulation associated with managing the "emotions, motivation, attention, and empathy" of caregiving behavior. Bartels and Zeki (2004), however, argued that these patterns are not unique to mothering, but are associated more generally with what they called "human attachment." They noted that the "brain reward system" and neuroregulatory patterns observed in their study of mothers was analogous to the activation patterns of women "deeply in love" (i.e., sexual system) described in their earlier research (Bartels & Zeki, 2000).

Only three neuroimaging studies in this thread investigated mothers from a well-defined attachment theory perspective. Noriuchi, Kikuchi, and Senoo (2008) showed 13 mothers (average age, 31 years) video clips without sound of their 16-month-old infants engaged in what they defined as two different forms of attachment behavior—smiling at or crying for their mother. They found specific brain activation patterns that they interpreted as associated with infant recognition (e.g., orbitofrontal cortex, anterior insula, specific areas of the putamen) and distress in response to their infants' cries (e.g., orbitofrontal cortex, caudate nucleus, right inferior frontal gyrus, prefrontal cortex, anterior cingulate, posterior cingulate, thalamus, substantia nigra, posterior superior temporal sulcus). Noriuchi et al. suggested that these unique patterns mediate maternal love and "vigilant protectiveness."

Strathearn et al. (2009) examined 30 first-time new mothers to test whether differences in brain reward and oxytocin responses were related to individual differences in adult attachment status. The AAI (George, Kaplan, & Main, 1984/1985/1996) was administered during pregnancy (time during pregnancy was not specified) and classified into secure, dismissing, and preoccupied groups using a poorly validated attachment classification system (Crittenden, 2004). Mothers viewed their own 7-month-old infants' smiling and crying faces without sound in the scanner 11 months following birth. Mothers judged secure showed greater activation of brain reward regions (e.g., ventral striatum, oxytocin-associated hypothalamus/pituitary region). Mothers' oxytocin response measured at 7 months after physical contact with their babies was also significantly higher in mothers judged secure than insecure mothers, and was positively correlated with brain activation patterns observed in the scanner. Mothers judged insecure-dismissing showed higher insular activation in response to their infants' crying faces than did secure mothers. These results suggest an important contribution of individual differences in maternal adult attachment in dopaminergic and oxytocinergic neuroendocrine systems responses to their infants.

Fraedrich, Lakatos, and Spangler (2010) examined the relation between adult attachment status and neural face processes and brain asymmetry in a sample of 17 mothers (average age, 40.5 years). The stimuli were a standardized set of images of infant facial expressions. Attachment status was determined using the AAP. Women judged secure showed stronger reactions to infants' faces as compared with mothers judged insecure. There was larger negativity in event-related potentials in mothers judged dismissing than secure mothers, suggesting different neural and cognitive mechanisms related to processing emotion in these two groups of mothers.

The third thread is the small set of studies that address the fundamental features of adult attachment outlined in this book. The paucity of research in this thread is remarkable, given the burst of interest in the neurobiology of attachment in the past decade. Similar to the mother–child studies described earlier, two studies reported adults' general responses to pictures of their own parents as compared with images of nonparents (e.g., friends, celebrities) in the scanner (Arsalidou, Barbeau, Bayless, & Taylor, 2010–6 women and 4 men, average age, 35.4 years; Ramasubbu et al., 2007–10 women, average age, 25 years). These studies reported greater activation in face recognition areas for parent than for nonparent images (e.g., ventral medial prefrontal anterior cingulated cortex; fusiform superior temporal, middle temporal, and inferior frontal and superior frontal gyri). The activation in prefrontal and cingulate cortices related to maternal face processing is consistent with their implicated roles in mother–infant interactions, personal familiarity, and emotional and self-relevant processing. Arsalidou et al. (2010) reported greater activation for mother, followed by father, as compared with the pictures of celebrities. They also reported caudate activity associated with parents' pictures, which they interpreted as evidence of the continued love and affection for our childhood attachment figures into adulthood.

Warren et al. (2010) examined the association between attachment security and brain activation patterns in response to an emotion-word Stroop task in a sample of 34 men and women (21 women, average sample age, 35.7 years). Attachment was evaluated prior to the Stroop task using the "secure base script" completion method. This method rates the capacity to develop a secure base script from standard prompt lists that involve words that describe parent–child dyads, demonstrated as having a .50–.60 correlation with AAI coherence ratings (Waters & Rodriguez-Doolabh, 2001). Low scores on this measure are conceived as evidence of attachment insecurity. Lower secure base knowledge was associated with heightened left-frontal activity and the anterior division of the cingulated gyrus (dACC) only for pleasant words. The authors interpreted their findings as indicating insecure individuals' relative difficulty and inflexibility in regulating negative emotion.

What all these recent "adult attachment" studies have in common is that they mostly studied intimate attachment or social relationships. The researchers showed that the neural underpinnings of these unique intimate emotional states are linked to functionally specialized areas in the brain. Studies that examined attachment-related stimuli showed that brain regions like the amygdala and orbito/prefrontal cortices are likely involved in processing when attachment is activated. Conceptualizing this work from a behavioral systems–attachment theory perspective, these studies demonstrate unique emotional states and brain activation patterns generally associated with important relationship behavioral systems—the caregiving behavior system and the sexual behavioral system (romantic partnerships).

In addition, there are convergent results in caregiving system studies suggesting that dopamine-associated regions of the reward system are active that differ from the neural correlates of the postulated "attachment circuitry." These studies especially help set the stage to test hypotheses regarding the neurological correlates associated with the activation of attachment. With the exception of Warren et al.'s (2010) study using attachment scripts, however, none of these studies directly addressed the developmental adult attachment system. The mothering studies are especially interesting because their results provide neurobiological information of the behavioral system that is conceived as reciprocal to attachment (George & Solomon, 2008).

Contemporary attachment theory and research has been built on the analysis of individual differences in attachment narratives to assess "attachment representation," the mental foundation of the attachment relationship (Bowlby, 1969/1982, 1973). Developmental attachment researchers assess this representation in adults by using measures that focus on the linguistic and mental organization of speech (as compared with self-report assessments). The above overview demonstrates that the field actually knows very little about the neurobiology of attachment in relation to adult mental representations of attachment. The secure-base script approach is a form of representational assessment, but it only assesses relative security and does not differentiate among the core attachment patterns.

Another issue that emerged in reviewing this set of adult attachment studies is that attachment, when assessed, was always measured outside of the scanner. Scanner performance was then correlated with earlier or subsequent measurement. We have shown in other chapters that the unresolved and preoccupied attachment groups are subject to instability. In order to better understand the individual pattern differences associated with attachment, we must be able to systematically observe the attachment system "in action."

In the following section, we summarize the use of the AAP in a neurobiological context, including two studies in which we used the AAP to activate and observe the attachment system in action in the scanner. The discussion that follows summarizes how we have applied the AAP methodology in neurobiological research in four different studies.[2]

STUDY 1: USING THE AAP IN AN fMRI ENVIRONMENT

We were interested in this first study to determine whether the AAP could be used to both assess and observe attachment "in action" in an fMRI environment (Buchheim, Erk, et al., 2006; Buchheim, George, Kächele, Erk, & Walter, 2006). Because of our interest in psychopathology and the prevalence of unresolved attachment in clinical groups (Dozier et al., 2008), we also wanted to determine whether there were differences between organized and unresolved/disorganized adults. This feasibility study posed two challenges. One was how to administer the AAP in the scanner with minimal brain processing confounding from auditory networks. We would need to modify the fMRI administration procedure so that participants were not guided with probes while in the scanner. It was not clear, therefore, whether individuals would produce narratives that would contain the linguistic information needed to apply the standard AAP coding and classification system (George & West, 2001). The second was that individuals typically do not speak while in the fMRI scanner because of concern that head movement may produce

[2] The specifications for neuroimaging and statistical treatment of the data collected are detailed in the original publications.

fMRI movement and susceptibility artifacts. However, several published fMRI studies had demonstrated that analysis of fMRI data acquired while speaking was possible, even in schizophrenic patients with severe formal thought disorder (Kircher, Brammer, Williams, & McGuire, 2000; Kircher et al., 2001, 2002).

With regard to the neurobiology of attachment, we hypothesized that unresolved individuals would demonstrate higher activation in limbic regions as compared with individuals with organized attachment (secure, dismissing, preoccupied) (Buchheim, Erk, et al., 2006; Buchheim, George, et al., 2006). Adult unresolved attachment status, described more fully in Chapter 9, is conceived in terms of segregated representational systems that monitor and navigate unintegrated attachment trauma. This present study concentrated on the unresolved form of attachment trauma that is characterized by sudden dysregulation of "unmetabolized" emergence of disorganized thought and emotional dysregulation that defines the unresolved attachment groups (loss and abuse). With regard to assessment, dysregulation risk should increase as individuals face increased threatening and stressful situations. We thus hypothesized that brain activation patterns in the unresolved group would demonstrate a significant gradually increasing activation pattern that paralleled the AAP measurement design—that is, the introduction of increasingly stressful attachment scenes over the course of the assessment (i.e., *Window* → *Corner*).

The study sample was comprised 11 healthy, right-handed women (mean age 29.45 years) recruited in southern Germany. Most participants completed the equivalent of North American high school or a year of college.[3] The participants had no history of major head trauma or significant medical, neurological, or psychiatric illness (Buchheim, Erk, et al., 2006).

In order to circumvent the necessity of using AAP probes in the fMRI apparatus, we "trained" participants in the AAP response procedure by practicing storytelling without probes using two non-AAP neutral pictures (i.e., non-attachment themes such as a horseback riding scene) before entering the scanner. This training procedure was repeated two more times if necessary in order to ensure the participants knew what to do when they entered the scanner. Immediately before scanning, participants were again given the standard set of verbal instructions on the AAP (see Chapter 3). They were also instructed to hold their head

[3] Five participants were excluded from the final sample because of either excessive head movement or insufficient number of words produced while telling the AAP stories.

still while speaking. Once in the scanner, participants were asked to tell stories to two additional neutral (i.e., non-attachment) stimuli. The AAP attachment stimuli were then presented. Note again there was no prompting in the scanner, even if a participant paused or stopped speaking. A short version of the standard instruction preceded presentation of the next AAP stimulus, which is optional in normal AAP administration but not unusual.

Instructions and pictures were presented with fMRI-compatible video goggles. Speech was digitally recorded by means of an fMRI-compatible microphone positioned closely to the mouth and saved digitally with respect to picture onset on a computer. The participants wore customized headphones, which reduced the noise of image acquisition and allowed communication with the experimenter before and after the fMRI procedure. Each picture (shown for 120 seconds) was preceded by an instruction (10 seconds) followed by a fixation cross (10 seconds). Then again, a fixation cross was shown for 15 seconds until the next instruction appeared. The whole procedure lasted about 25 minutes. Individual functional images were corrected for motion artifacts. Participants also filled out a state-anxiety questionnaire immediately before and after scanning in order to evaluate their emotional state.

The AAPs were classified from verbatim transcripts of the stories told in the scanner. The narratives were coded and classified by Anna Buchheim (in German) and Carol George (from English translation), who was blind to participant identity and coding only from translated transcripts. The attachment classification group distribution of the sample was six resolved and five unresolved. We had 91% interjudge reliability for classification groups of interest in this study. All narratives were similar in content and discourse style to the AAP narratives told in non-fMRI settings. We double-checked a random sample of 20 cases of native English-speaking AAP transcripts and there was no significant difference between the average length of that sample and the English translations of the AAPs in this study. For external concurrent validation, we had also administered the AAI (George et al., 1984/1985/1996; Main & Goldwyn, 1985/1988/1994) to these subjects several weeks prior to their scanner session as part of a larger study. Because of the strong reported AAP–AAI concordance in the AAP validity study, we wanted to determine whether we had similar concordance in this study. The AAIs were classified in German by blind certified AAI judges. There was 100% classification agreement. All of these indices together suggested to us that we had successfully assessed attachment using the modified scanner procedure and that the results were not influenced by the fMRI environment.

Summary of Results

One of our interests was to evaluate attachment-activation brain patterns during the AAP. State anxiety and number of words produced were not related to attachment classifications, which gave us confidence that we could observe attachment in action with minimal confounding by anxiety state and linguistic production.

The AAP is constructed such that the attachment system should be increasingly involved beginning with the *Window* stimulus and ending with the *Corner* stimulus. We were able to examine this at the neurobiological level by evaluating "increasing" and, conversely, "decreasing" attachment system effects. We also examined possible interactions by attachment group for the increasing attachment effects.

We indeed found a main effect for increasing activation of the attachment system; the effect was observed in the right inferior frontal cortex and the left occipital cortex. There was no main effect for "decreasing activation of the attachment system." There was an interaction effect for unresolved > resolved increasing activation of attachment system. Unresolved attachment showed a significantly stronger increasing activation in the right inferior frontal cortex, the left superior temporal gyrus, head of the left caudate nucleus, and in bilateral medial temporal lobe regions.

In summary, this study demonstrated that it is indeed feasible to use the AAP in a neuroimaging context. Our sample size was small, but no smaller than those typically used in neuroimaging studies. Unlike some of the studies reviewed earlier in this chapter, we controlled for gender and handedness. The attachment distribution was not regarded as representative of the general population of adults, nor was it necessary to the goals of this study to obtain a representative attachment sample.

The brain response patterns indicated that the order of AAP stimulus picture presentation (*Window* → *Corner*) does indeed increasingly activate attachment distress. Drawing from other neurobiological studies (e.g., Beauregard, Levesque, & Bourgouin, 2001; Ochsner, Bunge, Gross, & Gabrieli, 2002), increased activation of the right inferior frontal cortex demonstrates the increasing demand for emotional regulation control processes as distress and threat to the projected self increases over the course of the AAP. The inferior prefrontal cortex is associated with suppressing unwanted emotion and reappraising highly emotional stimuli to become unemotional.

We demonstrated for the first time in the neurobiological attachment literature specific brain activation patterns associated with unresolved attachment (Buchheim, Erk, et al., 2006). Unresolved participants showed significantly more activation of limbic areas in the course of the AAP than did organized participants. Heightened activation patterns were detected in the medial temporal regions including the amygdala and the hippocampus, central processing areas respectively associated with perception of fear and automatic autobiographic memory retrieval (Adolphs, Tranel, Damasio, & Damasio, 1995; Markowitsch, Vandekerckhovel, Lanfermann, & Russ, 2003; Phillips, Drevets, Rauch, & Lane, 2003; Piefke, Weiss, Zilles, Markowitsch, & Fink, 2003). Amygdala activation is also thought to be part a defense response control network (LeDoux, 1996). It appears, then, that the threatening situations in the AAP were emotionally more involving for the unresolved participants than for participants judged resolved, especially at the end of the AAP where the pictures were drawn to portray traumatic situations (*Cemetery, Corner*). The amygdala and hippocampal results also suggest that the AAP may reactivate "unresolved" traumatic or negatively valenced autobiographical memories.

STUDY 2: USING THE AAP TO STUDY THE NEURAL CORRELATES OF ATTACHMENT TRAUMA IN BORDERLINE PERSONALITY DISORDER

Building on our first study, we were next interested in examining the brain patterns associated with adult psychopathology, specifically borderline personality disorder (Buchheim et al., 2008a). Borderline personality disorder (BPD) is a heterogeneous constellation of symptoms characterized by severe and persistent problems across interpersonal, cognitive, behavioral, and emotional domains of functioning (Gunderson, 2009; Linehan, 1993). The main diagnostic symptoms include frantic efforts to avoid abandonment, patterns of unstable and intense interpersonal relationships, an unstable sense of self, chronic feelings of emptiness, stress-related paranoid ideation or severe dissociative symptoms, suicidal or other self-harm, and marked emotional instability and reactivity, especially difficulty with controlling intense anger (American Psychiatric Association, 2000).

There have been a fairly large number of BPD structural imaging studies, which indicate smaller hippocampal and amygdalar volumes in both the right and left hemispheres as compared with health control participants (Nunes et al., 2009). These studies suggest that BPD is associated with a network of brain regions involved in emotional regulation and impulsivity (e.g., amygdala, hippocampus, prefrontal cortex), including affect dysregulation (including the inability to control intense anger), dissociation, self-injury and pain processing problems, and social interaction problems (Mauchnik & Schmahl, 2010; Roth & Buchheim, 2010).

Every developmental attachment study and approximately half of the attachment-style studies reported a strong association between BPD and trauma (e.g., unresolved, fearful, preoccupied with trauma, angry/hostile attachment) (Aaronson, Bender, Skodol, & Gunderson, 2006; Agrawal, Gunderson, Holmes, & Lyons-Ruth, 2004; Bakermans-Kranenburg & van IJzendoorn, 2009; Critchfield, Levy, Clarkin, & Kernberg, 2009; Fossati et al., 2005; Levy et al., 2006; Minzenberg, Poole, & Vinogradov, 2006; Morse et al., 2009). Following the discussion of attachment trauma in Chapter 9, we believe that current situations and attachment figures (including adult romantic partners) likely activate past memories of abuse and aloneness for individuals diagnosed with BPD. We would expect, then, that attempts to organize current attachment relationships and current experience is derailed by chronic mourning of loss, abuse (i.e., unresolved state of mind), and a complex spectrum of assaults to attachment.

We were therefore interested in the neural patterns associated attachment trauma. In addition to the standard attachment classification groups, however, we used a trauma coding system to "look inside" participants' attachment representation (Buchheim et al., 2008a). Although we know that an individual is unresolved with regard to attachment, the classification group placement tells us little about the unique features that differentiate one unresolved individual from another. We applied the AAP trauma coding system after completing classifications in order to assess a more individualized level of attachment analysis.

The system was developed when Carol George noted, after blind-coding several hundred community and patient AAPs, that some segregated systems indicators in the AAP were unusual or distressing (see Chapter 4 for a description of AAP segregated systems coding). As a result, she developed a supplementary AAP coding scheme that differentiated between "normative" and "traumatic" markers. Normative markers were more typical and often seemed to be related to the stimulus "pull." For example, it was not unusual for AAP responses to include the theme of death in *Ambulance* response or discussions with the deceased in *Cemetery*. Traumatic dysregulation markers seemed particularly frightening or bizarre responses to the AAP stimulus. These included themes of severe abuse, entrapment, abandonment, murder, suicide, or incarceration. Some responses included descriptions of segregated material, including attachment trauma, in personal experience elements of the response, indicating flooding by autobiographical trauma (see Chapter 9).

We were especially interested in this study to examine a particular state of mind thought to be a key organizing feature associated with BPD called "intolerance of aloneness" (Gunderson, 1996). Attachment threat to the alone self is depicted in four AAP stimuli. Furthermore, the AAP permits evaluating differences in responses between the projected alone self and the self in potential attachment dyads (see Chapter 4). According to Bowlby (1973), aloneness is associated with extreme fear. In the AAP, we reasoned that extreme fear would not only be associated with the trauma attachment classifications described in Chapter 9, but perhaps more importantly by indices of dysregulated traumatic segregated systems in specific AAP responses.

We hypothesized in this study that AAP alone stimuli would elicit a significantly greater association with traumatic dysregulation indicators (and not necessarily normative markers) in individuals diagnosed with BPD than in community controls. On the neural level, we predicted that individuals diagnosed with BPD, as compared with controls, would show increased activation of brain regions associated with fear and pain (e.g., amygdala, anterior cingulate cortex) while responding to the AAP stimuli in the scanner. We were especially interested in responses to the alone and dyadic attachment scenes.

The BPD sample comprised 11 women diagnosed with BPD (average age, 27.8 years) and recruited from an inpatient psychiatric hospital in southern Germany. The control sample comprised the data collected for the 11 women who participated in the feasibility sample, to which we added six more healthy female volunteers, resulting in 17 women in the control group (average age, 28.4 years). All participants were right-handed. There were no differences in age or education in the BPD or control participants. Psychiatric diagnoses, including diagnostic criteria for BPD, were assessed by a trained psychiatrist using the Structured Clinical Interview I and II for DSM-IV (First et al., 1996).

We used the same experimental procedure in this study as described for the feasibility study above. The AAP classification distribution was as follows: controls—10 resolved, 7 unresolved; borderline patients—11 unresolved. Interjudge reliability for AAP classification was 95% (kappa = .88) and 100% agreement for differentiating between normative and traumatic markers evaluated using the AAPs in the entire sample. We again checked the validity of the scanner-generated AAP against externally administered AAIs. All AAIs were classified by independent trained reliable German AAI judges. There was an 88% correspondence rate between the AAP and AAI resolved versus unresolved categories (kappa = .70).

Summary of Results

We found distinct prevalence patterns of traumatic dysregulation indicators in the AAPs of patients with BPD, which provide a more detailed level of understanding of the organization and threats to attachment in BPD than exists in the literature to date (see Buchheim et al., 2008a). As we expected, the number of traumatic dysregulation markers in the response of patients with BPD to the AAP alone stimuli was significantly greater than for controls. Flooded and overwhelmed, the patients with BPD in this study failed to integrate organizing AAP narrative elements (i.e., internalized secure base, agency of self, connectedness to others) into their alone stories and they remained dysregulated when attachment was activated. Unresolved controls showed significantly more normative segregated systems markers, suggesting either story pull or perhaps an attachment state of mind that had integrated and was no longer flooded by attachment trauma. There were no significant differences between the groups for any of the dyadic stimuli. The alone responses were significantly different in the responses to the *Window, Bench*, and *Cemetery* scenes. Therefore, we selected these three alone stimuli for fMRI analysis.

On a neural level, the presentation of the AAP alone picture stimuli triggered traumatic dysregulation and was accompanied by activation in brain regions associated with pain and fear. Patients with BPD showed significantly more activation in the dorsal anterior cingulate cortex. We predicted and found increased activation of limbic brain regions associated with fear and pain during narration in response to these alone stimuli for patients with BPD, as associated with stronger activation of the dorsal anterior cingulate cortex, as compared with the controls. Anterior cingulate cortex activation has been associated in neurobiology research with pain and unpleasantness (Schnitzler & Ploner, 2000) and social exclusion and grief (Eisenberger, Lieberman, & Williams, 2003; GŸndel, O'Connor, Littrell, Fort, & Lane, 2003). In particular, the anterior cingulate cortex activation observed in this study has been linked to pain, especially fear avoidance (Vogt, 2005). We suggest that the pattern observed in this study is a neural signature of pain and fear associated with attachment trauma, which is also consistent with reports that abandonment fears are the most persistent long-term symptoms with BPD (Zanarini, Frankenburg, Hennen, & Silk, 2003). The activation of this brain region suggests unsuccessful coping with emotional pain, and may be related to repeated attempts at self-mutilation (following Schmahl et al., 2006). These findings may provide evidence on the possible mechanisms related to the fearful intolerance of aloneness in patients with BPD (Gunderson, 1996).

Clinical Outlook Using the BPD Study

This neurobiological study of attachment trauma in patients with BPD underscores the importance for therapists to think about BPD from an attachment theory perspective, especially in articulating aloneness in terms of "representational attachment isolation." We have discussed using the AAP as a diagnostic tool at the outset of therapy in a recent case study (Buchheim & George, 2011). The AAP can provide clinicians with a realistic and enriching analysis of different levels of trauma, evidenced in response to different AAP stimuli. This assessment can provide more specific information about what is "traumatizing" than attachment classification alone. It can lead to therapeutic hypotheses for examining the adverse childhood experiences that shape patients' styles of discourse, defense, and coping (especially elements of attachment agency, connectedness, and synchrony), and add a new level of understanding regarding patients' frightened and distressed behavior in transference. Based on assessment of traumatic dysregulation, treatment could focus on helping a patient to understand step by step the representational contexts associated with attachment dysregulation and the intense emotional reactions of helplessness.

STUDY 3: USING THE AAP IN PSYCHOANALYTIC TREATMENT OF DEPRESSION

At present, neuroscience is increasingly integrated into psychotherapy. We have initiated the first functional imaging study examining psychodynamic treatment with chronically depressed patients during psychoanalytic treatment at the beginning and after 15 months of treatment (Buchheim et al., 2008b). Walter, Berger, and Schnell (2009) have suggested a working definition of neuropsychotherapy that includes the identification of mediators and functional targets, determination of new therapeutic routes to such targets, and even the design of psychotherapeutic techniques. Walter et al. (2009) also showed that neuroimaging studies are increasingly used to study the effects and mechanisms of psychotherapy.

This ongoing study uses the AAP as one paradigm and a clinical interview as a second paradigm (operationalized psychodynamic diagnostic; Kessler et al., 2011) to capture individually relevant material that might be invaluable to the psychotherapeutic process. The experimental setting of the AAP paradigm we used here differed from the one we used in the study with the patients with BPD. Two to 4 weeks prior to the fMRI experiment, one trained judge conducted a standard AAP interview. Three core sentences representing a participant's unique attachment response were extracted verbatim from the responses to each AAP stimulus by two independent certified judges (e.g., "A girl is incarcerated in that big room," "My mother suffered until the end and the ambulance came often"). These unique statements were paired with each respective picture to constitute the "personally relevant" scanner trials. The same pictures were also paired with a standard set of sentences describing only the environment depicted by the AAP stimulus (e. g., "There is a window with curtains on the left and right," "There is a bed with a big blanket"). These pairings constituted the "neutral" scanner trials. Neutral trials were identical for all participants. Scanner presentations alternated between the personally relevant and neutral in groups of seven AAP picture stimuli. We expected and found neural changes in depressed patients during psychodynamic psychotherapy using these individually tailored stimuli. These data are about to be published elsewhere, and we cannot provide more detail at this time.

This study represents an innovative way of using the AAP, not only in treatment research, but also in neurobiological research more generally. Unlike the previous two studies, the AAP was not administered in the scanner. Yet the AAP material presented in the scanner, countered by neutral material, was just as unique and personally relevant as the scanner administration method. This alternate method may provide researchers with more flexibility in neurobiological research than the scanner administration method.

STUDY 4: USING THE AAP TO EXAMINE THE BIOCHEMISTRY OF ADULT ATTACHMENT

Like the feasibility study, we initiated this study to pilot a new AAP-derived methodology, this time to examine the biochemistry of adult attachment (Buchheim et al. 2009). Oxytocin enhances the experience of attachment security. We were interested in investigating whether increases in oxytocin would enhance feelings of attachment security. Our interest draws from an expansive literature that describes the role of oxytocin in fostering social relationships and intimacy, including maternal behavior in nonhuman mammals (Carter, 1998; Uvnas-Moberg, 1998; Young & Wang, 2004). Intranasal oxytocin administration in humans has been found to reduce endocrine and psychological responses to social stress, increase trust and social approach, capacity for mentalizing, and eye contact (Domes, Heinrichs, Michel, Berger, & Herpertz, 2007; Guastella, Mitchell, & Dadds, 2008; Heinrichs, Baumgartner, Kirschbaum, & Ehlert, 2003; Heinrichs & Domes, 2008; Kosfeld, Heinrichs, Zak, Fischbacher, & Fehr, 2005). We hypothesized that oxytocin might also promote the experience of secure attachment in humans. In particular, we expected that intranasal oxytocin administration would enhance the subjective perception of attachment security in insecurely attached individuals.

The participants for this study were a subsample of 26 healthy males (ages 21–33 years) recruited from a larger sample of college students in southern Germany. Only participants classified with an insecure attachment pattern using the AAP, and who were willing to have oxytocin administered nasally, were invited to participate because our aim was to examine oxytocin-induced shifts from attachment insecurity toward attachment security. Administering oxytocin during what is typically a 25–30 minute AAP administration period may not be feasible without introducing confounds. We addressed this problem by adapting a form of the AAP that was amenable to our double-blind, placebo-controlled within-subject (AB–BA) design.

We could have administered the AAP and used each participant's unique attachment statements, as we did in the depression therapy study described above. But first, we wanted to run a pilot study to see whether we could use the AAP to more generally enhance feelings of attachment security. So for this pilot study, we developed a set of 32 prototypical statements that captured the essential elements of each attachment group for each picture. We were able to do this because of our combined experience with hundreds of AAPs. We used the AAP stimuli, presenting the standard eight picture stimuli (one neutral; seven attachment) four times in the same order. Each of the 32 picture presentations was accompanied by four prototypical phrases (in German) representing one of the four established attachment categories: secure and three insecure categories (dismissing, preoccupied, unresolved).

The participants were instructed to rank these phrases from what they believed was the most to the least appropriate for each presentation. The phrases were presented in a randomized balanced sequence in order to minimize simple memory effects across test sessions. Each phrase placement was scored 3 to 0, with 3 indicating their first choice. The ranked scores were summed scores for each attachment scale ("secure," "dismissing," "preoccupied," and "unresolved trauma"). These sums were used to derive an attachment scale total.

Participants were randomly assigned subgroups to receive the oxytocin or placebo condition first. A single dose of 24 IU oxytocin (Syntocinon spray; Novartis, Basel, Switzerland) or placebo was administered intranasally 50 minutes before the attachment task at both testing sessions. The placebo contained all inactive ingredients except for the neuropeptide. Participants underwent both conditions in a 2–3 week range. Participants filled out questionnaires before the oxytocin administration and before the attachment task to assess potential confounding effects of arousal, wakefulness, and mood.

As predicted, we found that subjective perception of attachment security associated with oxytocin produced significantly more selections of the secure attachment phrases than in the control condition. This was indicated by increasing the rank of their selection of the secure phrases, which consequently decreased the preference rank of insecure phrases. The change was small but significant, and observed in the majority of participants (69%), as compared with change in the decreased preference direction in only 31% of participants. We examined the three insecure scales to determine whether any particular "form" of insecurity was being affected. The decrease in global insecurity was most associated with the preoccupied statements; there were no changes in ranked placement for the dismissing or unresolved statements. Comparisons of the first and second trials suggested no evidence of a practice effect.

This was the first study to show effects of a single dose of intranasally administered oxytocin on perceptions of attachment (Buchheim et al., 2009). The effect was small, but the intervention was similarly small—one nasal administration of a small doses of oxytocin. This seemed to produce a momentary mind change for insecure participants, especially related to reduced rankings of statements representing preoccupied state of mind. As described in Chapters 4 and 8, preoccupation is associated with cognitive disconnecting defenses that create tension and uncertainty, sometimes accompanied by depression and sadness, that undermines the ability to integrate attachment and feelings of security. We also saw in Chapter 8 how disconnecting defenses undermine representations personal agency, connectedness, and even functional synchrony in relationships. The oxytocin effect in this study might provide enhanced clarity about attachment figure availability. This may in turn accentuate felt security, either through deactivating defenses or integrating representational strategies. This result concurs with recent findings from neuroimaging studies in healthy humans, demonstrating that looking at pictures of significant others showed marked overlap with regions that show high densities of oxytocin receptors (e.g., striatum) (Bartels & Zeki, 2004).

CONCLUSION

The neurobiology of attachment behavior has been studied extensively in animal models and more recently in humans using fMRI. In this chapter, we summarized current state of the art neurobiological studies of adult attachment and then, summarizing our own studies, described the unique contribution of using the AAP in this research area.

We demonstrated three different ways to use the AAP in an experimental design. In the first two studies, the AAP was administered and adult attachment was assessed in the fMRI scanner (Buchheim, Erk, et al., 2006; Buchheim et al., 2008a), providing evidence for the feasibility of the AAP fMRI procedure. In the pilot study with healthy controls (Buchheim, Erk et al., 2006), we found a significant interaction effect between sequence of AAP pictures and attachment category. Only the unresolved participants showed increasing activation of medial temporal regions, including the amygdala and the hippocampus, in the course of the AAP task. This pattern was demonstrated especially at the end of the AAP, where the pictures are drawn to portray traumatic situations. We interpreted these results as confirming our hypothesis linking unresolved attachment to dysregulation of attachment.

In the clinical study with borderline patients (Buchheim et al., 2008a), we developed a more fine-grained way to differentiate unresolved subjects using a specific analysis on segregated systems markers. This study analyzed group differences in narrative and neural responses to alone (characters facing attachment threats alone) versus dyadic AAP picture stimuli (interaction between characters in an attachment context). Behavioral narrative data showed that alone pictures were significantly more traumatic for borderline patients than for controls. As hypothesized, borderline patients showed significantly more anterior midcingulate cortex activation in response to alone pictures than did controls. In response to dyadic pictures, patients showed more activation of the right superior temporal sulcus and less activation of the right parahippocampal gyrus as compared with controls. Our results suggested evidence for potential neural mechanisms of attachment trauma underlying interpersonal symptoms associated with BPD, that is, fearful and painful intolerance of aloneness, hypersensitivity to social environment, and reduced positive memories of dyadic interactions.

In the third study, we modified our fMRI paradigm to control better for movement artifacts in the scanner. The modified procedure presented individuals with "core sentences" from their own AAP stories. These personally relevant trials were contrasted with neutral sentences (Buchheim et al., 2008b). This paradigm was developed for using the AAP in a neurobiological psychotherapy study to examine neural changes during psychodynamic treatment in recurrent major depression. This more standardized paradigm seems to be a successful way to confront patients, compared to controls, with their own crucial attachment patterns to assess changes in their mental organization of attachment-relevant material on a neural level in the course of their psychotherapy. On the one side this paradigm avoided talking in the scanner and on the other side it suggested a procedure to give standardized and individually tailored stimuli at the same time.

The fourth study used the AAP in yet another way. Here we were interested to see whether healthy insecure participants will rate "prototypical secure sentences" from AAPs more often than "prototypical insecure ones" under the condition of oxytocin compared to placebo (Buchheim et al., 2009). This paradigm suggested a "compromise" to using a paper-and-pencil attachment measure ("what kind of attachment style I believe I have") to capture some "unconscious" parts of how individuals judge "prototypical" AAP statements as relevant for them or not without knowing what the attachment category the statements belong to. Here we used an experimental manipulation using oxytocin versus placebo using double-blind, placebo-controlled within-subject design. Indeed, the results gave first evidence that a single dose of intranasally administered oxytocin was sufficient to enhance the experience of attachment security. Oxytocin seemed to induce a *momentary* state-of-mind change in which insecure subjects shift to attachment security. Thus, under the oxytocin condition, the insecure-classified individuals experienced phrases as most appropriate associated with attachment-related comfort, secure base, and feelings of safety. Oxytocin might have provided these individuals with a sense of mental emotional integration with the capacity to connect to others.

In summary, these four AAP studies demonstrated that the AAP is a unique attachment measure combining pictures and stories, or crucial sentences extracted from a person's AAP stories relevant for their attachment category, to be assessed in different experimental situations in healthy participants and psychiatric patients to examine for neural and biological correlates of attachment in the moments when the attachment system is activated.

References

Aaronson, C. J., Bender, D. S., Skodol, A. E., & Gunderson, J. G. (2006). Comparison of attachment styles in borderline personality disorder and obsessive–compulsive personality disorder. *Psychiatric Quarterly, 77,* 69–80.

Abrams, K. Y., Rifkin, A., & Hesse, E. (2006). Examining the role of parental frightened/frightening subtypes in predicting disorganized attachment within a brief observation procedure. *Development and Psychopathology, 18,* 345–361.

Adolphs, R., Tranel, D., Damasio, H., & Damasio, A. R. (1995). Fear and the human amygdala. *Journal of Neuroscience, 15,* 5879–1591.

Agrawal, H. R., Gunderson, J., Holmes, B. M., & Lyons-Ruth, K. (2004). Attachment studies with borderline patients: A review. *Harvard Review of Psychiatry, 12,* 94–104.

Aikins, J. W., Howes, C., & Hamilton, C. (2009). Attachment stability and the emergence of unresolved representations during adolescence. *Attachment and Human Development, 11*(5), 491–512.

Ainsworth, M. D. S. (1964). Patterns of attachment behavior shown by the infant in interaction with his mother. *Merrill Palmer Quarterly, 10,* 51–58.

Ainsworth, M. D. S. (1967). *Infancy in Uganda.* Baltimore, MD: Johns Hopkins Press.

Ainsworth, M. D. S. (1989). Attachment beyond infancy. *American Psychologist, 44,* 709–716.

Ainsworth, M. D. S., Blehar, M., Waters, E., & Wall, S. (1978). *Patterns of attachment: A psychological study of the Strange Situation.* Hillsdale, NJ: Erlbaum.

Allen, J. P. (2008). The attachment system in adolescence. In J. Cassidy & P. R. Shaver (Eds.), *Handbook of attachment: Theory, research, and clinical applications* (2nd ed., pp. 419–435). New York: Guilford Press.

American Psychiatric Association. (2000). *Diagnostic and statistical manual of mental disorders* (4th ed.). Washington, DC: Author.

Ammaniti, M., & Stern, D. N. (1994). *Psychoanalysis and development: Representations and narratives.* New York: New York University Press.

Arnett, J. J. (2006). Emerging adulthood: Understanding the new way of coming of age. In J. J. Arnett & J. L. Tanner (Eds.), *Emerging adults in America: Coming of age in the 21st century* (pp. 3–20). Washington, DC: American Psychological Association Press.

Arsalidou, M., Barbeau, E. J., Bayless, S. J., & Taylor, M. J. (2010). Brain responses differ to faces of mothers and fathers. *Brain and Cognition, 74,* 47–51.

Bakermans-Kranenburg, M. J., & van IJzendoorn, M. H. (2009). The first 10,000 Adult Attachment Interviews: Distributions of adult attachment representations in clinical and non-clinical groups. *Attachment and Human Development, 11,* 223–263.

Bar-Haim, Y., Dan, O., Eshel, Y., & Sagi-Schwartz, A. (2007). Predicting children's anxiety from early attachment relationships. *Journal of Anxiety Disorders, 21,* 1061–1068.

Bartels, A., & Zeki, S. (2004). The neural correlates of maternal and romantic love. *NeuroImage, 21*(3), 1155–1167.

Bartholomew, K., & Horowitz, I. M. (1999). Attachment style among young adults: A test of a category model. *Journal of Personality and Social Psychology, 61,* 236–244.

Beauregard, M., Levesque, J., & Bourgouin, P. (2001). Neural correlates of conscious self-regulation of emotion. *Journal of Neuroscience, 21,* RC165.

Béliveau, M.-J., & Moss, E. (2005). Contribution aux validités convergente et divergente du projectif de l'attachement adulte. *La Revue Internationale de l'Éducation Familiale, 9,* 29–50.

Benetti, S., McCrory, E., Arulanantham, S., De Sanctis, T., McGuire, P., & Mechelli, A. (2010). Attachment style, affective loss and gray matter volume: A voxel-based morphometry study. *Human Brain Mapping, 31,* 1482–1489.

Benoit, M., Bouthillier, D., Moss, E., Rousseau, C., & Brunet, A. (2010). Emotion regulation strategies as mediators of the association between level of attachment security and PTSD symptoms following trauma in adulthood. *Anxiety, Stress and Coping, 23,* 101–118.

Berndt, T. J. (1996). Transitions in friendship and friends' influences. In J. A. Graber, J. Brooks-Gunn, & A. C. Petersen (Eds.), *Transitions through adolescence: Interpersonal domains and context* (pp. 57–84). Mahwah, NJ: Erlbaum.

Berndt, T. J. (2004). Children's friendships: Shifts over a half of century in perspectives on their development and their effects. *Merrill-Palmer Quarterly, 50,* 206–223.

Bernier, A., & Dozier, M. (2003). Bridging the attachment transmission gap: The role of maternal mind-mindedness. *International Journal of Behavioral Development, 27,* 355–365.

Bifulco, A., Moran, P., Jacobs, C., & Bunn, A. (2009). Problem partners and parenting: Exploring linkages with maternal insecure attachment style and adolescent offspring internalizing disorder. *Attachment and Human Development, 11,* 69–85.

Bowlby, J. (1951). *Maternal care and mental health.* Geneva, Switzerland: World Health Organization.

Bowlby, J. (1969/1982). *Attachment and loss: Vol. 1. Attachment.* New York: Basic Books.

Bowlby, J. (1973). *Attachment and loss: Vol. 2. Separation: Anxiety and anger.* New York: Basic Books.

Bowlby, J. (1980). *Attachment and loss: Vol. 3. Loss: Sadness and depression.* New York: Basic Books.

Bowlby, J. (1988). *A secure base.* New York: Basic Books.

Bowlby, J. (1991). Ethological light on psychoanalytical problems. In P. Bateson (Ed.), *The development and integration of behaviour: Essays in honour of Robert Hinde* (pp. 301–313). New York: Cambridge University Press.

Bretherton, I. (1985). Attachment theory: Retrospect and prospect. In I. Bretherton & E. Waters (Eds.), Growing points in attachment theory and research. *Monographs of the Society for Research in Child Development, 50* (1–2, Serial No. 209), 3–35.

Bretherton, I. (1992). The origins of attachment theory: John Bowlby and Mary Ainsworth. *Developmental Psychology, 28,* 759–775.

Bretherton, I. (2005). In pursuit of the internal working model construct and its relevance to attachment relationships. In K. E. Grossmann, K. Grossmann, & E. Waters (Eds.), *Attachment from infancy to adulthood: The major longitudinal studies* (pp. 13–47). New York: Guilford Press.

Bretherton, I., & Munholland, K. A. (2008). Internal working models in attachment relationships. In J. Cassidy & P. R. Shaver (Eds.), *Handbook of attachment: Theory, research, and clinical applications* (2nd ed., pp. 102–127). New York: Guilford Press.

Bretherton, I., Ridgeway, D., & Cassidy, J. (1990). Assessing internal working models of the attachment relationship: An attachment story completion task for 3-year-olds. In M. T. Greenberg, D. Cicchetti, & E. M. Cummings (Eds.), *Attachment in the preschool years* (pp. 273–308). Chicago: University of Chicago Press.

Britner, P. A., Marvin, R. S., & Pianta, R. C. (2005). Development and preliminary validation of the caregiving behavior system: Association with child attachment classification in the preschool Strange Situation. *Attachment and Human Development, 7,* 83–102.

Broberg, A. G. (2001). Can attachment theory, and attachment research methodologies, help children and adolescents in mental health institutions? *Attachment and Human Development, 3,* 330–338.

Brumariu, L. E., & Kerns, K. A. (2010). Mother–child attachment patterns and different types of anxiety symptoms: Is there specificity of relations? *Child Psychiatry and Human Development, 41,* 663–674.

Buchheim, A., Erk, S., George, C., Kächele, H., Kircher, T., Martius, P., et al. (2008a). Neural correlates of attachment dysregulation in borderline personality disorder using functional magnetic resonance imaging. *Psychiatry Research: Neuroimaging, 163,* 223–235.

Buchheim, A., Erk, S., George, C., Kächele, H., Kircher, T., Martius, P., et al. (2008b). Neural correlates of attachment trauma in borderline personality disorder: A functional magnetic resonance imaging study. *Psychiatry Research, 30,* 223–235.

Buchheim, A., Erk, S., George, C., Kächele, H., Ruchsow, M., Spitzer, M., et al. (2006). Measuring attachment representation in an fMRI environment: A pilot study. *Psychopathology, 39,* 144–152.

Buchheim, A., & George, C. (2011). The representational, neurobiological, and emotional foundation of attachment disorganization in borderline personality disorder and anxiety disorder. In J. Solomon & C. George (Eds.), *Disorganized attachment and caregiving* (pp. 343–382). New York: Guilford Press.

Buchheim, A., George, C., Gündel, H., Heinrichs, M., Koops, E., O'Connor, M.-F., et al. (2009). Oxytocin enhances the experience of attachment security. *Psychoendochronology, 34,* 1417–1422.

Buchheim, A., George, C., & Kächele, H. (2008). "My dog is dying today": Attachment narratives and psychoanalytic interpretation of an initial interview. In D. Diamond, S. J. Blatt, & J. D. Lichtenberg (Eds.), *Attachment and sexuality* (pp. 161–178). Hillsdale, NJ: Analytic Press.

Buchheim, A., George, C., Kächele, H., Erk, S., & Walter, H. (2006). Measuring adult attachment representation in an fMRI environment: concepts and assessment. *Psychopathology, 39,* 136–143.

Buchheim, A., Taubner, S., Fizke, E. & Nolte, T. (2010). Bindung und Neurobiologie: Ergebnisse bildgebender Verfahren. (Attachment and neurobiology: Neuroimaging results.) *Psychotherapie in Psychiatrie, Psychotherapeutischer Medizin und Klinischer Psychologie, 15,* 22–31.

Carlson, E. A. (1998). A prospective longitudinal study of attachment disorganization/ disorientation. *Child Development, 69,* 1107–1129.

Carter, C. S. (1998). Neuroendocrine perspectives on social attachment and love. *Psychoneuroendocrinology, 23,* 779–818.

Carter, C. S., Lederhendler, I., & Kirkpatrick, B. (Eds.). (1997). *Annals of the New York Academy of Sciences, Vol. 807: The integrative neurobiology of affiliation.* New York: New York Academy of Sciences.

Cassidy, J., & Berlin, L. J. (1994). The insecure/ambivalent pattern of attachment: Theory and research. *Child Development, 65,* 971–991.

Cassidy, J., & Kobak, R. R. (1988). Avoidance and its relation to other defensive processes. In J. Belsky & T. Nezworski (Eds.), *Clinical implications of attachment* (pp. 300–323). Hillsdale, NJ: Erlbaum.

Cassidy, J., Marvin, R. S., & the MacArthur Working Group (1987–1992). *Attachment organization in preschool children: Coding guidelines.* University Park, PA: Penn State University.

Cassidy, J., & Shaver, P. R. (Eds.). (1999). *Handbook of attachment: Theory, research, and clinical applications.* New York: Guilford Press.

Cassidy, J., & Shaver, P. R. (Eds.). (2008). *Handbook of attachment: Theory, research, and clinical applications* (2nd ed.). New York: Guilford Press.

Chopra, M. (2006). Delusional themes of penetration and loss of boundaries and their relation to early sexual trauma in psychotic disorder. *Clinical Social Work Journal, 34,* 483–497.

Cicchetti, D., & Schneider-Rosen, K. (1986). An organizational approach to childhood depression In M. Rutter, C. Izard, & P. Read (Eds.), *Depression in young people: Developmental and clinical perspectives* (pp. 71–134). New York: Guilford Press.

Coan, J. A. (2008). Toward a neuroscience of attachment. In J. Cassidy & P. R. Shaver (Eds.), *Handbook of attachment: Theory, research, and clinical applications* (2nd ed., pp. 241–265). New York: Guilford Press.

Coan, J. A., Schaefer, H. S., & Davidson, R. J. (2006). Lending a hand: Social regulation of the neural response to threat. *Psychological Science, 17,* 1032–1039.

Collins, N. L., & Read, S. J. (1990). Adult attachment, working models, and relationship quality in dating couples. *Journal of Personality and Social Psychology, 58,* 644–663.

Critchfield, K. L., Levy, K. N., Clarkin, J. E., & Kernberg, O. F. (2009). The relational context of aggression in borderline personality disorder: Using attachment style to predict forms of hostility. *Journal of Clinical Psychology, 64,* 67–82.

Crittenden, P. M. (1997). Toward an integrative theory of trauma: A dynamic-maturation approach. In D. Cicchetti & S. L. Toth (Eds.), *Developmental perspectives on trauma: Theory, research, and intervention* (pp. 33–84). Rochester, NY: University of Rochester Press.

Crittenden P. M. (2004). *Patterns of attachment in adulthood: A dynamic–maturational approach to analyzing the Adult Attachment Interview.* Unpublished manuscript.

Crowell, J., Fraley, R. C., & Shaver, P. R. (2008). Measurement of individual differences in adolescent and adult attachment. In J. Cassidy & P. R. Shaver (Eds.), *Handbook of attachment: Theory, research, and clinical applications* (2nd ed., pp. 599–634). New York: Guilford Press.

Crowell, J. A., & Treboux, D. (1995). A review of adult attachment measures: Implications for theory and research. *Social Development, 4,* 294–327.

Dallaire, D. H., & Weinraub, M. (2005). Predicting children's separation anxiety at age 6: The contributions of infant–mother attachment security, maternal sensitivity, and maternal separation anxiety. *Attachment and Human Development, 7,* 393–408.

Damasio, A. R. (2003). *Looking for Spinoza: Joy, sorrow and the feeling brain.* Orlando, FL: Harcourt.

de Haas, M. A., Bakermans-Kranenburg, M. J., & van IJzendoorn, M. H. (1994). The Adult Attachment Interview and questionnaires for attachment style, temperament, and memories of parental behavior. *Journal of Genetic Psychology: Research and Theory on Human Development, 155,* 471–486.

De Haene, L., Grietens, H., & Verschueren, K. (2010). Adult attachment in the context of refugee traumatisation: The impact of organized violence and forced separation on parental states of mind regarding attachment. *Attachment and Human Development, 12,* 249–264.

de Ruiter, C., & van IJzendoorn, M. H. (1992). Agoraphobia and anxious-ambivalent attachment: An integrative review. *Journal of Anxiety Disorders, 6,* 365–381.

de Wolff, M. S., & van IJzendoorn, M. H. (1997). Sensitivity and attachment: A meta-analysis on parental antecedents of infant attachment. *Child Development, 68,* 571–591.

Derogatis, L. R., & Cleary, P. A. (1977). Confirmation of the dimensional structure of the SCL-90: A study in construct validation. *Journal of Clinical Psychology 33,* 981–989.

Di Riso, D., Lis, A., Chessa, D., & George, C. (in press). Anorexia and attachment: Dysregulated defense and pathological mourning.

Domes, G., Heinrichs, M., Michel, A., Berger, C., & Herpertz, S.C. (2007). Oxytocin improves "mind-reading" in humans. *Biological Psychiatry, 61,* 731–733.

Dozier, M., Stovall-McClough, C., & Albus, K. E. (2008). Attachment and psychopathology in adulthood. In J. Cassidy & P. R. Shaver (Eds.), *Handbook of attachment: Theory, research, and clinical applications* (2nd ed., pp. 718–744). New York: Guilford Press.

Edelman, G. (1992). *Brilliant air, brilliant fire.* New York: Basic Books.

Eisenberger, N., Lieberman, M.D. & Williams, K.D., (2003). Does rejection hurt? An fMRI study of social exclusion. *Science, 302,* 290–292.

Feeney, J. A., & Noller, P. (1990). Attachment style as a predictor of adult romantic relationships. *Journal of Personality and Social Psychology, 58,* 281–291.

Finn, S. (2011). Use of the Adult Attachment Projective Picture System (AAP) in the middle of a long-term psychotherapy. *Journal of Personality Assessment, 93,* 427–433.

First, M. B., Spitzer, R. L., Gibbon, M., & Williams, J. B. W. (1996). *Structural Clinical Interview for DSM-IV Axis I Disorders. Clinical Version.* Washington, DC: American Psychiatric Press.

Fonagy, P., Steele, H., & Steele, M. (1991). Maternal representation of attachment during pregnancy predict the organization of attachment at one year of age. *Child Development, 62,* 891–905.

Fonagy, P., Leigh, T., Steele, M., Steele, H., Kennedy, R., Mattoon, G., et al. (1996). The relation of attachment status, psychiatric classification, and response to psychotherapy. *Journal of Consulting and Clinical Psychology, 64,* 22–31.

Fossati, A., Feeney, J. A., Carretta, I., Grazioli, F., Milesi, R., Leonardi, B., et al. (2005). Modelling the relationships between adult attachment patterns and borderline personality disorder: The role of impulsivity and aggressiveness. *Journal of Social and Clinical Psychology, 24,* 520–537.

Fraedrich, E. M., Lakatos, K., & Spangler, G. (2010). Brain activity during emotion perception: The role of attachment representation. *Attachment and Human Development, 12,* 231–248.

Fraley, C., & Spieker, S. J. (2003). Are infant attachment patterns continuously or categorically distributed? A taxometric analysis of Strange Situation behavior. *Developmental Psychology, 39,* 387–404.

Freud, A., & Dann, S. (1949). An experiment in group upbringing. In A. Freud, H. Hartmann, & E. Kris (Eds.), *The psychoanalytic study of the child. Vol. 3/4.* (pp. 127–168). Oxford, UK: International Universities Press.

Freud, S. (1895/1954). Project for a scientific psychology (J. Strachey, Trans.). In

M. Bonaparte, A. Freud, & E. Kris (Eds.), *The origins of psycho-analysis* (pp. 347–445). New York: Basic Books.

Freud, S. (1926/1959). Inhibitions, symptoms and anxiety. In J. Strachey (Ed. and Trans.), *The standard edition of the complete psychological works of Sigmund Freud* (Vol. 22, pp. 77–175). London: Hogarth Press.

George, C., Isaacs, M., & Marvin, R.M. (2011). The implications of attachment assessment in custody evaluation: The case of a two-year old and his parents. *Family Court Review, 48,* 438–500.

George, C., Kaplan, N., & Main, M. (1984/1985/1996). *The Adult Attachment Interview.* Berkeley: University of California.

George, C., & Solomon, J. (1996). Representational models of relationships: Links between caregiving and attachment. *Infant Mental Health Journal, 17,* 198–216.

George, C., & Solomon, J. (1999). Attachment and caregiving: The caregiving behavioral system. In J. Cassidy & P. R. Shaver (Eds.), *Handbook of attachment: Theory, research, and clinical applications* (pp. 649–670). New York: Guilford Press.

George, C., & Solomon, J. (2008). The caregiving system: A behavioral systems approach to parenting. In J. Cassidy & P. R. Shaver (Eds.), *Handbook of attachment: Theory, research, and clinical applications* (2nd ed., pp. 833–856). New York: Guilford Press.

George, C., & Solomon, J. (2011). The disorganized caregiving system: Mothers' helpless state of mind. In J. Solomon & C. George (Eds.), *Disorganized attachment and caregiving* (pp. 133–163). New York: Guilford Press.

George, C., & West, M. (1999). Developmental vs. social personality models of adult attachment and mental ill health. *British Journal of Medical Psychology, 72,* 285–303.

George, C., & West, M. (2001). The development and preliminary validation of a new measure of adult attachment: The Adult Attachment Projective. *Attachment and Human Development, 3,* 30–61.

George, C., & West, M. (2004). The Adult Attachment Projective: Measuring individual differences in attachment security using projective methodology. In M. J. Hilsenroth & D. L. Segal (Eds.), *Comprehensive handbook of psychological assessment, Vol. 2: Personality assessment* (pp. 431–447). Hoboken, NJ: Wiley.

George, C., & West, M. (2008). *The Adult Attachment Projective Picture System.* Unpublished coding and classification system, Mills College, Oakland, CA.

George, C., & West, M. (2009). *The Adult Attachment Projective Picture System.* Unpublished coding and classification system, Mills College, Oakland, CA.

George, C., West, M., & Pettem, O. (1997–2007). *The Adult Attachment Projective Picture System.* Unpublished coding and classification system, Mills College, Oakland, CA

George, C., West, M., & Pettem, O. (1999). The Adult Attachment Projective: Disorganization of adult attachment at the level of representation. In J. Solomon & C. George (Eds.), *Attachment disorganization* (pp. 462–507). New York: Guilford Press.

Gervai, J., Nemoda, Z., Lakatos, K., Ronai, Z., Toth, I., Ney, K., et al. (2005).

Transmission equilibrium tests confirm the link between DRD4 gene polymorphism and infant attachment. *American Journal of Medical Genetics Part B. Neuropsychiatric Genetics, 132B,* 126–130.

Gillath, O., & Schachner, D. A. (2006). How do sexuality and attachment interrelate?: Goals, motives, and strategies. In M. Mikulincer & G. S. Goodman (Eds.), *Dynamics of romantic love: Attachment, caregiving, and sex* (pp. 337–355). New York: Guilford Press.

Gillath, O., Bunge, S. A., Shaver, P. R., Wendelken, C., & Mikulincer, M. (2005). Attachment-style differences in the ability to suppress negative thoughts: Exploring the neural correlates. *NeuroImage, 28,* 835–847.

Guastella, A. J., Mitchell, P. B., & Dadds, M. R. (2008). Oxytocin increases gaze to the eye region of human faces. *Biological Psychiatry, 63,* 3–5.

Gündel, H., O'Connor, M. F., Littrell, L., Fort, C., & Lane, R. (2003). Functional neuroanatomy of grief: An fMRI study. *American Journal of Psychiatry, 160,* 1946–1953.

Gunderson, J. G. (1996). The borderline patient's intolerance of aloneness: Insecure attachments and therapist availability. *American Journal of Psychiatry, 153,* 752–758.

Gunderson, J. G. (2009). Borderline personality disorder: Ontogeny of a diagnosis. *American Journal of Psychiatry, 166,* 530–539.

Gunnar, M. R., Brodersen, L., Nachmias, M., Buss, K., & Rigatuso, J. (1996). Stress reactivity and attachment security. *Developmental Psychobiology, 29,* 191–204.

Hamilton-Oravetz, S. (1992). *Patterns of attachment and grief in primary care medicine patients.* Unpublished doctoral dissertation, California School for Professional Psychology, Alameda, CA.

Hamilton-Oravetz, S., & George, C. (1991). *Scale for rating absent grief-failed mourning and absent response to trauma.* Unpublished doctoral dissertation, California School for Professional Psychology, Alameda, CA.

Hazan, C., & Shaver, P. R. (1987). Romantic love conceptualized as an attachment process. *Journal of Personality and Social Psychology, 52,* 511–524.

Hazan, C., & Shaver, P. R. (1990). Love and work: An attachment-theoretical perspective. *Journal of Personality and Social Psychology, 59,* 270–280.

Hebb, D. (1980). *Essay on mind.* Mahwah, NJ: Erlbaum.

Heinrichs, M., Baumgartner, T., Kirschbaum, C., & Ehlert, U. (2003). Social support and oxytocin interact to supress cortisol and subjective responses to psychosocial stress. *Biological Psychiatry, 54,* 1389–1398.

Heinrichs, M., & Domes, G. (2008). Neuropeptides and social behavior: Effects of oxytocin and vasopressin in humans. *Progress in Brain Research, 170,* 337–350.

Hesse, E. (1996). Discourse, memory, and the Adult Attachment Interview: A note with emphasis on the emerging Cannot Classify category. *Infant Mental Health Journal, 17,* 4–11.

Hesse, E. (2008). The Adult Attachment Interview: Protocol, methods of analysis, and empirical studies. In J. Cassidy & P. R. Shaver (Eds.), *Handbook of attachment: Theory, research, and clinical applications* (2nd ed., pp. 552–598). New York: Guilford Press.

Hesse, E., & Main, M. (2000). Disorganized infant, child, and adult attachment: Collapse in behavioral and attentional strategies. *Journal of the American Psychoanalytic Association, 48,* 1097–1127.

Hesse, E., & Main, M. (2006). Frightened, threatening, and dissociative parental behavior in low-risk samples: Description, discussion, and interpretations. *Development and Psychopathology, 18,* 309–343.

Hilsenroth, M. J. (2004). Projective assessment of personality and psychopathology: An overview. In M. J. Hilsenroth & D. L. Segal (Eds.), *Comprehensive handbook of psychological assessment: Vol. 2. Personality assessment* (pp. 283–296). Hoboken, NJ: Wiley.

Hinde, R. A. (1982). *Ethology.* New York: Oxford University Press.

Hinde, R. A., & Stevenson-Hinde, J. (1991). Perspectives on attachment. In C. M. Parkes, J. Stevenson-Hinde, & P. Marris (Eds.), *Attachment across the life cycle* (pp. 52–65). New York: Routledge.

Hobson, R. P. (1994). On developing a mind. *British Journal of Psychiatry, 165,* 577–581.

Hofer, M.A. (1995). Hidden regulators: Implications for a new understanding of attachment, separation, and loss. In S. Goldberg, R. Muir, & J. Kerr (Eds.), *Attachment theory: Social, developmental, and clinical perspectives* (pp. 203–230). Hillsdale, NJ: Analytic Press.

Hoffman, K. T., Marvin, R. S., Cooper, G., & Powell, B. (2006). Changing toddlers' and preschoolers' attachment classifications: The Circle of Security intervention. *Journal of Consulting and Clinical Psychology, 74,* 1017–1026.

Holden, R. R., Starzyk, K. B., McLeod, L. D., & Edwards, M. J. (2000). Comparison among the Holden Psychological Screening Inventory (HPSI), the Brief Symptom Inventory (BSI), and the Balanced Inventory of Desirable Responding (BIDR). *Assessment, 7,* 163–175.

Holmes, J. (1993). Attachment theory: A biological basis for psychotherapy? *British Journal of Psychiatry, 163,* 430–438.

Iacouvou, M. (2002). Regional differences in the transition to adulthood. *Annals of the American Academy of Political Science Studies, 580,* 40–69.

Isaacs, M., George, C., & Marvin, R. S. (2009). Utilizing attachment measures in custody evaluations: Incremental validity. *Journal of Child Custody, 6,* 139–162.

Isabella, R. A., & Belsky, J. (1991). Interactional synchrony and the origins of mother–infant attachment: A replication study. *Child Development, 62,* 373–384.

Jackson, D. N. (1971). The dynamics of structured tests. *Psychological Review, 78,* 229–248.

Jacobvitz, D., Hazen, N., Curran, M., & Hitchens, K. (2004). Observations of early triadic family interactions: Boundary disturbances in the family predict symptoms of depression, anxiety, and attention-deficit/hyperactivity disorder in middle childhood. *Development and Psychopathology, 16,* 577–592.

Jacobvitz, D., Leon, K., & Hazen, N. (2006). Does expectant mothers' unresolved trauma predict frightened/frightening maternal behavior? Risk and protective factors. *Development and Psychopathology, 18,* 363–379.

Kerig, P. K. (2005). Introduction: Contributions of the investigation of boundary dissolution to the understanding of developmental psychopathology and family process. *Journal of Emotional Abuse, 5,* 1–4.

Kessler, H., Taubner, S., Buchheim, A., MŸnte, T. F., Stasch, M., KŠchele, H., et al. (2011). Individualized and clinically derived stimuli activate limbic structures in depression: An fMRI study. *PLoS ONE 6*, e15712.

Kircher, T. T., Brammer, M. J., Williams, S. C., & McGuire, P. K. (2000). Lexical retrieval during fluent speech production: An fMRI study. *Neuroreport, 11,* 4093–4096.

Kircher, T. T., Liddle, P. F., Brammer, M. J., Williams, S. C., Murray, R. M., & McGuire, P. K. (2001). Neural correlates of formal thought disorder in schizophrenia: Preliminary findings from a functional magnetic resonance imaging study. *Archives of General Psychiatry, 58,* 769–774.

Kircher, T. T., Liddle, P. F., Brammer, M. J., Williams, S. C., Murray, R. M., & McGuire, P. K. (2002). Reversed lateralization of temporal activation during speech production in thought-disordered patients with schizophrenia. *Psychological Medicine, 32,* 439–449.

Klagsbrun, M., & Bowlby, J. (1976). Responses to separation from parents: A clinical test for young children. *British Journal of Projective Psychology, 21,* 7–21.

Klopfer, B., Ainsworth, M. D., Klopfer, W. G., & Holt, R. R. (1954). *Developments in the Rorschach technique: Vol. I. Technique and theory.* Oxford, UK: World Book.

Kobak, R., & Madsen, S. (2008). Disruptions in attachment bonds: Implications for theory, research, and clinical intervention. *Handbook of attachment: Theory, research, and clinical applications* (2nd ed., pp. 23–47). New York: Guilford Press.

Kosfeld, M., Heinrichs, M., Zak, P. J., Fischbacher, U., & Fehr, E. (2005). Oxytocin increased trust in humans. *Nature, 435,* 673–676.

Kraemer, G. W. (1992). A psychobiological theory of attachment. *Behavioral and Brain Sciences, 15,* 493–541.

Lanyon, R. I., & Carle, A. C. (2007). Internal and external validity of scores on the Balanced Inventory of Desirable Responding and Paulhus Deception Scales. *Educational and Psychological Measurement, 67,* 859–876.

LeDoux, J. E. (1996). *The emotional brain: The mysterious underpinnings of emotional life.* New York: Simon & Schuster.

Leibenluft, E., Gobbini, M. I., Harrison, T., & Haxby, J. V. (2004). Mothers' neural activation in response to pictures of their children and other children. *Biological Psychiatry, 15,* 225–232.

Leichtman, M. (2004). Projective tests: The nature of the task. In M. J. Hilsenroth & D. L. Segal (Eds.), *Comprehensive handbook of psychological assessment: Personality assessment* (Vol. 2, pp. 291–314). Hoboken, NJ: Wiley.

Lemche, E., Giampietro, V. P., Surguladze, S. A., Amaro, E. J., Andrew, C. M., Williams, S. C., et al. (2006). Human attachment security is mediated by the amygdala: Evidence from combined fMRI and psychophysiological measures. *Human Brain Mapping, 27,* 623–635.

Levitt, M. J. (2005). Social relations in childhood and adolescence: The convoy model perspective. *Human Development, 48,* 28–47.

Levy, K. N., Meehan, K. B., Kelly, K. M., Reynoso, J. S., Weber, M., Clarkin, J. F., et al. (2006). Change in attachment patterns and reflective function in a randomized control trial of transference-focused psychotherapy for borderline personality disorder. *Journal of Consulting and Clinical Psychology, 74,* 1027–1040.

Lim, M. M., & Young, L. J. (2004). Vasopressin-dependent neural circuits underlying pair-bond formation in the monogamous prairie vole. *Neuroscience, 125,* 35–45.

Linehan, M. M. (1993). *Cognitive-behavioral treatment of borderline personality disorder.* New York: Guilford Press.

Liotti, G. (2004). Trauma, dissociation, and disorganized attachment: Three strands of a single braid. *Psychotherapy: Theory, Research, Practice, Training, 41,* 472–486.

Liotti, G. (2011). Attachment disorganization and the clinical dialog: Theme and variations. In J. Solomon & C. George (Eds.), *Disorganized attachment and caregiving* (pp. 383–413). New York: Guilford Press.

Lis, A., Mazzeschi, C., Di Riso, D., & Salcuni, S. (2011). Attachment, assessment, and psychological intervention: A case study of anorexia. *Journal of Personality Assessment, 93,* 434–444.

Loevinger, J. (1957). Objective tests as instruments of psychological theory. *Psychological Reports, 3,* 635–694.

Lorberbaum, J. P., Newman, J. D., Dubno, J. R., Horwitz, A. R., Nahas, Z., Teneback, C. C., et al. (1999). Feasibility of using fMRI to study mothers responding to infant cries. *Depression and Anxiety, 10,* 99–104.

Lutz, W. J., & Hock, E. (1995). Maternal separation anxiety: Relations to adult attachment representations in mothers of infants. *Journal of Genetic Psychology, 156,* 57–73.

Lyons-Ruth, K., Bronfman, E., & Parsons, E. (1999). Maternal frightened, frightening, or atypical behavior and disorganized infant attachment. In J. I. Vondra & D. Barnette (Eds.), Atypical paterns of early attachment: Theory, research, and current directions. *Monographs of the Society for Research in Child Development, 64*(3, Serial No. 67), 67–96.

Lyons-Ruth, K., & Jacobvitz, D. (2008). Attachment disorganization: Unresolved loss, relational violence, and lapses in behavioral and attentional strategies. In J. Cassidy & P. R. Shaver (Eds.), *Handbook of attachment: Theory, research, and clinical applications* (2nd ed., pp. 666–697). New York: Guilford Press.

Lyons-Ruth, K., & Spielman, E. (2004). Disorganized infant attachment strategies and helpless-fearful profiles of parenting: Integrating attachment research with clinical intervention. *Infant Mental Health Journal, 25,* 318–335.

Lyons-Ruth, K., Yellin, C., Melnick, S., & Atwood, G. (2003). Childhood experiences of trauma and loss have different relations to maternal unresolved and hostile-helpless states of mind on the AAI. *Attachment and Human Development, 5,* 330–352.

Maier, M. A., Bernier, A., Pekrun, R., Zimmerman, P., & Grossmann, K. E. (2004). Attachment working models as unconscious structure: An experimental test. *International Journal of Behavioral Development, 28,* 180–189.

Main, M. (1990). Cross-cultural studies of attachment organization: Recent studies, changing methodologies, and the concept of conditional strategies. *Human Development, 33,* 48–61.

Main, M. (1991). Metacognitive knowledge, metacognitive monitoring, and singular (coherent) vs. multiple (incoherent) models of attachment. In C. M. Parkes, J. Stevenson-Hinde, & P. Marris (Eds.), *Attachment across the life cycle* (pp. 407–373). London: Routledge.

Main, M. (1995). Recent studies in attachment: Overview, with selected implications for clinical work. In S. Goldberg, R. Muir, & J. Kerr (Eds.), *Attachment theory: Social, developmental, and clinical perspectives* (pp. 407–474). Hillsdale, NJ: Analytic Press.

Main, M., & Cassidy, J. (1988). Categories of response to reunion with the parent at age 6: Predictable from infant attachment classifications and stable over a 1-month period. *Developmental Psychology, 24,* 1–12.

Main, M., & George, C. (1985). Responses of abused and disadvantaged toddlers to distress in agemates: A study in the day care setting. *Developmental Psychology, 21,* 407–412.

Main, M., & Goldwyn, R. (1985/1988/1994). *Adult attachment scoring and classification system.* Unpublished rating and classification manual, University of California, Berkeley.

Main, M., Goldwyn, R., & Hesse, E. (2003). *Adult attachment scoring and classification system.* Unpublished rating and classification manual, University of California, Berkeley.

Main, M., & Hesse, E. (1990). Parents' unresolved traumatic experiences are related to infant disorganized attachment status: Is frightened and/or frightening parental behavior the linking mechanism? In M. T. Greenberg, D. Cicchetti, & E. M. Cummings (Eds.), *Attachment in the preschool years* (pp. 161–182). Chicago: University of Chicago Press.

Main, M., Kaplan, N., & Cassidy, J. (1985). Security in infancy, childhood, and adulthood: A move to the level of representation. In I. Bretherton & E. Waters (Eds.), Growing points in attachment theory and research. *Monographs of the Society for Research in Child Development 50*(1–2, Serial No. 209), 66–104.

Main, M., & Morgan, H. (1996). Disorganization and disorientation in infant Strange Situation behavior: phenotypic resemblance to dissociative states. In L. Michelson & W. Ray (Eds.), *Handbook of dissociation* (pp. 107–137). New York: Plenum Press.

Main, M., & Solomon, J. (1986). Discovery of a new, insecure disorganized/disoriented attachment pattern. In T. B. Brazelton & M. Yogman (Eds.), *Affective development in infancy* (pp. 95–124). Norwood, NJ: Ablex.

Main, M., & Solomon, J. (1990). Procedures for identifying infants as disorganized/disoriented during the Ainsworth Strange Situation. In M. T. Greenberg, D. Cicchetti, & E. M. Cummings (Eds.), *Attachment in the preschool years* (pp. 121–160). Chicago: University of Chicago Press.

Markowitsch, H. J., Vandekerckhovel, M. M., Lanfermann, H., & Russ, M. O. (2003). Engagement of lateral and medial prefrontal areas in the ecphory of sad and happy autobiographical memories. *Cortex, 39,* 643–665.

Marvin, R. S. (1977). An ethological-cognitive model for the attenuation of mother-child attachment behavior. In T. M. Alloway, L. Krames, & P.

Pliner (Eds.), *Advances in the study of communication and grief: Vol. 3 Attachment behavior* (pp. 25–60). New York: Plenum Press.

Marvin, R. S., & Britner, P. (2008). Normative development: The ontogeny of attachment. In J. Cassidy & P. R. Shaver (Eds.), *Handbook of attachment: Theory, research, and clinical applications* (2nd ed., pp. 269–294). New York: Guilford Press.

Marvin, R. S., Cooper, G., Hoffman, K., & Powell, B. (2002). The Circle of Security project: Attachment-based intervention with caregiver–pre-school child dyads. *Attachment and Human Development, 4,* 107–124.

Mauchnik, J., & Schmahl, C. (2010). The latest neuroimaging findings in borderline personality disorder. *Current Psychiatry Reports, 12,* 46–55.

McClelland, D. C., Atkinson, J. W., Clark, R. A., & Lowell, E. L. (1953). *The achievement motive.* East Norwalk, CT: Appleton-Century-Crofts.

Meins, E., Fernyhough, C., Fradley, E., & Tuckey, M. (2001). Rethinking maternal sensitivity: Mothers' comments on infants' mental processes predict security of attachment at 12 months. *Journal of Child Psychology and Psychiatry, 42,* 637–649.

Meyer, G. (2004). The reliability and validity of the Rorscach and Thematic Apperception Test (TAT) compared to other psychological and medical procedures: An analysis of systematically gathered evidence In M. J. Hilsenroth & D. L. Segal (Eds.), *Comprehensive handbook of psychological assessment: Vol. 2. Personality assessment* (pp. 315–342). Hoboken, NJ: Wiley.

Millon, T. (1969). *Modern psychopathology: A biosocial approach to maladaptive learning and functioning.* Philadelphia: Saunders.

Minzenberg, M. J., Poole, J. H., & Vinogradov, S. (2006). Adult social attachment disturbance is related to childhood maltreatment and current symptoms in borderline personality disorder. *Journal of Nervous and Mental Disease, 194,* 341–348.

Modell, A. (1990). *Other times, other realities.* Cambridge, MA: Harvard University Press.

Moles, A., Kieffer, B. L., & D'Amato, F. R. (2004). Deficit attachment behavior in mice lacking the m-opioid receptor gene. *Science, 304,* 1983–1986.

Moran, G., Bailey, H. N., Gleason, K., DeOliveira, C. A., & Pederson, D. R. (2008). Exploring the mind behind unresolved attachment: Lessons from and for attachment-based interventions with infants and their traumatized mothers. In H. Steele & M. Steele (Eds.), *Clinical applications of the Adult Attachment Interview* (pp. 371–398). New York: Guilford Press.

Morse, J. O., Hill, J., Pilkonis, P. A., Yaggi, K., Broyden, N., Stepp, S., et al. (2009). Anger, preoccupied attachment, and domain disorganization in borderline personality disorder. *Journal of Personality Disorders, 23,* 240–257.

Moss, E., & St-Laurent, D. (2001). Attachment at school age and academic performance. *Developmental Psychology, 37,* 863–874.

Nitscke, J. B., Nelson, E. E., Rusch, B. D., Fox, A. S., Oakes, T. R., & Davidson, R. J. (2004). Orbitofrontal cortex tracks positive mood in mothers viewing pictures of their newborn infants. *NeuroImage, 21,* 583.

Noruchi, M., Kikuchi, Y., & Senoo, A. (2008). The functional neuroanatomy of maternal love: Mother's response to infant's attachment behaviors. *Biological Psychiatry, 63,* 415–423.

Nunes, P M., Wenzel, A., Borges, K T., Porto, C. R., Carminha, R. M., & de Oliveira, I. R. (2009). Volumes of the hippocampus and amygdala in patients with borderline personality disorder. *Journal of Personality Disorders, 23,* 333–345.

Nunnally, J. C. (1978). *Psychometric theory.* New York: Mc-Graw-Hill.

Ochsner K. N., Bunge, S. A., Gross, J. J., & Gabrieli, J. D. (2002). Rethinking feelings: An fMRI study of the cognitive regulation of emotion. *Journal of Cognitive Neuroscience, 14,* 1215–1229.

O'Shaughneessy, R., & Dallos, R. (2009). Attachment research and eating disorders: A review of the literature. *Clinical Child Psychology and Psychiatry, 14,* 559–574.

Panksepp, J., Siviy, S. M., & Normansel, L. A. (1985). Brain opioids and social emotions. In M. Reite & T. Field (Eds.), *The psychobiology of attachment and separation* (pp. 3–50). Orlando, FL: Academic Press.

Parkes, C. M. (2006). *Love and loss.* New York: Routledge.

Patrick, M., Hobson, R. P., Castle, D., & Howard, R. (1994). Personality disorder and the mental representation of early social experience. *Development and Psychopathology, 6,* 375–388.

Paulhaus, D. L. (1998). *The Balanced Inventory of Desirable Responding.* Toronto: Multi-Health Systems.

Pederson, D. R., & Moran, G. (1995). A categorical description of infant–mother relationships in the home and its relation to Q-sort measures of infant-mother interaction. *Monographs of the Society for Research in Child Development, 60,* 111–132.

Peter, H., BrŸckner, E., Hand, I., & Rufer, M. (2005). Childhood separation anxiety and separation events in women with agoraphobia with or without panic disorder. *The Canadian Journal of Psychiatry/La Revue canadienne de psychiatrie, 50,* 941–944.

Peris, T. S., & Emery, R. E. (2005). Redefining the parent–child relationship following divorce: Examining the risk for boundary dissolution. *Journal of Emotional Abuse, 5,* 169–189.

Perry, B. D., Pollard, R. A., Blakley, T. L., Baker, W. L., & Vigilante, D. (1995). Childhood trauma, the neurobiology of adaptation, and "use dependent" development of the brain: How "states" become "traits." *Infant Mental Health Journal, 16,* 271–289.

Phillips, M. L., Drevets, W. C., Rauch, S. L., & Lane, R.(2003). Neurobiology of emotion perception I: The neural basis of normal emotion perception. *Biological Psychiatry, 54,* 504–514.

Piefke, M., Weiss, P. H., Zilles, K., Markowitsch, H. J., & Fink, G. R. (2003). Differential remoteness and emotional tone modulate the neural correlates of autobiographical memory. *Brain, 126,* 650–668.

Pierrehumbert, B., Torrisi, R., Glatz, N., Dimitrova, N., Heinrichs, M., & Halfon, O. (2009). The influence of attachment on perceived stress and cortisol response to acute stress in women sexually abused in childhood or adolescence. *Psychoneuroendocrinology, 34,* 924–938.

Ramasubbu, R., Masalovich, S., Peltier, S., Holtzheimer, P. E., Heim, C., & Mayberg, H. S. (2007). Neural representation of maternal face processing: A functional magnetic resonance imaging study. *Canadian Journal of Psychiatry, 52,* 726–734.

Riggs, S. A. (2010). Childhood emotional abuse and the attachment system across the life cycle: What theory and research tell us. *Journal of Aggression, Maltreatment and Trauma, 19,* 5–51.

Riggs, S. A., Paulson, A., Tunnell, E., Sahl, G., Atkison, H., & Ross, C. A. (2007). Attachment, personality, and psychopathology among adult inpatients: Self-reported romantic attachment style versus Adult Attachment Interview states of mind. *Development and Psychopathology, 19,* 263–291.

Rokach, A. (2000). Perceived causes of loneliness in adulthood. *Journal of Social Behavior and Personality, 15,* 67–84.

Roth, G., & Buchheim, A. (2010). Neurobiology of personality disorders. In J. F. Clarkin, P. Fonagy, & G. O. Gabbard (Eds.), *Psychodynamic psychotherapy for personality disorders: A clinical handbook* (pp. 89–124). Washington, DC: American Psychiatric Publishing.

Ruby, P., & Decety, J. (2004). How would you feel versus how do you think she would feel?: A neuroimaging study of perspective taking with social emotions. *Journal of Cognitive Neuroscience, 16,* 988–999.

Sagi-Schwartz, A., Koren-Karie, N., & Joels, T. (2003). Failed mourning in the Adult Attachment Interview: The case of Holocaust child survivors. *Attachment and Human Development, 5,* 398–409.

Schafer, R. (1992). *Retelling a life: Narration and dialogue in psychoanalysis.* New York: Basic Books.

Scharfe, E., & Bartholomew, K. (1995). Accommodation and attachment representations in young couples. *Journal of Social and Personal Relationships, 12,* 389–401.

Schmahl, C. G., Bohus, M., Esposito, F., Treede, R. D., Salle, F., Greffrath, W., et al. (2006). Neural correlates of antinociception in borderline personality disorder. *Archives of General Psychiatry, 63,* 1–9.

Schnitzler, A., & Ploner, M., 2000. Neurophysiology and functional neuroanatomy of pain perception. *Journal of Clinical Neurophysiology, 17,* 592–603.

Schneider-Rosen, K. (1990). The developmental reorganization of attachment relationships: Guidelines for classification beyond infancy. In M. T. Greenberg, D. Cicchetti, & E. M. Cummings (Eds.), *Attachment in the preschool years: Theory, research, and intervention* (pp. 185–220). Chicago: University of Chicago Press.

Schore, A. N. (2001). Attachment and the regulation of the right brain. *Attachment and Human Development, 2,* 23–47.

Schore, A. N. (2002). Dysregulation of the right brain: a fundamental mechanism of traumatic attachment and the psychopathogenesis of posttraumatic stress disorder. *Australian and New Zealand Journal of Psychiatry, 36,* 9–30.

Schuengel, C., & van IJzendoorn, M. H. (2001). Attachment in mental health institutions: A critical review of assumptions, clinical implications, and research strategies. *Attachment and Human Development, 3,* 304–323.

Shaver, P. R., & Clark, C. L. (1996). Forms of adult romantic attachment and their cognitive and emotional underpinnings. In G. G. Noam & K. W. Fischer (Eds.), *Development and vulnerability in close relationships* (pp. 29–58). Hillsdale, NJ: Erlbaum.

Shaver, P. R., Papalia, D., Clark, C. L., & Koski, L. R. (1996). Androgyny and attachment security: Two related models of optimal personality. *Personality and Social Psychology Bulletin, 22,* 582–597.

Siegel, D. J. (1999). *The developing mind: Toward a neurobiology of interpersonal experience.* New York: Guilford Press.

Slade, A., Grienenberger, J., Bernbach, E., Levy, D., & Locker, A. (2005). Maternal reflective functioning, attachment, and the transmission gap: A preliminary study. *Attachment and Human Development, 7,* 283–298.

Smith, J., & George, C. (1993, March). *Working models of attachment and adjustment to college: Parents, peers, and romantic partners as attachment figures.* Paper presented at the biennial meeting of the Society for Research in Child Development, New Orleans, LA.

Smith, J. D., & George, C. (in press). Therapeutic assessment case study: Treatment of a woman diagnosed with metastic cancer and attachment trauma. *Journal of Personality Assessment.*

Solomon, J., & George, C. (1996). Defining the caregiving system: Toward a theory of caregiving. *Infant Mental Health Journal, 17,* 183–197.

Solomon, J., & George, C. (1999a). The development of attachment in separated and divorced families: Effects of overnight visitation, parent and couple variables. *Attachment and Human Development, 1,* 2–33.

Solomon, J., & George, C. (1999b). The effects on attachment of overnight visitation in divorced and separated families: A longitudinal follow-up. In J. Solomon & C. George (Eds.), *Attachment disorganization* (pp. 243–264). New York: Guilford Press.

Solomon, J., & George, C. (2000). Toward an integrated theory of caregiving. In J. Osofsky & H. Fitzgerald (Eds.), *WAIMH handbook of infant mental health* (pp. 323–368). New York: Wiley.

Solomon, J., & George, C. (2006). Intergenerational transmission of dysregulated maternal caregiving: Mothers describe their upbringing and childrearing. In O. Mayseless (Ed.), *Parenting representations: Theory, research, and clinical implications* (pp. 265–295). New York: Cambridge University Press.

Solomon, J., & George, C. (2008). The measurement of attachment security in infancy and childhood. In J. Cassidy & P. R. Shaver (Eds.), *Handbook of attachment: Theory, research, and clinical applications* (2nd ed., pp. 383–416). New York: Guilford Press.

Solomon, J., & George, C. (2011a). The disorganized attachment–caregiving system: Dysregulation of adaptive processes at multiple levels. In J. Solomon & C. George (Eds.), *Disorganized attachment and caregiving* (pp. 25–51). New York: Guilford Press.

Solomon, J., & George, C. (2011b). Dysregulation of maternal caregiving across two generations. In J. Solomon & C. George (Eds.), *Disorganization of attachment and caregiving* (pp. 3–24). New York: Guilford Press.

Solomon, J., George, C., & De Jong, A. (1995). Children classified as controlling at age 6: Evidence of disorganized representational strategies and aggression at home and at school. *Development and Psychopathology, 7,* 447–463.

Solomon, J., George, C., & Melamed, S. (2007, April). *Intergenerational patterns of representation and interaction: Threat, helplessness, and controlling patterns in mother and child.* Paper presented at the biennial meeting of the Society for Research in Child Development, Boston, MA.

Solomon, J., George, C., & Silverman, N. (1990). *Maternal caretaking Q-sort: Describing age-related changes in mother-child interaction.* Unpublished manuscript.

Spence, D. (1982). *Narrative truth and historical truth.* New York: Basic Books.

Spieker, S., Nelson, E. M., DeKlyen, M., Jolley, S. N., & Mennet, L. (2011). Continuity and change in unresolved classifications of Adult Attachment Interviews with low-income mothers. In J. Solomon & C. George (Eds.), *Disorganized attachment and caregiving* (pp. 80–109). New York: Guilford Press.

Sroufe, L. A., Egeland, B., Carlson, E. A., & Collins, A. W. (2005). *The development of the person.* New York: Guilford Press.

Sroufe, L. A., & Fleeson, J. (1986). Attachment and the construction of relationships. In W. Hartup & Z. Rubin (Eds.), *The nature and development of relationships* (pp. 51–71). Hillsdale, NJ: Erlbaum.

Strathearn, L., Fonagy, P., Amico, J., & Montague, R. P. (2009). Adult attachment predicts maternal brain and oxytocin response of infant cues. *Neuropsychopharmacology, 34,* 2655–2666.

Stern, D. N. (1985). *Interpersonal world of the infant.* New York: Basic Books.

Subic-Wrana, C., Beetz, A., Langenbach, M., Paulussen, M., & Beutel, M. (2007). Connections between unresolved attachment trauma and retrospectively remembered childhood traumatisation in psychosomatic inpatients. *Journal of Psychosomatic Research, 61,* 399.

Suslow, T., Kugel, H., Rauch, A. V., Dannlowski, U., Bauer, J., Konrad, C., et al. (2009). Attachment avoidance modulates neural response to masked facial emotion. *Human Brain Mapping, 30,* 3553–3562.

Swain, J. E. (2008). Baby stimuli and the parent brain: Functional neuroimaging of the neural substrates of parent–infant attachment. *Psychiatry, 5,* 28–36.

Swain, J. E., Lorberbaum, J. P., Kose, S., & Strathearn, L. (2007). Brain basis of early parent–infant interactions: Psychology, physiology, and in vivo functional neuroimaging studies. *Journal of Child Psychology and Psychiatry, 48,* 262–287.

Szajnberg, N., & George, C. (2011). *Attachment in Ethopian immigrants living in Israel: A three-year study of children and their parents.* Manuscript in preparation.

Thompson, R. A. (2008). Early attachment and later development: Familiar questions, new answers. In J. Cassidy & P. R. Shaver (Eds.), *Handbook of attachment: Theory, research, and clinical applications* (2nd ed., pp. 348–365). New York: Guilford Press.

Tronick, E. Z. (1989). Emotions and emoitional communication in infants. *American Psychologist, 44,* 112–119.

Turton, P., Gauley, G., Marvin-Avellan, L., & Hughes, P. (2001). The Adult Attachment Interview: Rating and classification problems posed by nonnormative samples. *Attachment and Human Development, 3,* 284–303.

Uvnas-Moberg, K. (1998). Oxytocin may mediate the benefits of positive social interaction and emotions. *Psychoneuroendocrinology, 23,* 819–835.

Van Ecke, Y. (2006). Unresolved attachment among immigrants: An analysis using the Adult Attachment Projective. *Journal of Genetic Psychology, 167,* 433–442.

Van Ecke, Y., Chope, R. C., & Emmelkamp, P. M. G. (2005). Immigrants and attachment status: Research findings with Dutch and Belgian immigrants in California. *Social Behavior and Personality, 33,* 657–673.

van IJzendoorn, M. H., & Bakermans-Kranenburg, M. J. (1996). Attachment representations in mothers, fathers, adolescents, and clinical groups: A meta-analytic search for normative data. *Journal of Consulting and Clinical Psychology, 64,* 8–21.

van IJzendoorn, M. H., & Bakermans-Kranenburg, M. J. (2006). DRD47-repeat polymorphism moderates the association between maternal unresolved loss or trauma and infant disorganization. *Attachment and Human Development, 8,* 291–307.

van IJzendoorn, M. H., Vereijken, C. M. J. L., Bakermans-Kranenburg, M. J., & Riksen-Walraven, J. M. (2004). Assessing attachment security with the Attachment Q Sort: Meta-analytic evidence for the validity of the observer AQS. *Child Development, 75,* 1188–1213.

Vogt, B.A. (2005). Pain and emotion interactions in subregions of the cingulate gyrus. *Nature, 6,* 533–544.

Vrticka, P., Andersson, F., Grandjean, D., Sander, D., & Vuilleumier, P. (2008). Individual attachment style modulates human amygdala and striatum activation during social appraisal. *PloS One*, *3*, e2868.

Wallis, P., & Steele, H. (2001). Attachment representations in adolescents: Further evidence from psychiatric residential settings. *Attachment and Human Development, 3,* 259–268.

Walter, H., Berger, M., & Schnell, K. (2009). Neuropsychotherapy: Conceptual, empirical, and neuroethical issues. *European Archives of Psychiatry and Clinical Neuroscience, 259,* 173–182.

Warren, S. L., Bost, K. K., Roisman, G. I., Silton, R. L., Spielberg, J. M., Engels, A. S., et al. (2010). Effects of adult attachment and emotional distractors on brain mechanisms of cognitive control. *Psychological Science, 21,* 1818–1826.

Waters, E. (1995). Appendix A: The Attachment Q-Set (version 3.0). In E. Waters, B. E. Vaughn, G. Posada, & K. Kondo-Ikemura (Eds.), Caregiving, cultural, and cognitive perspectives on secure-base behavior and working models: New growing points of attachment theory and research. *Monographs of the Society for Research in Child Development, 60* (2–3, Serial No. 244), 234–246.

Waters, E., & Beauchaine, T. (2003). Are there really patterns of attachment? Theoretical and empirical perspectives. *Developmental Psychobiology, 39,* 417–422.

Waters, E., Crowell, J., Elliott, M., Corcoran, D., & Treboux, D. (2002). Bowlby's secure base theory and the social/personality psychology of attachment styles: Work(s) in progress. *Attachment and Human Development, 4,* 230–242.

Waters, E., & Deane, K. E. (1985). Defining and assessing individual differences in attachment relationships: Q-methodology and the organization of behavior in infancy and early childhood. In I. Bretherton & E. Waters (Eds.), Growing points in attachment theory and research. *Monographs of the Society for Research in Child Development, 50*(1–2, Serial No. 209), 41–65.

Waters, E., Merrick, S., Treboux, D., Crowell, J., & Albersheim, L. (2000). Attachment security in infancy and early adulthood: A twenty-year longitudinal study. *Child Development, 71,* 684–689.

Waters, H. S., & Rodriguez-Doolabh, L. (2001, April). *Are attachment scripts the building blocks of attachment representations?* Paper presented at the biennal meeting of the Society for Research in Child Development. Retrieved from *www.psychology.sunysb.edu/attachment/srcd2001/scrd2001.htm.*

Waters, H. S., & Waters, E. (2006). The attachment working models concept: Among other things, we build script-like representations of secure base experiences. *Attachment and Human Development, 8,* 185–197.

Webster, L., & Hackett, R. K. (2007). A comparison of unresolved and resolved status and its relationship to behavior in maltreated adolescents. *School Psychology International, 28,* 265–278.

Webster, L., & Hackett, R. K. (2011). An exploratory investigation of the relationships among representation security, disorganization, and behavior in maltreated children. In J. Solomon & C. George (Eds.), *Disorganized attachment and caregiving* (pp. 292–317). New York: Guilford Press.

Webster, L., Hackett, R. K., & Joubert, D. (2009). The association of unresolved attachment status and cognitive processes in maltreated teens. *Child Abuse Review, 18,* 6–23.

Webster, L., & Joubert, D. (2011). The use of the Adult Attachment Projective Picture System with assessments of adolescents in foster care. *Journal of Personality Assessment, 93,* 417–426.

Webster, L., & Knoteck, S. (2007). Attachment in high-risk populations: Implications and practice for schools. *School Psychology International, 28,* 259–263.

Wechsler, D. (1981). *The Wechsler Adult Interview Scale–Revised.* New York: Psychological Corporation.

Weinfield, N. S., Sroufe, L. A., Egeland, B., & Carlson, E. (2008). Individual differences in infant–caregiver attachment. In J. Cassidy & P. R. Shaver (Eds.), *Handbook of attachment: Theory, research, and clinical applications* (2nd ed., pp. 78–101). New York: Guilford Press.

Weiss, R. S. (1982). Attachment in adult life. In C. M. Parker & J. Stevenson-Hinde (Eds.), *The place of attachment in human behavior* (pp. 171–184). New York: Basic Books.

West, M., & George, C. (1999). Abuse and violence in intimate adult relationships. New perspectives from attachment theory. *Attachment and Human Development, 1,* 137–156.

West, M., & George, C. (2002). Attachment and dysthymia: The contributions of preoccupied attachment and agency of self to depression in women. *Attachment and Human Development, 4,* 278–293.

West, M., Rose, S., Spreng, S., & Adam, K. (2000). The adolescent unresolved attachment questionnaire: The assessment of perception of parental abdication of caregiving behavior. *Journal of Genetic Psychology, 161,* 493–503.

West, M., Rose, S., Spreng, S., Sheldon-Keller, A., & Adam, K. (1998). Adolescent Attachment Questionnaire: A brief assessment of attachment in adolescents. *Journal of Youth and Adolescence, 27,* 661–673.

West, M., & Sheldon-Keller, A. E. (1994). *Patterns of relating: An adult attachment perspective.* New York: Guilford Press.

West, M., Sheldon, A., & Reiffer, L. (1987). An approach to the delineation of adult attachment: Scale development and reliability. *Journal of Nervous and Mental Disease, 175,* 738–741.

Westen, D. (1992). Social cognition and social affect in psychoanalysis and cognitive psychology. In J. W. Barron, M. N. Eagle, & D. L. Wolitzky (Eds.), *Interface of pschoanalysis and psychology* (pp. 375–388). Washington, DC: American Psychological Association.

White, R. W. (1959). Motivation reconsidered: The concept of competence. *Psychological Review, 66,* 297–333.

Winnicott, D. W. (1965). *The family and individual development.* Oxford, UK: Basic Books.

Wood, J. M., Nezworski, M. T., & Stejskal, W. J. (1996). The comprehensive system for the Rorscach: A critical examination. *Psychological Science, 7,* 3–10.

Woodhouse, S. S., Dykas, M. J., & Cassidy, J. (2009). Perceptions of secure base provision within the family. *Attachment and Human Development, 11,* 47–67.

Yamakawa, K., & Takahashi, K. (2007, April). *A validating study of the Attachment Doll Play among Japanese preschool children.* Paper presented at the biennial meeting of the Society for Research in Child Development, Boston, MA.

Young, L. J., & Wang, Z. (2004). The neurobiology of pair bonding. *Nature Neuroscience, 7,* 1048–1054.

Zajac, K., & Kobak, R. (2009). Caregiver unresolved loss and abuse and child behavior problems: Intergenerational effects in a high risk sample. *Development and Psychopathology, 21,* 173–187.

Zanarini, M. C., Frankenburg, F. R., Hennen, J., & Silk, K. R. (2003). The longitudinal course of borderline psychopathology: 6-year prospective followup of the phenomenology of borderline personality disorder. *American Journal of Psychiatry, 160,* 827–832.

Zeifman, D., & Hazan, C. (2008). Pair bonds as attachments: Reevaluating the evidence. In J. Cassidy & P. R. Shaver (Eds.), *Handbook of attachment: Theory, research, and clinical applications* (2nd ed., pp. 436–455). New York: Guilford Press.

Index

Page numbers followed by *f*, *t*, or *n* indicate figures, tables, or notes.

B

M

N

O

P